Hack Yourself Healthy

Reclaim your health
to boost your energy,
clear your mind and
live a long, vibrant life

JULIA BRADBURY
WITH SARAH OLIVER

Hack Yourself Healthy

Reclaim your health
to boost your energy,
clear your mind and
live a long, vibrant life

PIATKUS

PIATKUS

First published in Great Britain in 2025 by Piatkus

1 3 5 7 9 10 8 6 4 2

Copyright © Julia Bradbury 2025
Written with Sarah Oliver

The moral right of the author has been asserted.

Illustrations by Emil Dacanay / D.R. ink

Poem on page ix: 'Perspective', originally published in *To the Women* by Black & White
London, an imprint of Bonnier Books UK. Text copyright © Donna Ashworth 2025

A CIP catalogue record for this book is available from the British Library.

ISBN: 978-0-349-43625-8

Typeset in Sabon MT by Hewer Text UK Ltd, Edinburgh
Printed and bound in Great Britain by Clays Ltd, Elcograf S.p.A.

Papers used by Piatkus are from well-managed forests and
other responsible sources.

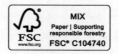

Piatkus
An imprint of
Little, Brown Book Group
Carmelite House
50 Victoria Embankment
London EC4Y 0DZ

The authorised representative
in the EEA is
Hachette Ireland
8 Castlecourt Centre
Dublin 15, D15 XTP3, Ireland
(email: info@hbgi.ie)

An Hachette UK Company
www.hachette.co.uk

www.littlebrown.co.uk

To my parents, Chrissi and Michael, who have given me and my sister, Gina, unwavering support and love throughout our lives. To be loved unconditionally provides an invaluable foundation of sureness and security. Thank you for being amazing parents.

'Stir well the cocktail of life, but make sure you avoid the dregs.'

Michael Bradbury

Contents

Introduction   1

1   Hooke, Line and Thinker: Time to
    Rethink our Health   9
2   Becoming Wonder Woman   29
3   Bite-Size Science: Why Food is the Best Biohack of All   47
4   When Cheers Turns to Tears   65
5   Spit Happens   83
6   Snooze or Lose   91
7   Air Apparent   103
8   Untamed: Rewilding People and the Planet   121
9   Saunas – Sweat, Stretch, Chat   135
10   Fifty Shades of Green   155
11   Ananda: The Healing Himalayas   167
12   The Two-Way Street: Mind–Body Health   189
13   Emotional Adulting   205
14   Flex Appeal   227
15   Breast Cancer, Drugs and DNA   251
    Appendix: Testing, Testing 1, 2, 3 –
    The Science of Self   285

Acknowledgements   319
References   321

Perspective

I climbed the biggest hill I could find
each step evacuating
my over cluttered mind

breath falling into rhythm
lungs billowed full sized
like sails at full mast
to ride with the tide

and with each step
and with each breath

I scaled further away
from my life and its worry
until perspective shifted
and cropped out the hurry

until this life looked very small
and I could *see*

the only thing which needs
to be moved, is me

everything I truly need
grows amidst the leafy trees
and ebbs and flows

in carefree breeze.

by Donna Ashworth

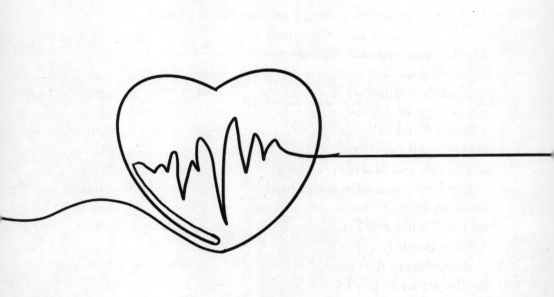

Introduction

My name is Julia and I'm dying.

So are you, dear reader.

There's nothing we can do about that. But the human body is a marvel of biological engineering, constantly renewing itself by killing off old cells and generating new ones. This continuous cycle of cell death and regeneration is crucial for maintaining our health and function, and it's something we *can* influence.

I've had cancer, I'm a mother to three young children and I couldn't be more invested in staying alive and living my healthiest life. That's why I've set out to improve my healthspan, which, I think, is subtly different from longevity.

According to the *Oxford Dictionary*, longevity means 'long life' or 'the ability to last for a long time'. (The word comes from the Latin *longaevitās*.) But I don't just want to endure, I want to be able to run around after my children for decades to come and, if I'm lucky, after my grandchildren too. I want to be able to lift and carry things and continue to leap up the stairs two at a time. I want to get better at tennis, not worse, and be strong enough so that if I stumble or fall, I can steady myself or get up relatively unscathed.

That's healthspan, not lifespan: being strong enough to handle life's knockbacks with resilience, hopefully well into older age (or the wisdom years, as I like to call them).

Running to my publishers recently (late again!), I tripped on the voluminous legs of my floaty silk trousers in Regent Street in central London. I slammed down onto the pavement, sliding forwards on my stomach in an ungainly kind of football dive, but I managed to put out an arm to save myself – and my teeth – from serious damage. I was bruised and embarrassed but able to get up and gallop on. My shins were turning blue with new bruises but I wasn't seriously hurt.

If that happens when I'm 80, I want the same outcome. I don't want to end up in hospital with a broken hip, destined to become an old-age statistic: someone who never fully recovers and dies within a year. The charity Age Concern says that falls are the most common cause of injury-related deaths in people over 75 in the UK. The government estimates the cost to the country of fractures from falls at £4.4 billion annually, with a quarter of that spent on the social care people need afterwards. In human terms, it's the end of your independence – but enough scaremongering.

Here in *Hack Yourself Healthy* I'm putting myself up as a 'crash test mummy' to trial lifestyle changes that promise to extend healthspan. I'll be taking you through them with experts who, I promise, have an excellent bedside manner. Most are things that you can try at home, in the gym, or outside in your garden or local green space. There will be tests you can have on the NHS, plenty of stuff that's free and, yes, some bits and pieces that you might want to invest in, but which don't cost the earth. (Actually, some of them *do* cost the earth, because they're niche and pioneering. I'll be telling you about those too, because they're the future of this kind of preventative medicine.)

In Chapter 6 I talk to Professor Satchin Panda, a world-renowned expert on circadian rhythms and sleep, and in Chapter 3 you can find age-defying Dr Kara Fitzgerald telling us what we should be eating to turn back our biological clocks.

I've travelled to the Himalayas to find a sanctuary called Ananda and learn more about Ayurveda, the oldest medical system in the world (practised for the last 10,000 years), to ask what it can offer the West. Read about that in Chapter 11. Here in the UK, I have sat on a machine I nicknamed the 'orgasma-tron' to strengthen my pelvic floor (and, no, it doesn't do anything more exciting), gone naked (apart from a hat and gloves) in Europe's coldest cryotherapy chamber (-140°C, since you ask), and exercised to my body's fail point, wearing a mask that makes me look like Mrs Hannibal Lecter, to test my VO2 max. VO2 max is one of the best predictors of longevity we have, and you can learn how I got on at London's pioneering personalised health clinic, Hooke, in Chapter 1.

Lots of me have been examined and analysed, from my brain-waves to my breasts: I have been poked, prodded and stuck with needles; I have given plenty of blood (I'm blood type A RhD positive, which is not rare) and I've shared my poo; a saliva test enabled specialists to decode my DNA – not to trace my ances-try, but to work out what diseases I'm susceptible to; and even my emotional health and psychological resilience – both surpris-ingly significant in human healthspan – have been picked apart. There really has been nowhere to hide.

As always, I've been heartened to reaffirm how important it is to have nature in our lives, every day. It has a tangible impact on our well-being that must not be overlooked. Feeling the sunlight on your face, breathing in fresh air, hugging trees, walking, look-ing at the colour green: these all create proven physiological change for the better in our bodies.

My physical and mental responses to 'vitamin N' have been measured in a series of experiments specially conducted for *Hack Yourself Healthy* by Ben Wheeler, a professor at the European Centre for Environment and Human Health at the University of Exeter. You'll be staggered by the amount of money I save the NHS because of the time I spend in nature – and you could too. In a London park, I managed to uplift my HRV levels (heart rate variability) to Jedi status, leveraging the power of birdsong. And in North Yorkshire, on the 2,500-acre estate of Broughton Sanctuary, I learned more about the spiritual connection we all have to nature, and how it's possible for land and people to be rewilded together, nourishing the body, mind and soul.

All the how-tos and the why-tos are laid out in this book so that you can join me on this quest to 'make the best of the rest'. I hope my experiments and enquiries will serve as a blueprint for you as you think about what healthspan means in terms of your own life.

In terms of my own, it has produced a stunning revelation: I have a cyst deep in tiger country: smack bang in the centre of my brain.

Head case

OK, so I wasn't expecting that.

My decision to become the 'crash test mummy' and have myself examined all over, inside and out, including a state-of-the-art body and brain MRI scan, revealed a cyst smack bang in the centre of my brain. It was ironic really, because they were focusing on my breast region, given my cancer diagnosis in 2021.

It's a pineal cyst located in what the neurosurgeon, Kevin O'Neill, described as 'tiger country', after looking at my scan.

These cysts are rare but usually benign guests in the pineal gland. The epiphysis cerebri, as it's also known, is connected to our eye function and plays a role in the production of melatonin, the hormone that regulates our sleep–wake cycle. Mine has a lump in it, approximately 6mm (millimetres) by 10mm, and the shape of a 'half-sucked Murray mint', apparently.

I was every bit as terrified as you might expect to discover this, but in the two years that it's taken me to write *Hack Yourself Healthy*, there's nothing – nothing – that has come closer to proving to me that preventative medicine is the way forward. There isn't a better path to building a longer, healthier life than getting to know your own body.

For me, that means having a second MRI scan in six months' time to ensure that there has been no change in my cyst's size or characteristics. (It's currently a smooth and well-defined lozenge.) If that's the case, I can relax and accept that it's stable and symptomless, and there's every chance that I can live safely with a cough sweet inside my head.

Apparently, 1 per cent of us do – it's just that we don't know until and unless they start to cause trouble.

If you think of your brain as a 3-D dartboard, the pineal gland is situated at the bullseye. 'This central location means that it's near a lot of critical neurological structures, so you don't want to do anything to it unless you really, really have to,' says Kevin, who is best known as the hero surgeon who operated on the brain tumour of my friend and fellow TV presenter, Davina McCall.

If my cyst grows, it could potentially:

- Block my cerebrospinal fluid pathways.
- Create pressure on my surrounding brain structures.
- Cause me headaches or neurological symptoms.

Surgery to remove it risks leaving me with movement-control issues, visual disturbances, deficits to my motor skills (and we all know I'm already so clumsy that I can trip over my own trousers) and, in very rare cases, neurological damage.

Kevin, however, stresses that there is zero need to panic or intervene, because, for me, this is a natural part of my anatomy: I was born with it. When I have my follow-up, he will check for any tiny changes that might ring an alarm bell and ensure that there's baseline data for future comparisons.

He doesn't prescribe any lifestyle modifications – but he does warn me to take the best care I can of my brain. That means prioritising good-quality sleep, taking regular exercise, maintaining a balanced diet and taking targeted supplements. (In my case omega-3s and vitamin D3 with K2.) Lots of exercise, a good diet and supplements are part of my life already, the first one, sleep, I'm working on.

If anything is going to make me redouble my efforts, however, it's finding out that I have a hard-to-reach cyst in my brain.

Kevin is a huge believer in preventative medicine. 'Ignoring your health is like leaving unopened bills on the kitchen counter,' he says. The problems don't disappear, they just grow larger and more complicated. Just as those unopened envelopes accumulate interest and penalty charges, unaddressed health issues can silently escalate, transforming minor concerns into major medical challenges.

So, er, yes, I have a cyst in my brain, but I know that I have the measure of it, literally: I can monitor it, optimise my health to protect my grey matter and take action in the future if I need to.

Thanks to my neighbour, Lizzie, for suggesting the scan. No, really. I don't know about you, but I'm definitely in the 'What you know empowers you' camp, not the 'I don't wanna know' faction. As Benjamin Franklin once said, 'An ounce of prevention is worth a pound of cure.'

As you read through *Hack Yourself Healthy* I'll be describing all the different ways that we can build healthspan, as introduced above, and each chapter ends with some simple ways that you can help yourself: my Happy Hacks.

I hope you'll enjoy the journey with me.

Julia

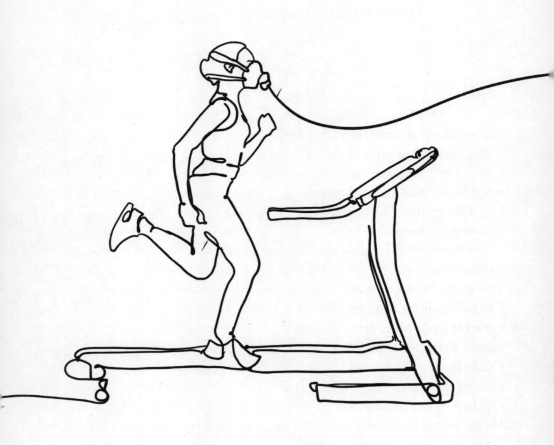

Chapter 1

Hooke, Line and Thinker: Time to Rethink our Health

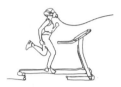

The mask is clamped, airtight, over my nose and mouth. Beneath it I'm sucking in air as hard as I can and exhaling great gales of CO_2. My lungs are burning and so are my thighs as my legs pound the treadmill. I'd started at a brisk walk, now I'm sprinting. The gradient has been increasing. I am nearing my fail state (when you exercise to failure).

Do I have another minute in me? Another 30 seconds? Am I going to throw up or give up first? In my head I picture my chicks: my three little ones. I'm not running in a gym, masked and wired to a machine, I'm racing along a sunny beach with them happy and free. It buys me a bit more time, and I can see the clock tick over the 12-minute mark. 'Keep pushing, Julia,' instructs trainer, Aaron Parsley. 'Push! Come on . . .' He can see I'm fading. 'Do an emergency stop if you need to, drop your feet off the sides.' And then . . . I'm done.

There is no official end to this test, no finish line, no tape to break. Just the certainty that my mind and body have reached their limit. My heart is pounding at 169bpm (beats per minute). I wobble off the treadmill, my arms too numb to unclip the Velcro straps of the mask, shaking with fatigue. I need some water, a sit down and a towel to mop the sweat running down my face, which is now the same colour as my pink top. I know why people wee themselves when they do marathons. I don't have a lot of control left.

Whatever my score, I'm proud of myself.

I gave it everything I've got. And now we'll see what it says about my longevity.

I'm at a pioneering personalised health clinic called Hooke in London's Mayfair, and I'm doing a VO2 max test, my first ever. It's a way of measuring maximum aerobic capacity (how efficiently our body uses oxygen during high-intensity exercise) and it is, without a doubt, the gold-standard marker for health and fitness. People with higher VO2 max levels live longer. It's that simple.

I have been both looking forward to this and dreading it. Running 'to failure' is not fun. But now I have done it, I am delighted: my score is 47.7ml of oxygen consumed in a minute, per kilo of bodyweight (ml/kg/min), well above the average for someone in their fifties, which is 30–33 ml/kg/min. This puts me in the 'excellent' category; better still, I'm in the 99th percentile for my age. Later, I learn that this is probably because of all the steady-state cardiovascular exercise I do every day, notably walking (I told you it was good for you!) and rebounding. This kind of continuous exercise at a moderate intensity has long been shown to help the body use its oxygen well.

My self-care self portrait

It's been quite the day here at Hooke, where I've given a lot of blood, urine and saliva, and I've been examined inside and out, from my brainwaves to my breasts, from the strength of my puff to the health of my gut. The outcome is a 76-page report, the Hooke Bioportrait, on the machine that is me. This bioportrait will be the foundation of my work with the clinic over the coming months, a baseline from which any improvements (or deteriorations) can be measured as I try to improve my own healthspan.

I have found a 3cm (centimetre) pelvic cyst that I didn't know I had, and a bony lump on my left collarbone. I will have to have a trans-vaginal ultrasound to check out the cyst, and I'll keep an eye on the nobbly bit on my clavicle. (Note: this is a really important area to check when you're doing your monthly breast checks and under the armpits.) Also, I now know that I have an unwelcome guest in my stomach called *Helicobacter pylori*, which comes with an increased risk of peptic ulcers and stomach cancer. That'll have to be eradicated. Plus, I have a bothersome issue relating to my iron levels, which I'll share with you later.

There are other things of note as well: my balance is bad when I have to do it in controlled circumstances rather than leaping onto a tree stump in some woods (I think I had stage fright in the gym). Being able to balance is crucial to your spatial orientation and stability, and it improves the plasticity of your brain, so it's pretty important. At my age (54 at the time of writing), I should be able to do 41 seconds with eyes open and 8 seconds with my eyes closed. I managed 11 seconds on both my left and right legs, with my eyes closed, which places me in the 81st percentile. My balance is something I work on every day, and I've never considered it a strength.

My olive-toned skin, courtesy of my Greek heritage, is technically known as Fitzpatrick skin-type III, which means that my skin burns moderately and tans gradually to light brown. The Fitzpatrick skin type classification scale is described by some as outdated and subjective, but it can be used alongside personal history and other information to assess skin cancer risk and whether certain skin procedures such as laser therapy might be suitable. My beneficial omega-3 levels at the time of testing were a bit low, my omega-6 levels, on the other hand, were a bit high – it should be the other way around. (After supplementing for four months with omega-3s, I corrected this.) One of my cholesterol markers was slightly elevated, but because other markers are well within range and I'm physically fit and not overweight it's not deemed to be an issue.

The good bits: if you want me to jump from standing still, I have 24.4cm of spring, which is well above average, in the 89th percentile for people my age doing this particular test; as for my grip, I can manage 39kg with my right hand and 37.6kg with my left, which also puts me into the 'excellent' category. (The clinicians were looking for better than 30kg.) Press ups? I can bang out 25, which is again 'excellent', although I suspect I would get no points for elegance. I'm in the top 10 per cent of the population for fitness in terms of my age and sex, and very well 'fat adapted', which means my body has a high capacity for using fat as fuel instead of glucose (sugar). This is a win in terms of age-related decline, as it lowers my risk of the chronic diseases that will shorten my lifespan.

I'm certain I'm looking at the future of healthcare. It's data-driven, completely personalised and about being proactive, not reactive. In short, Hooke believes in optimising good health rather than waiting until someone is sick and then trying to fix them.

Shouldn't this be national policy rather than something a bit niche? People hate it when I say so, but around 40 per cent of cancers are preventable.

Your body's SOS

In the UK, it's estimated that around one in four adults may have metabolic syndrome, which can increase the risk of heart disease, stroke and even dementia. (See the box below for a detailed look at metabolic health.) In the USA some estimates suggest that more than 87 per cent of the population is metabolically unhealthy. Contributing factors include high blood pressure, high blood sugars, unhealthy cholesterol levels and a larger waist circumference.

In England, 64 per cent of adults are either overweight or obese; in the USA that figure is closer to 71 per cent. The reason for these worrying statistics? In many instances it's lifestyle, which is something you can hack, starting right now, for free.

How bad food, poor sleep and stress impact your metabolism

You're going to hear a lot more about metabolic health in this book (there's even an annual International Metabolic Health Day on 10th October), so I asked Dr Nasha Winters, who's a pioneer in the field of integrative and metabolic oncology, and who helped guide me through my breast-cancer diagnosis in 2021, to explain it for us.

The silent saboteurs – my conversation with Dr Nasha Winters

What is metabolic health, and why should we be concerned about it?

Nasha: Metabolic health isn't just the absence of disease; it's a state where our body's energy systems function optimally, supporting every cell, tissue and organ. When we speak of metabolic health, we are referring to our body's ability to efficiently process nutrients, maintain balanced blood sugar levels, regulate cholesterol, and manage blood pressure – all while minimising inflammation and oxidative stress (when energy production produces unstable molecules that damage cells – more about this on page 147). Achieving metabolic health is a cornerstone of disease prevention and longevity, and it forms the basis of resilience against chronic illnesses, including cancer.

Why do metabolic markers matter?

Nasha: Several key metabolic markers serve as our 'vital signs' for metabolic health. These include blood pressure, blood glucose levels, waist circumference, triglyceride levels, and HDL cholesterol. Each one tells us a story about the body's current state, with deviations often hinting at underlying imbalances that could increase the risk of chronic diseases.

Metabolic markers

1 Blood pressure High blood pressure indicates that the heart is working harder than it should, often due to imbalances in electrolytes (essential minerals), stress or dietary factors. Elevated blood pressure can damage the blood vessels over time, leading to heart disease, kidney issues, and even certain cancers. Simple lifestyle changes – such as reducing sodium (salt), practising stress-management techniques such as deep breathing or meditation, and engaging in regular physical activity – can have a significant impact.

2 Blood glucose levels When our blood sugar levels remain consistently high, the risk of insulin resistance increases, meaning that your muscles, fat and liver don't respond correctly to the hormone insulin, thereby setting the stage for diabetes, cardiovascular disease and cancer. By managing our carbohydrate intake (a major source of sugar in the blood), focusing on nutrient-dense foods (such as meat, seafood and vegetables), and incorporating regular physical activity, we can support better control of our blood sugar.

3 Waist circumference Fat around the waistline, especially visceral fat (the fat that is wrapped around your internal organs), indicates metabolic imbalance and inflammation, which can disrupt hormonal function and increase the risk of disease. Monitoring your waist circumference, staying active and focusing on anti-inflammatory foods, rich in fibre, can make a difference.

4 Triglyceride levels Elevated triglycerides in the blood reflect an imbalance in how our body processes fat, and they are often linked to a high sugar intake, refined carbohydrates and/or excessive alcohol. Incorporating healthy fats such as those found in nuts, seeds and fatty fish (such as mackerel) can help to reduce triglyceride levels.

> **5 HDL cholesterol** Often called 'good' cholesterol, HDL helps to clear other forms of cholesterol from the bloodstream. Low levels are associated with a higher risk of heart disease. Increasing HDL involves embracing a balanced diet with healthy fats as mentioned above and taking regular exercise.

The pioneers of preventative medicine

No. 86 Brook Street in London's Mayfair is a vast white stuccoed house, which looks so glamorous that it could be a set in the Netflix Regency drama *Bridgerton*. But look harder, turn your gaze skywards to the decorations above the portico, and you'll see a serpent, the globally known symbol of medicine. (Snakes have represented doctors and healing since the time of the Ancient Greeks, representing life and renewal in the same way that a snake sheds its skin.)

The house itself has been there since 1725, but it was taken over by medics in 1922 as consulting rooms for a group of distinguished doctors who arranged it to suit their needs. A large 'muniment room' for patients' notes was built in the basement, with waiting rooms and consulting rooms on the ground and first floors. The decoration was smart and fresh throughout: blue for the sky, yellow for the sun, and another room left with its treated plaster showing to resemble green and lapis marbling – ocean colours, I guess.

Today it looks rather different, more like a gorgeous boutique hotel, but it's still a place of healing and medical inquiry. And that's why I found myself walking up those elegant steps one day in early spring 2024 to meet founder, Lev Mikheev, and his daughter Kate Woolhouse, the CEO.

From Moscow to Mayfair

Lev was brought up in Moscow. He was a theoretical physicist who became a hedge funder and lived a high-octane kind of life until he developed prostate cancer at the age of 49. (He is 62 at the time of writing.) He had a radical prostatectomy which, like my mastectomy in 2021, was a wake-up call. Lev started to read up on longevity, and then, stubborn as a mule in the face of a potentially deadly disease, turned himself into an endurance athlete.

Next, he created Hooke to share what he had learned.

The clinic brings a multi-disciplinary team under one roof: doctors, health and fitness experts and a scientific advisory board. It's the epitome of personalised medicine with cognitive-function testing and emotional analysis built in as standard. There's even psychometric profiling. As Lev points out, 'You need to know people's weak points if you are to help them achieve their healthspan and longevity goals.'

Hooke is small and exclusive, but it's determined to shift the perception that this kind of *preventative* healthcare will always be inaccessible to the majority. Their mission is to educate people about what can be done by themselves, for themselves. You will see at the end of this chapter that they have created a guide they're calling 'Hooke at Home' outlining tests you can ask for on the NHS and others you can reasonably source yourself.

Lev Mikheev and Kate Woolhouse on prevention not cure

'In the health-care sector, the only area that looks to maximise health – rather than fix you when you are broken – is professional sports medicine,' Lev tells me as I sit with him in Hooke's sunny meeting room. 'It's not the content but the method; a multi-disciplinary team: a doctor with a nutritionist, a fitness person with a psychologist. They don't wait until bad things happen. They test periodically, collect data, and try to improve things, to achieve your maximum potential based on objective observation. Why not work with this model instead of accepting that decline is inevitable from your forties onwards?

'It's about optimisation. Positive health care, not negative. At this point, we do it for the wealthy because that's where you have to start, the same as it was with the car industry and jet travel. It is expensive initially, but you go on to create a prototype which can be made more widely available and effective.'

Future proof

'On a big ethical level,' Lev goes on, 'I think humanity needs a new model for healthcare, and I don't think it needs to take that long; for example, the NHS is not efficient with the data it could be collecting, and what it does with that data. There are some basic inefficiencies in the system. If they run a blood sample, for example, they could be getting more blood markers from that same sample. There's no extra time involved. There's not even any extra blood that needs to be taken. Think how much more they could learn about a patient, and how that snapshot would help.'

The father–daughter team at Hooke is also curious about what putting an onus on employers and education establishments might achieve in future. 'Schools are criticised if pupils don't learn to read and write,' says Lev, 'but don't they also need to learn to move? I would throw in physical education as a much more substantive chunk of the school curriculum, not least because children learn better when they're not at their desk sitting down for six or seven hours a day.'

'I think you have to look at policy making and regulation: what are we doing about ultra-processed food, what is our

> urban planning like?' adds Kate. 'I'm a big fan of Japan, where the employers measure their employees' waistlines. In China they go on cross-country runs before they start work in the morning. I love stuff like that, but as a society in this country we are too squeamish about discussing it.'

I'm not sure how that would go down here, but I certainly agree that employers should focus more on the health of their employees. You'll see why in Chapter 10, where I do a productivity test based on the power of nature.

The Bradders bioportrait

I start by giving 14 vials of blood. (Tip: if you are giving blood, make sure you are fully hydrated, so drink plenty of water beforehand.) Tests will be done for, among other things, inflammation, the presence of metals, my various vitamin levels, my liver and kidney function and the strength of my immune system. They'll be scouting for any cancer markers too. There will be lipid tests to give advance warning of heart conditions, a glucose test for signs of future diabetes, and another one checking the health of my joints.

Next, I hop onto some intelligent scales, which measure various bits of me using electrical impulses. I am 58.9kg (9 stone 3lb – and within the normal range for my height of 173cm/5ft 8in) with a skeletal muscle mass of 27.5kg (also normal); my body fat is 14.8 per cent, which is at the lower end (18–28 per cent is usual). My visceral fat (the internal fat stored around our organs) is comfortably within safe margins. They're looking for a score beneath 100cm squared and I'm 41.6cm squared. My resting metabolic rate – the number of calories I need per day just to function without exercise or activity – is 1341, similar to other people of my height and weight.

Other tests done throughout the course of the day will show my pulse is 58 beats per minute and my blood pressure is a respectable 102/65. All the electrics in my heart are sparking properly and, as for my lungs, I take 17 breaths a minute and have a blood oxygen level (from room air) of 96 per cent, which is normal. My hip-to-waist ratio – a better health marker than body mass index (BMI) – is 0.85, also healthy.

Once we have established my baselines, it's into the gym with Aaron. He's a surfer and hiker, 40 at the time of writing. He looks outdoorsy – I can easily see him dragging his board out into the Atlantic swell on the west coast of France where he surfs with his brother. Squats, jumps, pulls, pushes, grips – all are analysed as he promises to make me strong enough to fulfil my fifty-something ambition of being able to do pull-ups. His attention is laser focused, and after each exercise he charts my performance on his laptop so that he can keep track of my progress in the months to come.

Top fitness kit

I asked Aaron which two bits of kit would top his list for home use, if you had the budget. Here they are:

1 Intelligent scales (that measure body composition, muscle and bone mass as well as weight) so that you understand your own body composition and how to improve it.
2 A wearable fitness tracker to help you keep track of yourself 24 hours a day.

Food, but with homework

Next, it's nutrition with Hooke's in-house expert, Aaron Deere. He's a tall, brawny Australian with a shaven head and neatly trimmed silver stubble, so big he fills the sofa opposite me.

One of the things Aaron will be addressing is the iron issue revealed by my blood tests. I have low transferrin saturation, which means the amount of iron that is bound to transferrin, the protein that transports it around the body. A normal range for this marker is between 20 per cent and 55 per cent, I have come in with just 18 per cent. Among other things, low transferrin can impact sleep patterns, as it's involved in regulating our sleep–wake cycles. It makes me wonder if it's been contributing to the insomnia I have been trying so hard to eradicate with bedtime rituals and breath work.

Aaron has written me a food prescription to up my iron (meat, more beans, peas, lentils, dark leafy greens like kale and watercress, wholegrains such as brown rice, and nuts and seeds). He also wants me to take on more calcium since I don't drink dairy milk. (That means sardines, soya beans, figs, almonds, white beans and oranges.) I also need to improve my ratio of omega-6s to omega-3s. A perfect score would be between 1.5 and 3 (meaning that you should take in no more than three times more omega-6 than omega-3). Mine is 7.78. It's a function of the modern Western diet and very common, but it increases our overall risk of inflammation, allergies and auto-immune reactions. He recommends a supplement to increase my omega-3 from its current low level and even out my ratio.

I have always thought that I ate a respectable amount of good-quality protein, but he's also crunched those numbers and apparently it's not enough to support my recovery from exercise and maintain my muscle mass. I'm going to need it if I want to do the pull-ups I've promised Aaron Parsley. That means bigger portions of beef and salmon, prawns, eggs, cottage cheese and my favourite Greek sheep's milk yoghurt, Oraia. The recommended amount of protein to consume each day in a normal diet is 0.8–1g (gram) per kilogram of body weight.

Mind games

Next, it's time for a bit of brainstorming with GP Dr Ummer Qadeer who's overseeing something called the Weschler Adult

Intelligence Scale, or WAIS for short. It's the world's leading test of intelligence for adults aged 16 to 90, designed to check my brain health and functioning power.

It was my idea of hell. 'They're going to get nasty aren't they?' I asked as a blur of arrows and dots and hexagons, in blue and red and yellow colour combinations, began flowing over a screen. I wasn't wrong. Mercifully, the tests end themselves if you get enough wrong – take from that what you will.

These things are important because our working memory – how much you can hold in your mind – is very sensitive to ageing and the corresponding decline in brain function. Comfortingly, what matters is your overall trend. You might only be in the 25th percentile in the first place, but it's the staying there that matters.

Here are my results:

1 Working memory, attention and ability to mentally manipulate information: 58th percentile, which was lower than I expected – do they know what it takes to do live TV?!
2 Processing speed, visual-motor co-ordination and attention to detail: 64th percentile.
3 Fluid intelligence (problem solving without relying on prior knowledge): 79th percentile.

Neuro nudges

After that, I took my poor, tired brain for a WAVi brain scan. I put on something that looked like a cycle helmet covered in electrodes, hooked myself up to a laptop and pretended I was in *The Matrix* for a series of reaction tests. (This was more for research than any diagnosis, by the way.)

The outcome was a colour map of activity in the brain – like a circular rainbow. Everyone's is different, apparently, like a fingerprint. Mine proved to be boringly normal. (I suspect if you could translate the brainwaves into words they were probably saying, 'This helmet is doing nothing for my hair.') What did I learn? That my ratio of theta brainwaves to beta brainwaves shows that my mind wanders more than it focuses, and that my frontal brain symmetry is at the upper limit of normal, which could indicate decreased efficiency associated with stress.

Stress will be a recurring theme for me, you'll notice.

Inside out

'Right, we know what you look like on the outside, but what do you look like on the inside?' asks Dr Pierre-Marc Bouloux as he prepares to give me a top-to-toe ultrasound. It's fascinating to watch his screen as he talks me through this grand tour from my salivary glands and the carotid artery in my neck down to my pancreas and out to my kidneys, where the fat running through them shows up as a little white line. When my gall bladder pops into view, Dr Bouloux rightly tells me that it's been a while since I ate. 'It fills overnight and between meals, but as soon as you eat, especially fatty food, it contracts and expels the bile to break down the fat, like squirting fairy liquid onto your pots and pans,' he says.

He was surprised by the discovery of a cyst in my ovary, which I've since had checked out with a vaginal ultrasound. Everything is OK – in fact, by the time I got to the follow up, there was nothing to see. It's not uncommon for ovarian cysts to come and go, but they are less common if you're post-menopausal, so it's always worth getting them monitored.

And top to bottom

Finally, it's time for the outside (mostly) of me to be scrutinised, and that's the job of Clare Nieland, a GP who divides her time between her NHS practice in Maidenhead and her work as a Longevity doctor here at Hooke London.

She's been practising lifestyle medicine for the last eight years. 'Working in the NHS, you start to realise that a pill doesn't cure every ill, and actually there is little point in giving medication if you're not addressing the root cause. Type-2 diabetes was a light-bulb moment for me. It's a chronic lifestyle-related illness, which is both reversible and preventable using a real-food, low-carb approach. I used to see one or two people a week with what we used to call "sugar diabetes". Today, I see four or five a day at least, and there are a lot of people walking around with type-2 diabetes who don't even know they've got it. If only we could empower people to look after themselves.'

Clare is a walking advert for her own health philosophy. When I met her, she was just about to head to the Lakes to celebrate her fiftieth birthday with a wild swim and a hill climb. But she could have passed for a decade younger with her dark blonde hair in a loose bun at the nape of her neck, a casual white T-shirt, white Vivo barefoot plimsolls and a tan belt around the trim waist of her navy suit trousers.

I'm telling you what she's wearing because I'm feeling a little underdressed in comparison, sitting wrapped in a blanket on a medical bed wearing only my pants and a pair of sports socks. The socks are particularly grim since they've recently been subjected to Aaron's VO2 max test.

Clare begins by mole mapping, and then there's a breast exam and a smear test, an eye and an ENT (ear, nose and throat) test and some spirometry, which is a bit like blowing into a megaphone, and is a test of lung function. I come back as normal, normal, normal, but what's brilliant about Hooke is that every element feeds into my bioportrait; this is the health of my whole self, body and mind, the bits I can see for myself and the things that would stay a secret, symptomless, until it was too late to course correct.

It's the prevention model, rather than the cure, the one we need in order to build healthspan.

Clare is the author of the mini guide we're calling 'Hooke at

Home', which will help you to be proactive and take control too (see opposite). But before we get there . . .

Inside my mind

(A lovely scenic route with the occasional outburst of anger.)

I have one final session at Hooke to tell you about, with psychologist Professor Aneta Tunariu. Here is what I learned about my mind that day.

1 Well-being index: 35 per cent, showing that I am navigating challenge alongside anxiety.
2 Satisfaction index: with health, 60 per cent; feeling part of a community, 60 per cent; life achievements, 80 per cent.
3 Meaning index: a sense that life is broadly interesting and exciting, 71 per cent; a sense of meaning in daily activities, 42 per cent; giving me an average of 58 per cent.
4 Positive vision index: for the self, 51 per cent, suggesting confidence in my abilities and a good self-regard; for life, 55 per cent, indicating a positive world view and hope for the future.
5 Health and vitality index: only 34 per cent; subjective health, my sense of myself as a healthy person, just 17 per cent.
6 Stress scale: an above-average 74 per cent.
7 Positive use of time index: my work–life balance came out at 83 per cent, which suggests harmony in how I combine my daily activities with my life goals. I was surprised, but I'll take the win.
8 Resilience index: 79 per cent, that's my ability to thrive in the face of a challenge, of which there have been several in the last few years.

Could do better

And here's the thing I was worst at:

- Using my imagination and being able to visualise things: 8 per cent.

Well, this blew my mind, and I want a re-do! I make up stories for my kids a lot, I draw and write. I'm abysmal at those horrible non-verbal reasoning tests where you have to imagine how an unravelled cube fits back together, but I visualise every day when I meditate too.

Hooke at Home, with Dr Clare Nieland

The following tests are all available on the NHS. (Do consult your own doctor if you have any immediate concerns.)
Dr Nieland writes:

Screening tests
- Cervical smear: people aged 25 to 49 receive invitations every three years. People aged 50 to 64 receive invitations every 5 years. Cervical screening is not recommended for anyone under 25 years old who has not been invited.
- Mammogram: the NHS Breast Screening Programme invites all women from the age of 50 to 70 registered with a GP for screening every 3 years.
- NHS health checks: for people who are aged 40 to 74 who do not have any significant pre-existing conditions. The check takes about 20–30 minutes and usually includes: height and weight; waist circumference, blood pressure, cholesterol test, and possibly a blood sugar level test. In addition, questions about health.
- Bowel cancer screening: home test kits (FIT test) for people aged 60–74 every 2 years, now being expanded to include those aged 50–59.

- Prostate cancer: no routine screening, but men over 50 can request a PSA blood test to detect prostate issues, including cancer.
- Sexual health screening: tests for STIs such as chlamydia, gonorrhoea and HIV are available free at sexual health clinics.

General tests:

Blood tests can be organised at your GP surgery on the NHS if you have concerns. Your doctor can organise tests such as Hba1c (this measures your average blood sugar levels over the past two to three months), lipids, full blood count, ferritin, folate and vitamin D.

If you have specific concerns, other investigations will be decided upon depending on your symptoms.

Other tests that are available include:

- Dexa scan: to assess your bone health, if you are in an at-risk group.
- Spirometry, for those with asthma/COPD or other respiratory concerns.
- ECG: to check the electrical activity of the heart.
- Brain health: the doctor can perform some tests on your memory, such as the GPCOG or MMSE if you have memory concerns.
- CGM (continual glucose monitor): available to buy or via Freestyle Libre Free trial for 2 weeks, to get an understanding of how certain foods affect your blood sugar (we use Dexcom here at Hooke). Wear it for a few weeks to get an understanding of which food affects your blood sugar control – you may be surprised!

Allied healthcare practitioners

The NHS now employs other practitioners who can help. Examples include:

- Health coaches: these work with individuals and in groups to help patients with behavioural change, working towards improving fitness, losing weight, addressing health issues through lifestyle measures and so on, group walking sessions, food and nutrition advice.

- Social prescribers: can help with falls prevention, gym referrals, exercise on prescription, social connection through local groups and clubs, and so on.
- Clinical pharmacists: they monitor blood pressure, advise on lipids and treatment, and some manage type-2 diabetes.
- Group consultations: some practices, such as the Cedars Surgery in Maidenhead where I work, run group sessions for those with certain conditions such as obesity and type-2 diabetes.
- Menopause and hormone health: some GP surgeries (again like mine) have doctors or specialist nurses, so ask to see what help is available.

Happy hacks

- **Speak to your GP** about any tests you might be entitled to – they will help you to build your own equivalent of the Hooke bioportrait.
- **Invest in some intelligent scales** to learn more about your own body and its daily, weekly and monthly trends. (If you can't access intelligent scales, you can use ordinary bathroom scales with skin calipers and a measuring tape for body circumference measurements such as waist, hips and thighs – www.wikihow.com/Use-Body-Fat-Calipers has some easy-to-follow instructions. There are loads of websites you can search – many of them full of muscle-bound men!)
- **Think about the right wearable fitness tracker** for you – it's like having a dashboard on your wrist.
- **As I write, the NHS is trialling** a new blood test developed by the University of Southampton and British start-up Xgenera called the miONCO-Dx. Using AI, it aims to detect up to 12 types of cancer, including bowel, lung, breast, ovarian and pancreatic cancers. Expect a version of this coming to a biohacking lab near you soon.

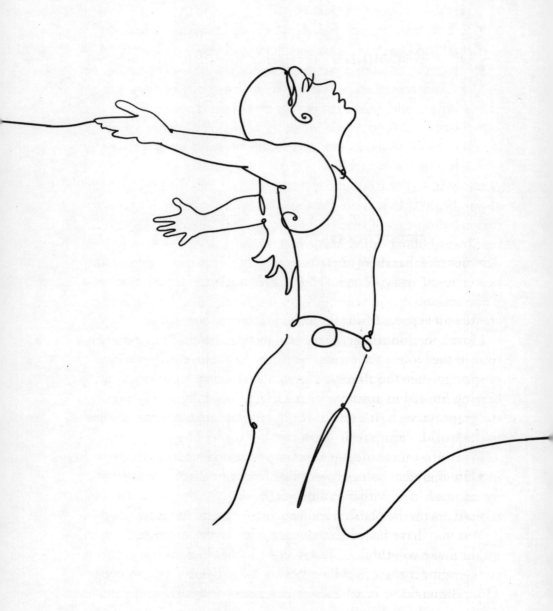

Chapter 2

Becoming Wonder Woman

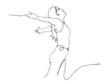

A few years ago, I bought a tiny holiday home in Portugal for about €7,000. It was in a cobblestoned village in the Guarda region (south-east of beautiful Porto), and it was for an ITV show that I was filming called *My 10k Holiday Home*. The idea was to demonstrate that there are still some bargains if you search off the beaten track and you're not looking for glitz. My little house was a one-up-one-down, with pull-out beds that hung off the wall to create more space. It was the size of a postage stamp.

I loved my months in Portugal, and right now I'm back, this time in the Douro Valley, a gorgeous place that is green and pink in spring, when the almond blossom bursts into bloom, and then blazing fire-red in autumn for the sacred weeks of the *vendimia*, the grape harvest. (It's one of the oldest demarcated wine regions in the world, dating from 1756.)

In my pre-cancer life, I would have been enjoying a glass or two in a late-night bar somewhere. Post-cancer I'm lacing up my boots for an epic hike with Ben Greenfield, one of the most famous biohackers on the planet. And I'm definitely not on holiday.

You may have heard the word 'biohacking', in which case it might make you think of tech tycoons spending millions trying to re-engineer their middle-aged bodies so that they can live to 150. (Biohacking is when someone uses data-driven lifestyle changes and often high-tech protocols and gadgets to improve their health and extend their lifespan.) In the case of Ben, it's

true that he is a man of extremes, what with his red-light therapy and cryotherapy, his cranial electrotherapy stimulation
and his pulsing-compression recovery boots, his brain-enhanc-
ing supplements and bi-weekly coffee enemas. He has even had
stem cells injected into his penis 'to go from good to great';
and uses a penis gym (a weighted penis ring and magnetic
weight) to work out every inch of his body. Don't worry if none
of this sounds familiar to you or in any way enticing – as I said
in the Introduction, some parts of the path to healthspan are
still *very* niche! For me, however, Ben has plenty to offer us all
on a simpler level, as I hope you will soon discover – so do read
on.

Who is Ben Greenfield?

Ben is a force of nature, memorably described by *The Sunday
Times* as 'the alpha male's alpha male'. He's a former competi-
tive athlete, now a health consultant, speaker, bestselling author,
podcaster and coach, who's his own biohacking guinea pig,
constantly pushing his body and his mind in a quest to live better,
for longer. He weighs 13 stone (82.5kg) with just 6 per cent
body fat. He looks like he's made of granite, the same as the
hills of the Douro. 'For you to be able to live with maximum
impact doing whatever it is that God put you on this planet to
do,' says Ben, 'you gotta make yourself strong, hard to kill, resilient, and with a well-functioning body and mind.'

For more: see bengreenfieldlife.com

Greenfield(s) and pastures new

Ben *likes* walking. Almost as much as me. He walks every day and
thinks it's the foundation of good health. It's October 2023 and
the sun is shining. I'm in a pack of Greenfield fans, trying to keep

pace with him. He's all wide shoulders and bare-chested-ness, capitalising on daylight, a one-man super-ripped solar panel.

The birds are singing from the branches of the holm oak, juniper and olive trees that surround us. It's not the dawn chorus, because it's early, but not that early. Ben protects his mornings. 'If I start accepting phone calls at 7am, beginning the work day, I get more of the signs and symptoms of stress,' he tells me. 'I gotta keep my morning protected until at least 9.30am. I get up at 3.45am or 4am just to be able to get my peace and quiet in, you know?'

I do (except for the 4am starts, which are still beyond me).

'When did it switch for you from just optimising your health to what we now call biohacking?' I ask.

'Never,' he says bluntly. 'Really it was just a gradual journey from podcasting and blogging. Back in my triathlon-racing days I used all sorts of computers, so I was accustomed to self-quantification from an exercise standpoint. But from a health standpoint, the increasing realisation that exercise and eating healthy does not solve all your . . .,' he can't quite find the word, 'it's not issues or problems, it's more about targets and aspirations,' he clarifies.

'A lot can be done using technologies and science, in addition to all the ancestral stuff, to move the dial, to be healthy.'

By ancestral stuff Ben means the things that we are going to discuss in *Hack Yourself Healthy*: food, breath, sleep and circadian rhythms, movement patterns, cold exposure and heat therapy, emotional well-being and social fitness.

Life in reverse

Ben believes in walking backwards – so do I, and you should try it too. Some physiotherapists swear by it to ease back pain, bad knees and arthritis. And even if you don't struggle with those physical issues, your bio-mechanics benefit from the switch-up. It's also believed to be good for cognitive skills, such as memory and reaction time, and for firing up your pre-frontal cortex, which is responsible for decision making and problem solving. The non-scientific way of putting it is that your brain pathways grow as your co-ordination and spatial awareness are challenged.[1]

Reverse walking, also known as retro-walking, was first documented in Ancient China, but it's finding renewed popularity in the 21st century, as we seek simple ways to lengthen and improve our lives. Whenever I post videos of me walking backwards on social media, people fill the comments section underneath with their experiences of how it has helped with stress and anxiety too. Reverse walking makes you be in the moment, because you have to be more alert to your movements and what's around you, creating a sense of calm.

I have been talking to Ben not because I want to be like him, but because he demonstrates the art of the possible. What really interests me in biohacking terms is the more user-friendly version, which will be coming to a high street near you soon.

Obviously, I've already tried it.

Bio hacking for you and me

It's an unexpectedly warm day in the middle of November 2024, and I am heading down a quiet residential street in London's Chelsea. Around me, well-heeled women are strolling with bags of what look like expensive Christmas gifts. There's just over a month to go. Aargh! I haven't even started my shopping yet! If only I was Wonder Woman.

Fortunately, I am on Ixworth Place outside Dr Mohammed Enayat's HUM2N Clinic where he's going to have a go at turning me into her.

Inside, there's a biohacking lab, which includes a hyperbaric oxygen chamber (HBO), one of the coldest cryotherapy chambers in the whole world (which uses extreme cold to support and improve certain health conditions) and a device called LungStrong. The LungStrong offers intermittent hypoxic hyperoxic treatment to improve cardiorespiratory function by varying oxygen levels. Think altitude training without the mountain.

In the adjacent body lab, there's the 'orgasmatron' like the one in the movie *Barbarella* with real-life Wonder Woman, Jane Fonda. The orgasmatron gives you 11,000 pelvic twitches in a single 28-minute session to strengthen your nether regions. It's like Kegels (the pelvic-floor exercises that we often forget to do) on steroids with the machine doing all the hard work.

This is the friendly face of biohacking, and Mo – or Dr E, as he is known to everybody – is at the forefront of it in the UK. Spaces such as his HUM2N clinic are still exclusive, but they are becoming more common at the time of writing, and I believe they'll be widespread soon. In 2024 John Mackey, the entrepreneur behind Whole Foods – the company that brought natural and organic food into the mainstream – opened his first Love.Life clinic in El Segundo California. He's now set to give healthspan the treatment he once gave groceries. (He took Whole Foods from a single store in Texas to a chain of 540 in the US and the UK.)

Mo is an NHS GP from Luton with a passion for preventative medicine. His parents were first-generation economic migrants – his dad owned a launderette in East London. They remortgaged their house to help him get this clinic off the ground. That's how much he believes in this.

Under pressure

My first stop is the hyperbaric oxygen chamber. I climb in and take a seat on one of the four forest-green chairs. It's a bit like being in a cosy space capsule as we're sealed shut and pressurised. An oxygen mask is clamped over my nose and mouth, and air, which is 98 per cent oxygen, starts to flow, pushed deep into my body by all that extra pressure. How does it feel? Like take-off on a plane without the speed but with the feeling of pressure in your ears. I wiggle my jaw to relieve it, start breathing deeply and regularly, and enjoy the 'ride'. Some people like to work in here without the interruption of their phone, others come in with a friend and chat from beneath their masks, others consider it a meditative experience.

However you choose to enjoy it, HBOT (hyperbaric oxygen therapy) is very good for you, supporting your body's ability to generate energy, reducing inflammation and helping you to heal if you've been injured or had surgery, or if you have been on a long flight. Fifty minutes later I emerge feeling peaceful and very refreshed.

The IV league

I move out of the 'arrivals lounge' into the IV area where a nurse expertly feeds an IV into a vein in my left forearm and hooks me up to a bag of golden liquid. It's the same colour as the nectar of the gods. This is NAD+ which is, wait for it, nicotinamide adenine dinucleotide. There's a shot of vitamin C, some minerals and amino acids in there too.

NAD is a compound found in all living things, and it plays an essential role in energy production, DNA repair and immune health – so, calling it the 'nectar of the gods' isn't far off. I drink plenty of water and then semi-snooze for 40 minutes while 150ml (millilitres) drips into me. It's odd: you can feel it arriving in your body. For me, that meant a gentle but distinct buzzing sensation in my upper body. (A full longevity course would be one infusion daily for five days, and then one once a month for maintenance.)

Next, I'm off to the orgasmatron, more accurately known as an Emsella. I perch with my knees and ankles apart to allow my undercarriage to make contact and allow the high-intensity focused electromagnetic technology to zap my pelvic floor for around half an hour. It tickles and tingles, and it makes my legs twitch madly, but it isn't unpleasant – you can have a scroll on your phone or a chat, though you have to stop giggling first.

'Thousands of little fairies underneath my bottom and my nether regions,' is what I said at the time, and, trust me, there's no amount of Kegel exercises going to do that for you.

I wish it had been around a decade ago when I carried and delivered my twin girls naturally.

Breathe easy

Finally, I'm masked and hooked up to the LungStrong machine, which I'm told will enhance my cardiovascular and respiratory health. You clamber into something that looks a bit like a dentist's chair, clamp on another oxygen mask, and let LungStrong go about its business. The machine is programmed to challenge you with varying oxygen levels to stimulate your body's adaptive response. It gives live biofeedback to ensure that I stay within safe ranges, but it drops and raises my blood oxygenation, forcing my heart to pump better, my lungs to expand, and my blood vessels to open. It's good for all of us, and in Mo's experience, particularly for those suffering from long-COVID.

He wishes LungStrong was available to everyone from the age of 40. It's not, yet, but the whole point of HUM2N is to show us what the future looks like.

I ask Mo what inspired him to do what he's doing. He tells me, 'I remember as a child listening to people saying, "When it's my time, it's my time", and having a fatalistic approach to their own health. They just handed responsibility for themselves over to the healthcare system, saying, "Oh, doctor knows best." These days we know that how you are living right now, this minute, is determining your future with regards to your health. If you layer advanced diagnostics on top of that, and the right clinical expertise, you can control a lot more of your own health journey.'

This personalised care is where we're heading, and I'm certain that soon enough biohacking clinics full of this kind of healthful wizardry will be as common as gyms, beauty parlours and nail salons on our high street.

(For more, see: hum2n.com)

Numb and number

I thought jumping into 0°C water on a recent adventure to Antarctica to save the whales was hardcore. It turns out, it's peanuts in the world of cryotherapy. The cryotherapy chamber at the HUM2N clinic (which looks like a giant and very expensive vertical freezer) is set to anywhere between -100 and -140°C – brrrrr!

I was given a scanty pair of sports shorts and a bra to wear, with a matching headband, and bright blue socks and gloves. I felt as if I was auditioning for 'Mother of Wonder Woman' in the next Marvel movie rather than Wonder Woman herself, but you have to have as much skin bared as possible for maximum expo-sure. All my jewellery has to come off too (in case it freezes to my skin) and I have an aggressive encounter with a body massage gun which pummels my shoulders, neck and glutes to prepare tissues for the cold.

Why, exactly, am I freezing my one good tit (and my implant) off? Well, it's because this kind of extreme cold triggers a fight-or-flight response, causing blood to flow to the core to protect the vital organs. When you leave the chamber, oxygenated blood then rushes back to the rest of the body, a process which is said to trigger our natural healing response.

I get in – it's . . . intense. The cold creeps into every fold of my body, it's as if icicles are forming on my skin, and I can see the blue spider veins on my legs popping to the surface, like a SatNav display. Strangely, the most powerful sensa-tions are inside my nostrils and on my inner thighs. I jump up and down on the spot, repeating a favourite Buddhist chant to distract myself from the cold, clapping and rubbing my hands together.

'Nam-myoho-renge-kyo'
'Nam-myoho-renge-kyo'

It's a pledge not to yield to difficulties, and I'm pretty sure it helps me through the next 180 challenging seconds. Stepping out I feel awake and exuberant – and suddenly famished too, because being massively cold for 3 minutes burns between 500 and 700 calories, which gives you a real measure of the changes your body undergoes.

Hacking your hormones

There are two things we can't ignore in a book about hacking our body systems: one is poo (search for 'Bristol Stool Chart', which categorises stool types on a scale of 1 to 7. Ideally, you have healthy sausage-shaped type-3s characterised by cracks on the surface as well as the shape); and the other is hormones, which we'll talk about now.

In the last decade, the once uncomfortable subject of the menopause has been the subject of a mini revolution. Discussions about how to meet its challenges with hormone replacement therapy (HRT) and lifestyle changes are everywhere. In Ayurvedic medicine, this stage of life (elderhood) is looked upon as an age of empowerment and a chance to realign values and let go of the need to achieve. The Ayurvedic way, which I learned more about when I stayed at Ananda in the Himalayas (more about that in Chapter 11), is to balance chaotic hormones with nutrition, exercise and breathwork.

This doesn't seem so very different to the approach of globally known hormone expert, Dr Sara Szal, whose book *The Hormone Cure*, written under the name Dr Sara Gottfried, I'd recommend: it's been supporting women for more than a decade now. It is such a huge topic, I can't do it justice in only one section of this book, but I did want to talk to Sara to get a few things out there.

'Hormones are chemical messengers, like a text message in the body,' she explains. 'They are released by various glands (your thyroid and ovaries, among many others) into the bloodstream and then travel on to all parts of your body, communicating with your cells. Hormones influence behaviour, emotion, brain chemicals, the immune system, and how you turn food into fuel. Each hormone has many jobs; for example, the hormone oestrogen has over 300 functions or biological tasks in the female body.'

For women, the top three hormones to pay attention to are: cortisol, thyroid and oestrogen:

- **Cortisol**, the main stress hormone, governs blood sugar, blood pressure and immune function.
- **Thyroid** affects metabolism and energy. It's like the gas pedal for your body.
- **Oestrogen** regulates menstruation and keeps women lubricated everywhere from their joints to their vagina.

Keeping on track, with Dr Sara Szal

What can we do to keep things on track throughout our lives?

Hormone imbalances develop over years, and it takes time for them to show up as fertility problems, for example, or as an increased cardiovascular risk. Get baseline measurements done before any problems occur.

The tests below can be performed via your GP, if they are willing to do them, or you could pay privately for them.

Alternatively, female hormone expert Pippa Campbell suggests testing on the following days (via your gynaecologist, GP or women's healthcare provider). 'Ideally, do a blood test and DUTCH Complete 24-hour test (see Appendix at the back of the book for a description) seven days before the start of your next period, on one day during days 19 to 22 of your cycle. If the DUTCH test is not an option, just have a blood test to measure oestrogen, progesterone and testosterone. Testosterone is pretty much the same all month. During days 19 to 22 of your cycle you have a progesterone peak and can catch the second rise of oestrogen.'

Sara's test suggestions.

In your twenties and thirties Benchmarking for sex hormones is best performed during your twenties and thirties. Begin tracking oestrogen, progesterone, testosterone, and DHEA levels. Look at the tango between oestrogen and progesterone. If there are polycystic ovarian symptoms, such as infrequent periods with increased facial hair or acne, consider checking androgens and insulin to check if you are outside the normal ranges.

Thirty to thirty-nine The more you know about your hormonal phenotype when you're in your thirties, the more you will be prepared as you move through the perimenopause and menopause. If you need HRT later in life, it is extremely important to know what your base case is in terms of the levels you want to replace and maintain.

Forty to fifty Perimenopause can start up to ten to fifteen years before menopause, so the forties can be a roller coaster if you're not in tune with your body. Look in depth at all sex-hormone levels. Cortisol levels become more important again. (Sara describes cortisol as a bully and says that if this hormone is out of balance, its influence on other hormones will be felt.) Oestrogen, progesterone and testosterone are declining and more vulnerable to the effects of cortisol. If cortisol levels are high, once medical reasons are excluded, try addressing the root cause, such as learning how to address chronic stress in a new way, for example by doing yoga, meditation or exercise. Consider tracking your blood sugar at this age too.

A fasting blood sugar level of 70–99 mg/dL (milligrams per decilitre)/3.9–5.5mmol/L (millimoles per litre) is considered normal for a woman in her fifties, but remember that the normal range is not necessarily the optimal range. I aim for as close to 4mmol/L, or under, as possible. You can buy finger-prick blood glucose meters from about £35 at most chemists and online. Our body's ability to balance blood sugar declines during perimenopause and even more so after menopause. Also, we lose muscle as we age, which alters the body's composition; the ratio of muscle to fat changes. Muscle acts like a sponge for blood sugar and, as muscle declines, you become more insulin resistant. Keeping blood sugar in range is more of a challenge.

Fifties and beyond Check your sex hormone levels, including your testosterone. Conventional medical doctors tend to focus on oestrogen, but women are exquisitely sensitive to testosterone. Ten years post-menopause is the optimal window to take bioidentical hormone replacement therapy to protect brain health, although this demands a detailed conversation with your doctor about your individual risks, your family history and your genetics before embarking on any regime. I would also advise checking your insulin and glucose levels, perhaps wearing a continuous glucose monitor, as both women and men become more insulin resistant as they age. Finally, do a cardiometabolic panel (a comprehensive blood test that evaluates risk factors for cardiovascular disease and type-2 diabetes); a bone-density check and a cortisol test.

How Sara Szal hacked her own hormones

Sara: When I was 32, I was struggling with high stress, low libido, weight gain, and raging premenstrual syndrome. I had a classic case of over-functioning, a pattern of behaviour where a person takes on excessive responsibility – physically, emotionally or mentally – often at the expense of their own well-being. It may appear as competence or strength, but over-functioning often leads to hormones that are haywire.

I took myself to my physician looking for help. He prescribed the birth-control pill, an antidepressant, and told me to eat less and move more to shed the extra pounds. (Sounds familiar?)

I left his office humiliated, then I got angry, because I just knew he was wrong. He had that knee-jerk response of a pill for every ill. Anger drove me to the lab to check my hormones. I was shocked to find my cortisol was three times what it should be, causing belly-fat deposits, irritability, and a short fuse. My insulin was too high, so I was storing fat and feeling hungry all the time. My thyroid was borderline slow, leading to hair loss and fluid retention.

Changes to my food plan got my insulin back to normal in three days. I learned that meditation and phosphatidyl serine (a supplement that seems to help with stress reception and mood regulation) dropped my cortisol. I started taking vitex (a Mediterranean shrub also known as agnus-castus, whose berries are used to help with symptoms of premenstrual syndrome (PMS) and menopause) to get my oestrogen and progesterone back on track.

It took me six weeks to correct most of my hormones. I lost weight more easily, and my mood also improved. I was more generous and patient with my kid. I wanted to go to yoga at night instead of to a wine bar. I reconnected to my essential nature, felt like myself again, back home in my body.

Sara's quick hormone-hack checklist

1. Measure your hormones to establish your baseline for oestrogen, progesterone, testosterone, thyroid and cortisol.
2. Pick up some weights. I recommend a minimum of six hours' exercise a week, which is two-thirds heavy weights and one-

  third cardio or aerobic activity. This will support your mito-chondria (the powerhouses of your cells), especially in terms of post-exercise fatigue, which worsens during perimeno-pause and menopause.

3 Check your insulin and glucose levels, as they tend to go sideways in perimenopause leading to an average of 5 pounds (2.25kg) of fat gain and 5 pounds (2.25kg) of muscle loss each decade after 40, unless you are specifi-cally doing something about it!

Sara's protocols for managing hormones mainly revolve around lifestyle, nutrition (including the use of herbs), exercise and – finally – bioidentical hormones.

  Most of her recommendations are available without a prescrip-tion, and she says that when women put an earnest effort into these initial steps, they find that most of their symptoms disap-pear. 'After completing steps one and two, few women need bioidentical hormones, but for those who do, the doses and duration of treatment are often lower than if they'd skipped the lifestyle design and herbal therapies.'

  Lastly, a warning from Sara about oral birth control pills, which she believes are the number one cause of hormone disor-ders globally. The oral contraceptive pill makes the hypotha-lamic-pituitary-adrenal-thyroid-gonadal axis (HPATG axis) less flexible, and so for the most part your stress response, mood, digestion and immune function are impacted.

  Additionally, when you go on the pill, it raises sex hormone bind-ing globulin (SHBG), the key protein that binds testosterone and keeps it from causing trouble. If levels of SHBG rise, the amount of free testosterone that women have is reduced. As a result, women can see a decrease in their libido and vaginal dryness. What trou-bles Sara is that the increase in SHBG does not go back to normal when you stop taking the pill. Studies show that, even a year later, SHGB levels are still elevated. 'That really troubles me,' she says.

There's a hormone-balancing protocol in Sara's book, *The Hormone Cure*, which also contains multiple helpful questionnaires, or you can find a modified version free on Sara's Instagram. @saragottfriedmd

Biohacking: where science meets self-experiment

Ben Greenfield's life is about optimising fitness and experimenting with some of the most cutting-edge longevity procedures and health protocols out there. He's a marvel of human mechanics and biology, but there will undoubtedly be a trickle-down effect on us all in the decade to come.

As for Dr Mohammed Enayat, he's a forward-thinking GP who wants to expand our idea of what's normal so that we can all live longer, healthier lives.

Dr Sara Szal is a perfect example of someone who took their health into their own hands because she wasn't satisfied with the answers her GP gave her. She hacked her hormones and has gone on to change the way millions of women approach their menstrual and menopausal health.

What all three have in common is their curiosity and their commitment to this new kind of health care – the one in which you get to take charge of your own healthspan. So let's now look at the easiest biohack of all – what and when you eat.

Happy hacks

- **Try your own cryotherapy** by easing in gently with a cold shower, or a bath full of ice, if you're brave enough. Deliberate cold exposure stimulates the long-lasting release of catecholamines: dopamine, adrenaline and noradrenaline. These hormones and neurotransmitters play a crucial role in the body's stress responses to make you feel great, so they're brilliant for mental health. Nobody enjoys it, but you shift states, and it helps you to manage those shifts better in the long term, in my opinion. How long should you do it for? Not to excess, but I always say to stay in for as long as you can and then, when you want to get out, push through that barrier and stay a little longer. Cover your shoulders and back with the water, and your head, if you can (although I don't always!). Cold-water exposure also activates brown fat (which burns energy in the body to make heat), which is found close to the bone, around our necks, under the breast bone and around our shoulder blades. When brown fat is activated, it burns white fat – the jiggly fat that we want to reduce. (See the note on page 212 about the negatives of cold bathing for some people.)

- **Walk backwards** from time to time to ease back pain and boost cognitive function.

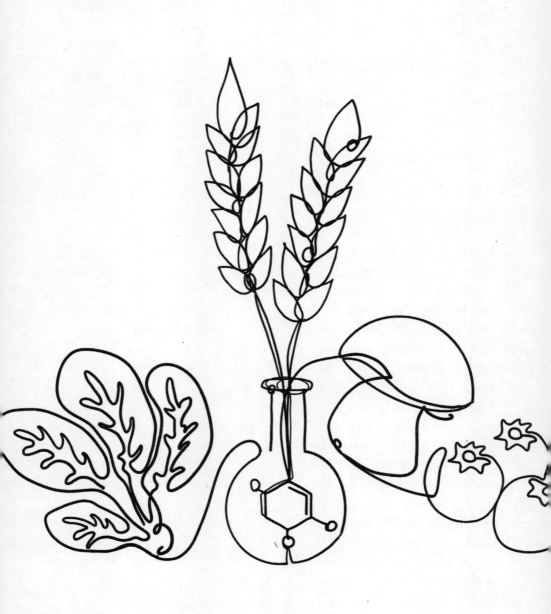

Chapter 3

Bite-Size Science: Why Food is the Best Biohack of All

What we eat can be the easiest and often most impactful thing that we can do to build healthspan. We eat three times a day, sometimes more, occasionally less. And every mouthful is an opportunity to do better.

Let's be honest, though – most of us don't want to see it that way because we are SSS: sedentary, stuck, stubborn. We're moving less than ever before, spending less time outside in nature than at any point in history, and eating ultra-processed foods that are pushed on us at the supermarket and via constant ads, which didn't exist a few decades ago.

We are trapped in a loop of bad food habits that we've drifted into, utterly distracted by screens, algorithms and relentless schedules. And that's how slippage starts. At least, it did for me. Out and about filming, I'd grab a sandwich and a bag of crisps on the run with the crew, or tuck into a pub lunch. Getting back late from work, it would be something that looked good from a box that took 20 minutes at 180°C, or a bowl of pasta, with veggies, of course (I'm healthy, right?), followed by half a tub of ice-cream, because I don't put on weight.

Before you know it, more than half the food you're eating is 'ultra-processed'. (That's anything containing preservatives, emulsifiers, colourings or sweeteners: ingredients that you wouldn't find in your kitchen cupboard at home, like xantham gum and polysorbates.) Bread, crisps, chocolate bars, ready meals, pies and pastries, nuggets, even a lot of fruit yoghurts, they're all UPFs, and together they now account for more than 50 per cent of the calories eaten in the UK and US, with other countries fast catching up.

The French phrase '*Dis-moi ce que tu manges, je te dirai ce que tu es*', translates as 'Tell me what you eat and I will tell you what you are'. It's attributed to French gastronome Jean Anthelme Brillat-Savarin, who published it in his 1825 book *The Physiology of Taste*. In the case of whole, fresh foods versus chemically preserved, flavour-enhanced, packable, stackable, bland UPFs, which turn to mush in your mouth, it's absolutely true.

I am not going to pretend that changing the contents of your kitchen cupboards and overhauling your diet is going to be easy. You might have to batch cook at weekends and swerve a lot of cafés, canteens and convenience stores while eating on the run, but alongside regular exercise (a recommended minimum of three hours across the week), it is one of the most important things you can do to live a healthier life, for longer.

(It's important to mention that not all processed foods are 'bad'. Pasta, canned vegetables, frozen veggies and fruit, are all 'processed'. For a much deeper dive into this topic, I would recommend the book *Ultra Processed People* by Dr Chris van Tulleken.)

Turning back time

It's scientifically possible to eat yourself younger, as Dr Kara Fitzgerald explained to me on a video call from her home in Mexico one day in the autumn of 2024. You can't change your chronological age, but your biological age – that's a different story.

Dr Kara came to global prominence with a 2021 study showing that an eight-week diet and lifestyle programme had the power to turn back the biological clock of middle-aged men by more than three years. She subsequently conducted the same trial on women with even stronger results: a reduction of more than four and a half years. You can read about her work in her bestselling 2022 book, *Younger You*. Her thesis is this: ageing is the greatest risk factor in chronic disease, which is itself the leading cause of morbidity and mortality in the world. If you can influence the trajectory on which you age, you can have a better quality of life, for longer. In other words: you gain healthspan.

Younger You food – nutrition with Kara Fitzgerald

Kara's clear that this is about lifestyle as a whole: sleep, stress, exercise, breath, hydration, as well as food. But nutrition is something you can tweak multiple times a day. A typical day's Younger You food might include: dark leafy greens, cruciferous veggies, colourful veggies, pumpkin seeds, sunflower seeds, beetroot, eggs, liver, some probiotics and a couple of supplements. According to her research, it's enough to encourage your body to behave differently.

This is an emerging science called epigenetics, which basically means how your genes express themselves. Dr Kara describes it as 'the layer of code written on top of your genes that regulates their expression and therefore the behaviour of your cells and organs. Within this epigenetic code,' she says, 'lie the instructions for your ageing journey.'

Kara: When we mapped out the human genome, when we figured out the 23,000 plus genes that each of us have as humans, in the early 2000s, we thought we would be able to create a Rosetta Stone of chronic disease. You know, 'this gene causes this disease, and that gene causes that disease'. But what really happened was this incredible awakening of 'No, in fact, that's not how it is.' Collections of genes can influence *trends* toward diseases, but ultimately, it's how these genes are being expressed that matters. So even if you see a trend in your family – my dad had this, my grandfather

had that – our *choices* will dictate whether this is our fate
too. Our genes are not our destiny. Maybe 10 per cent of our
genome really influences longevity – the rest is up to us.

Dr Kara's dynamic dozen

Dr Kara has created what she calls the 'dynamic dozen', hero
foods that we should all be eating to slow the hands of time.
Here they are:

• Turmeric, rosemary, green tea, beetroot, shiitake
  mushrooms, eggs, blueberries, seeds, liver, cruciferous
  vegetables, spinach and salmon.

Kara: I am a huge fan of nutrients called polyphenols. This
would include turmeric (or curcumin), veggies, greens (and the
darker green the better), are all packed with them. EGCG (a
powerful antioxidant and polyphenol) is in green tea and
rosemary. Our spice cabinet is a hotbed of these epinutrient
superfoods that are so important. Cruciferous vegetables have
something called sulforaphane, which is a key player for optimal
epigenetics. I think seeds have an important role to play – in
particular, pumpkin seeds. I'm a huge fan of sunflower seeds as
well. Nuts: walnuts are fabulous, and almonds!

Mushrooms are rock stars. You know, they're an epinutrient
extraordinaire. We highlight shiitake as one of the players in
the dynamic dozen, but any mushroom, including the lowly
button mushroom, is beneficial.

Salmon – any clean, fatty-fish protein – animal protein in
general. Eggs! Eggs are rockstars too. They have a nutrient
called choline. And finally, liver, which no one likes to eat (or
hardly anyone anyway).

Julia: That's not quite true! I take supplements, but I enjoy
organic chicken livers. A farmer friend, called Peter Piper,

told me never to eat them unless they are from free-range chickens. His grandfather was involved in the creation of factory-farmed chickens, a practice that he abhors.

The omega equation

Next, I ask Dr Kara about the fatty acids omega-3 and omega-6, because although they're both good for us, we're out of whack, eating loads of omega-6s and not nearly enough omega-3s. (You might remember that the blood tests at Hooke on page 20 showed mine were out of balance.)

How bad is that for our biology, and therefore our likely healthspan?

Kara: We evolved with an almost one-to-one relationship of omega-6 and omega-3. But when the industrial food complex kicked in, we started making tons of omega-6s because they're cheap and they're easy: you can get them from corn, seeds, grains and veggies, and so forth. This took over our diet, radically skewing the balance, so now we eat up to 25 omega-6s to one omega-3.

Omega-3s make potently anti-inflammatory compounds that act all over the body – they're just exquisitely important. Omega-6 likewise is essential. They tend to make compounds that are pro-inflammatory, so we want some, because we want to generate a nice, robust immune response if we get COVID, for example, but we don't want this overwhelming, dominant, inflammatory response without the control or the balance of the omega-3s. We should be looking at our diet so that we're eating somewhere in the neighbourhood of four omega-6s to one omega-3.

For reference, omega-6 foods include: eggs, peanut butter, sunflower seeds, tofu, walnuts and avocado oil. Omega-3 foods include: anchovies, salmon, mackerel, sardines, trout, herring, flaxseeds, walnuts, chia seeds and rapeseed oil.

Search online for a fuller list, but basically: eat more fatty fish! For vegetarians, there is promising research that microalgal oil (microscopic, single-celled algae) and ahi flower oil could be as beneficial as marine sources of omega-3. Up until recently this has been the subject of some dispute.

Do you dare take the test?

If you'd like to know more about the work of Dr Kara Fitzgerald, visit her website drkarafitzgerald.com. On it you can find a fascinating free online test, her 'Biological age self-assessment', which will tell you your own biological age. Mine came out as 48 years old, which, given I was actually 54 at the time, gave me an entry for my gratitude journal the following day. (Feeling gratitude is also good for your health, so hopefully that'll have knocked a few extra minutes off too.)

As with the tests available in the 'Hooke at Home' section in Chapter 1, and data from a wearable fitness tracker or intelligent scales, you can use it to build a baseline knowledge of your own body; it's a guide to what you're already doing right and what you can improve.

A fork in the road

For me, cancer was a turning point. I'd been gambling with my gut health my entire adult life, thinking slim equalled safe. It took me a year to reorganise my kitchen, but I managed to reorganise my attitudes and opinions before that.

How?

I stopped thinking about what I couldn't eat and started thinking about all the lovely things that I could, the foods that would power my health, one mouthful at a time. As a cancer survivor, I was also determined to learn more about eating to protect myself from any recurrence, which is why I found myself in a darkened lecture hall in London one gloriously hot day in June 2024 listening to Dr William Li who had flown in from America to speak.

Dr Li is a renowned cancer researcher, physician and scientist, and the author of two *New York Times* bestselling books, *Eat to Beat Disease* and *Eat to Beat Your Diet*. His 2010 Ted Talk 'Can we Eat to Starve Cancer?' has been watched over 11 million times, and his ground-breaking research has led to the development of more than 40 new medical treatments for 70-plus diseases.

He was immaculately dressed in a tailored navy suit, charming with a firm and friendly handshake. Anyone would want him as their doctor. I certainly would. (Although, I feel fortunate with all my doctors, thank you!) Originally a vascular biologist, he believes in what he calls a 'whole person' approach to disease, which means that our diet doesn't just affect our microbiome (gut bacteria), it also affects our immune system, our circulation and our blood vessels. It follows that if what you eat makes a difference to every cell of your body, from your blood cells to your fat cells, from your immune system to your gut, then nutrition is an essential part of the treatment of disease, even a cancer, like mine.

Can we really eat to beat cancer?

Dr William Li explains, 'What you should know is that with a scientific approach, integrated with a more holistic approach that is tailored around the whole person, including diet and lifestyle, and guided by scientific evidence, we can tip the odds against cancer, in some cases even turning stage-four cancer to stage-zero,' he tells the audience.

I am stunned. But his 40-minute lecture is crammed with case histories – including a compelling story about his own mother.

The first was about a woman diagnosed with colon cancer at the age of 22. (Currently, the number of young adults with colo-rectal cancer is up 22 per cent in the UK, part of the worrying upward trend in younger people being diagnosed with cancer.[1]) She had surgery followed by chemotherapy, but the tumour returned, and by the time she was 24, she had stage-four colorectal cancer. She was sent home on palliative care and morphine (to which she became addicted), to die.

Following this death sentence, she received a treatment that enabled her immune system to be strengthened. By activating that microenvironment, and kick starting her own body's anti-cancer defences, she was able to defeat her cancer, and she's alive and thriving today with no evidence of disease, Dr Li revealed.

His own mother was diagnosed with endometrial cancer at the age of 80. An emergency scan identified a large tumour in her uterus, which was surgically removed. She had radiation treatment, but within a year she was diagnosed with stage-four cancer. Her medical team suggested that Dr Li take his mum on a farewell cruise before she died.

If I was in his shoes, I think it would be perfectly acceptable to use the phrase 'Do you know what I do for a living?!' at this point. He didn't take her on a cruise. He cured her.

Now you want to know how, don't you?

One of the most common forms of cancer treatment is to target cancer cells and kill them. Dr Li says, 'We say we want to find "weapons to destroy them", and this is why cancer treatment has been so feared. But this is an old, historic way of thinking about cancer – we've changed.'

What he means is that we have evolved from killing to healing, looking at the body as an ecosystem (as in nature). Instead of a farewell cruise, Dr William Li treated his mother by boosting her immune system. He tailored her diet, adjusted her microbiome, and, within three treatments, using immunotherapy, her own body was able to eliminate all signs of cancer.

When I followed up with Dr Li almost a year later, his mum had just celebrated her ninetieth birthday, and there was no evidence of the disease.

(Please note: every one of us is different, every cancer is different. I am not suggesting that we can all eat to beat cancer, and you should not pursue this without speaking to your own medical team.)

From poison to prescription

You may not know that the origins of chemotherapy are partly found in a wartime scandal, something Dr Li shared with us during his lecture.

On 2 December 1943, at the height of World War II the American battleship *John Harvey* was charged with bringing supplies from Algeria to Bari, Italy. But the ship contained, hidden in its cargo, 2,000 mustard-gas bombs, in contravention of the Geneva Convention.

German aircraft intercepted and bombed the ship. The gas killed everyone on board, and many people in the town of Bari. The smuggled chemical weapons were revealed by a physician sent to investigate. His decision to save tissue samples from the dead would then contribute to the earliest knowledge of chemotherapy. Basically, victims of mustard gas die with low numbers of white cells, immune system cells, in their blood. The hypothesis therefore ran that, expertly targeted, the gas should be able to kill cancerous cells too. Nitrogen mustard, the compound used to make the gas, was the first experimental chemotherapy.

That's the origin story of chemo, and Dr Li thinks it's why we talk about cancer recovery as a battle. He also thinks it's time to stop – to stop talking about killing cancer cells and to start talking about healing the individual.

Edible armour

Is your microbiome in proper defensive form? If you are a cancer patient, Dr Li thinks you should be asking your oncologist this question, and if you're an oncologist, you should be asking it of your patient.[2]

The tools to assess the microbiome now exist. (I have given many, many stool samples in the name of science for *Hack Yourself Healthy*!) And this information can be used over time (just like scans and X-rays) to assess how well it's doing; whether it has lost or gained good bacteria, and to establish what can be done to improve your response to treatment.

I like to think of the microbiome as a garden: there are weeds, but you don't want to kill them with a toxic herbicide that will be harmful to all the good bacteria/good flora as well. Imagine feeding the goodies, allowing them to flourish and outgrow the bad.

In his talk, Dr Li mentioned a bacterium called *Akkermansia*.[3] Researchers have shown that if it is present in your gut, you're likely to respond favourably to immunotherapy. If you don't have any, there's a dramatic downturn in your prospects.[4] 'The remarkable thing is that science is showing that the presence of a single beneficial bacteria can literally make the difference between life and death,' he says. 'This is not about gut health and exercise, and longevity and anti-aging, this is about cancer therapy. The gut microbiome and the foods we eat that can influence it should be part of the thinking of every oncologist.'[5]

There's an *Akkermansia* probiotic available – but you can also grow your own. Here's a list of foods as recommended by Dr Li:

- Pomegranates contain ellagitannins, which help your gut secrete mucin (mucus). *Akkermansia*'s full name is *Akkermansia mucinophila* (it loves mucin).
- Cranberries – if you can't find fresh ones, dried cranberries will do. They also contain dietary fibre but be wary – most dried ones are sweetened so read your labels and avoid that extra sugar.
- Concord grapes – this sweet grape also creates *Akkermansia*, but moderate your intake, because they're high in fruit sugars.
- Peach juice and peach flesh (which contains dietary fibre) are helpful.
- Zhejiang vinegar, a black vinegar from China, has also been shown to grow *Akkermansia* in the gut.

As I type, one of the latest microbiome tests that I've taken has shown that I have no *Akkermansia* in my own gut.

I'm working on it.

Kathryn Lukas Damer's culture club

Kathryn is a master fermenter. Originally from California, she fell in love with fermented foods back in the early 1990s in a farm cellar in Stuttgart, Germany, when she ate a freshly fermented, unpasteurised sauerkraut. It tasted mild, tart and crunchy, and it fizzed on her tongue; it was unlike anything she had ever tried before. 'My body had a very different reaction to it,' she told me, when I sat down to tea with her one afternoon in August 2024.

A cook and restaurateur, Kathryn eventually perfected her own fermenting techniques, circling the world from South Korea to Peru. She came to understand that ultra-processed food, the over-use of antibiotics, widespread pesticides, chlorinated water, and, as she puts it, 'anti-bacterial everything' had depleted the human microbiome, but that eating foods rich with living micro-organisms, including bacteria, yeast and good mould, could replenish it.

Why is this important? Because a healthy composition of gut microbes (they must be both plentiful and diverse) is essential for good metabolic health and immunity. Microbes, she says, are 'our allies'. She launched a live-culture food and drink company and, along with her son Shane Peterson, wrote what's basically the American fermenting bible, *The Farmhouse Culture Guide to Fermenting*, published in 2019. It's a kitchen guide to creating your own kimchi, krauts and pickles, as well as hot sauces, preserved fruits, yoghurt, kombucha and delicious drinks such as a blueberry ginger beet sour.

There's no denying that buying fermented foods can be expensive. (The global market was expected to exceed £516 billion in 2025, according to the BBC.) In addition, not everything available on the supermarket shelf offers the maximum benefit: if it's been pasteurised, it's lost a lot of what is supposed to make it good for us. You might want to think about a DIY make-at-home option, just like the world's gut health guru, Professor Tim Spector, professor of genetic epidemiology at King's College London and author of *Ferment*.

Tim believes, 'everyone would be healthier if they had some fermented foods every day of their lives'. He certainly does, and you can find him online performing simple fermentations; for example, sticking peeled garlic cloves into a jar of raw honey. You screw the lid back on, give the jar a good shake and put it somewhere dark, remembering to flip it every day to keep the cloves submerged. Open it every 48 hours so that it can 'burp' and then, after a week or two, you have something which can be used as either a cold remedy or a salad dressing.

The sugar shock

If you read my last book, *Walk Yourself Happy*, you'll be all too familiar with my fondness for sugar. Big puffy pastries for breakfast, cake for elevenses, biscuits in my backpack for a snack on the go, and no meal complete without a pudding. On the road, I'd raid whatever sweeties the kids had stashed in the glove compartment of our car, and in front of the telly I would munch on a bucket of microwaved popcorn. I might even have tossed a bag of Maltesers into it. I never met a flapjack that I didn't want to eat and, as a walker, I was a connoisseur of a proper sugar-laden high tea at many a rural tea shop.

Quitting sugar was the hardest thing I did to change my diet – and also the best. You can still find me in a tea shop – just not eating the cake – because I have mentally and physically weaned myself off it.

If you think that I am using the language of dependence here, then yes, I am, and with good reason, because sugar acts like a drug on our brains and bodies, and many of us are hooked. I know I was. I'm not talking about the sugar that occurs naturally in vegetables, wholegrain foods and dairy products. I mean 'added sugar', the extra teaspoons of the stuff we eat for pleasure in biscuits and sweets, or worse still, without really noticing, because it's in something we think is healthy: fruit-flavoured yoghurts, breakfast cereals, honey, maple syrup, fruit juices and, er, smoothies.

Sugar is sugar, whatever it's wearing – and too much of it is toxic and will hurt your healthspan.

Broadly, there are two types – glucose and fructose – which we digest and metabolise differently. Glucose is the sugar naturally found in grains, nuts, veggies, spuds, rice and milk. Fructose is what makes fruit, honey and root veg sweet. The real problem comes when we eat them as 'dietary sugars', in other words, in sweet treats, many of which are UPFs – and all of which are calorie laden.

To talk about this, I hopped on a Zoom call with Professor Robert Lustig, who I've got to know fairly well over the past few years. He's incredibly smart, and can switch from topics such as molecular mimicry to global food chains in a single conversation. His 2009 lecture 'Sugar: The Bitter Truth' went viral, bringing the science of sugar out of the lab and into the mainstream. He's a professor emeritus of endocrinology at the University of California, San Francisco, with a degree in science from Massachusetts Institute of Technology, and a doctorate in medicine from Cornell. He went on to take a master's in studies in law, as his interest in health policy and how to make top-down change grew. His book, *Fat Chance: Beating the Odds Against Sugar, Processed Food, Obesity, and Disease,* was a *New York Times* bestseller.

Today, he is a leading – sometimes controversial – global voice in public health, arguing that sugar is fuelling what he calls our 'diabetes, obesity, and metabolic syndrome epidemics'. (By 'metabolic syndrome', just to remind you, we mean things like high blood pressure, high cholesterol and insulin resistance, as explained in Chapter 1.)

'Sugar's not dangerous because of its calories, or because it makes you fat,' Robert likes to say. 'Sugar is dangerous because it's sugar.'

It was a long conversation. Here are the headlines:

Robert Lustig in conversation

Fructose – the stealth toxin

Central to Robert's argument is the distinction between glucose and fructose. 'The food industry often misconstrues words and, for obfuscation purposes, makes it so that the public doesn't understand,' he tells me. 'One of those words is sugar. They will tell you a sugar's a sugar and that is absolutely not correct. The reason they say that is because all sugars are 4 calories per gramme, so they explode the same amount of heat in a bomb calorimeter [something that measures the heat of combustion]. But we're human beings, not bomb calorimeters. The glucose in dietary sugar is not great, but it's not terrible. Dietary fructose, however, is completely vestigial to all animal life on this planet. There's just no biochemical reaction that requires it.' Fructose, which is half of 'high fructose corn syrup', is a common ingredient in sauces, sugary drinks, fast food and flavoured yoghurt, so check your food labels. They're all calorie- and fructose-laden, he reminds us.

Fibre: the unsung hero when it comes to eating sugar

I tell Robert that readers will automatically say, 'but what about the sugar in my fruit, what about all my apples and my pears and my bananas, aren't they supposed to be good for me?'

'Everybody always asks that,' he chuckles. 'And the answer is fibre. Fibre is removed from ultra-processed food because you can't freeze it. Put an orange in your freezer overnight, take it out in the morning, let it thaw and all you get is mush. The food industry knows that, so they squeeze it and freeze it, and turn fruit into a storable commodity: juice. It's a great way to decrease depreciation and increase profit.' In contrast, eating a whole fruit, complete with its fibre, makes you feel full, slows fructose absorption in the gut and feeds your microbiome. (The same applies even if you make smoothies at home and include the skin, says the British Heart Foundation. Blending still releases the sugar from within the cell walls of the fruit, making it the equivalent of added sugar. Putting in vegetables such as spinach or kale doesn't help either.)

Your brain and liver: hardwired to be hurt by sugar

This is the most complex part, but basically, says Robert, 'all the chronic diseases of Western society – type-2 diabetes hypertension, cardiovascular disease, cancer, dementia, fatty liver disease – are diseases of mitochondrial dysfunction. Mitochondria are the powerhouses of every cell, and the brain has the most because it's the most energy-intensive organ. Yet [dietary] fructose actually shuts down mitochondrial function – it's a mitochondrial toxin.' This is why researchers are looking at links between Alzheimer's disease and dietary sugar. 'I'm not saying that this is the only thing that happens in Alzheimer's,' Robert goes on, 'but it's been shown with numerous animal models, and there's certainly epidemiological data that suggests the more sugar consumed, the more risk there is for Alzheimer's – that's very clear.' In your liver too, dietary fructose acts as a mitochondrial toxin. The liver gets overwhelmed by all that extra sugar in the gut and re-routes it from making energy into making fat, driving insulin resistance and non-alcoholic fatty liver disease.

The sugar paradox: awareness versus action

Sugar: The Bitter Truth ignited public awareness of sugar's dangers, but 15 years later we still eat far too much it. 'Left to their own devices, people can't break the biochemical drive to consume,' says Robert. 'That's why we need regulation for tobacco, that's why we need regulation for alcohol, that's why we need regulation for opiates. For sugar, we have no regulation. We know it's the right thing to do, but breaking the habit is hard. The criteria for regulation established by the public-health community are four things: ubiquity – you can't get rid of it; toxicity – it's bad for you; abuse – you can't stop; and finally, externalities – that is, your consumption hurts someone else. For alcohol, this is drunk driving, for tobacco it's second-hand smoke. The question is what's the externality for sugar? And the answer is – eventually – no healthcare. If you can't treat chronic diseases, and the patients keep piling up, you're going to be behind the eight ball pretty quick. [Eight ball is an American version of pool where the balls have to be potted in order. 'Behind the eight ball' is not where you want to be stuck.] It's what's happening all over the world.'

Policy and practice: the root of the crisis

Robert is angry that food subsidies make sugar cheap. What he'd like is for the price of the stuff on our supermarket shelves to be realigned with the downstream health costs of eating it. He's also bewildered by the pushback he still gets from some doctors. 'We have to re-educate the medical establishment,' he tells me. 'I'm trying to do that, but it's unbelievably complicated, because you can't tell a doctor anything. Whatever they learn in medical school, that's all they ever believe. It's like the priesthood, God forbid that you should have a thought of your own.'

Talking to Robert has been illuminating, but he knows what he is up against when it comes to the war on sugar. He reminds me of the old adage that science progresses 'one funeral at a time'. It dates from 1902 when Max Planck, a Nobel prize-winning German theoretical physicist, wrote: 'A new scientific truth does not triumph by convincing its opponents and making them see the light, but rather because its opponents eventually die, and a new generation grows up that is familiar with it.'

As I said, I'm not waiting for this. I have already quit sugar, and I'm certain that in time we will have a sugar tax (currently, in the UK it's only applied to soft drinks) in the same way that we eventually accepted a tax on tobacco and seatbelts being made mandatory too. Robert Lustig is not a lone voice speaking out against sugar. Michael Ash (Chapter 9) and almost every nutritionist I know gives me stern advice about over-consuming sugar. As I write, a research group from the University of Vienna have been able to prove that certain immune cells (monocytes) react more strongly to bacterial toxins after fructose consumption. That's good, right? No, actually. This reaction makes the body more susceptible to inflammation, infections and even food intolerances.[6]

Happy hacks

- **Make a list** of Dr Kara's dynamic dozen on your phone, and buy and eat them regularly.
- **Eat more omega-3s.** I supplement, because I can only manage so much oily fish.
- **Have a go** at simple home fermenting.
- **Cut down on sugar** – you'll be surprised at how quickly your taste buds adjust. Watch out for hidden sugars; there are at least 60 different names used on labels for refined sugar including high-fructose corn syrup, barley malt, dextrose and maltose. I found that eliminating snacking (I don't eat in between meals at all anymore) helped me cut out the sugar habit.
- **Eat your fruit bowl** and your veg box – don't drink it.

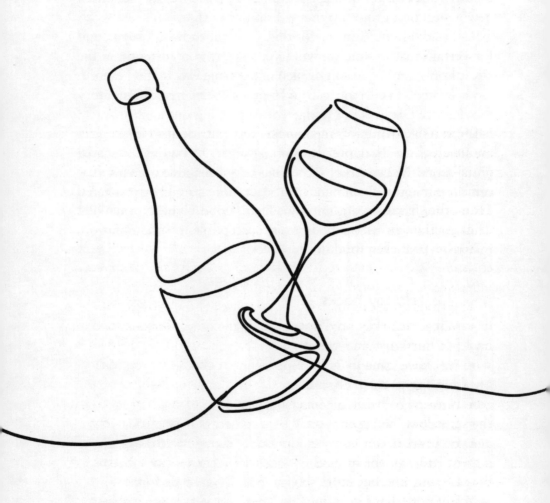

Chapter 4

When Cheers Turns to Tears

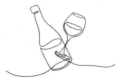

Is the sun over the yardarm? Good. That means it's time to talk about alcohol. That phrase is nautical, believed to have originated in the North Atlantic, where the sun would rise above the upper spars (yards) of a mast on a square-rigged ship at about 11am, the signal for officers and men to nip off and have the first drink of the day.

You're probably thinking: *Huh! I never drink before lunch/cocktail o'clock/dinner time; and I do not therefore have an issue with alcohol, so bottoms up, Bradbury!*

The thing is, though, alcohol is a toxin, and although lots of us love it – me in my pre-cancer life included – it doesn't love us back. It hurts us, and it's time to reconsider our relationship with it. I have gone from being the last of the rock-steady crew on a big night out to living an alcohol-free life as part of my commitment to being a cancer thriver. I'm not insisting you do the same, but I am going to tell some stories for you and encourage you to work out how the gorgeous plum and tobacco leaf of a great Rioja or the honeysuckle spice of a Viognier can still be part of your life, but more safely.

You'll note that I described my own life as alcohol-free rather than teetotal. I would not deny myself a glass of something delicious if I wanted one – it's just that normally I don't any more, and I am fine with that. Polymath Galileo Galilei said that 'Wine is sunlight, held together by water', but when Professor Gareth

Evans told me that my risk of breast cancer recurrence would increase by 28 per cent if I consumed four units of alcohol a day, I knew my days of boozing were behind me.

Sadly, it doesn't matter what shape or flavour you consume it in, alcohol itself is the poison. The World Cancer Federation (which links alcohol to seven types of cancer) is very cross about the messaging around alcohol consumption in adverts, and thinks that tag lines such as 'drink responsibly' and 'in moderation' should be banned because they are misleading. The federation's stark message is that alcohol harms every organ of the body and there is no safe limit when it comes to healthspan and longevity.

Gulp.

You might be reading this and screaming at the page, 'Jools, it's too much! I'm going to drink, I don't have a problem with alcohol, I enjoy it occasionally.' So here's what our friendly biohacker, Ben Greenfield, advises if you've got a big (or small) night on the sauce planned, and a few tips I picked up along the way.

Ben and Jools's boozy rules

1 **Get plenty of sleep** before you indulge. If you know you're going to a party or have a big birthday coming up, get those sleep miles in the bag. Despite feeling knocked out by booze, it disrupts sleep, and we don't get the same quality or duration when we drink alcohol.

2 **Exercise** Strength training or HIT before a drinking session can improve glycaemic response (how much a food or drink raises blood sugar), and exercise also increases antioxidant activity, which can reduce liver damage.

3 **If you follow me on social media, you'll know that I drink a shot of extra-virgin olive oil** every morning. It turns out that the polyphenols in olive oil and avocado oil can protect against

alcohol-induced oxidative stress, and the monounsaturated and saturated fats protect the liver too.

4 **Eat a light meal** before you drink. Anything colourful and pungent is good for alcohol metabolism, such as a beetroot salad with some fish and nuts, or scrambled eggs with ground turmeric, and a handful of berries afterwards. Some food in the stomach will slow the absorption of alcohol, to reduce the risk of flooding your body with too much ethanol too fast.

5 **Supplements** that can help the body cope include vitamin C, NAC or glutathione, and magnesium (which gets depleted by alcohol). A probiotic can also aid the gut. There are some out there now created especially for the drinkers' market.

6 **The after-party** When you're done, before bed, make sure you're hydrated. You can take some electrolytes (I have my preferred brand, which I travel with because they're good for more than just a hangover), or make your own: mix half a teaspoon of salt with the juice of a lime or lemon, add a cup and half of water and stir. Ben suggests adding black-strap molasses as well. It's a rich source of antioxidants and contains plenty of iron, calcium, magnesium, potassium and phosphorus. (A little factoid here: blackstrap molasses contains more iron than eggs, more calcium than milk, and more potassium than any other food. I use it sparingly as a sweetener at home, because it's more nutritious than refined sugar.)

7 **Take some activated charcoal** to mop up any toxins in the gut. Contrary to popular belief, charcoal does not absorb alcohol, but it does absorb toxins. I take activated charcoal, or a binder that contains humic and fulvic acid, if I've eaten anything that I'm uncertain about (for example, the oil that a food has been cooked in, or pesticides/herbicides, and so on, that might have been added). These are available from all good health-food shops.

The doctor will see you now

Let's move to the Integrative and Personalised Medicine Conference in London in 2024. The conference rooms are in the Queen Elizabeth II centre in London, opposite the centuries-old sanctuary of Westminster Abbey and the Houses of Parliament. Not that the QEII centre is part of that historical cityscape, no, it's a product of 1970s design and 1980s build. A bit like me, really.

I'm here on a warm June day, as a speaker. One of the attendees is GP Matthew Dennison who comes to find me for a chat while I am signing copies of *Walk Yourself Happy*. He is in his early fifties, tall and gleaming with good health. He lives in Devon with his wife of almost 30 years, their three kids and their family Labrador Daisy, a blonde.

Matt is evangelical about living well; he eats food from local farms, and he paddleboards and surfs in his free time, prioritises sleep and starts his mornings with stillness and breathing exercises. He's also a practising Christian and belongs to a church congregation that meets on a Devon farm. (Interestingly, research suggests that people who have a faith might live longer, potentially by several years.) Basically, he's the kind of human being who ticks all the typical boxes for physical and mental wellness. Even in his consulting room he stays active, using resistance bands and a standing desk.

If you ask him about his own alcohol consumption, he'll tell you that he has the very occasional glass of red, or perhaps a cold beer on a hot day, and that's it. It's partly because he doesn't like the loss of focus and the interrupted sleep that alcohol causes, but mostly it's because, as a GP on the front line of community care, he sees what happens to people who drink.

Matthew Dennison's sobering truth

Matthew: In every shift working for the NHS urgent-care service, I witness first-hand how alcohol quietly undermines health.

It's not always a crisis, but rather alcohol exacerbating the very issues my patients are trying to manage. Take Steve [not his real name], a 55-year-old engineer who came in with a leg wound that wouldn't heal. He's overweight, has type-2 diabetes and now requires daily insulin due to poor blood sugar control. Yet Steve didn't link his significant daily alcohol intake to these problems. He's going to work and taking care of his responsibilities at home, so his drinking feels harmless. But alcohol is worsening his diabetes, leading to slow wound-healing and damage to his kidneys, eyes and brain.

Steve's story is far from unique. Drinking habits are deeply ingrained and, for many, alcohol is woven into the fabric of daily life. In today's fast-paced world, especially for those juggling careers, families and endless to-do lists, a glass of wine or a beer can feel like a well-deserved reward or a way to unwind. But how many of us are quietly slipping into 'danger drinking' without even realising it?

What's more, the health issues connected to drinking are not always obvious: fatigue, high blood pressure, poor sleep – these are examples of the more hidden problems I regularly see in my patients.

For some, alcohol becomes a kind of anaesthetic – a way to numb stress, worry or sadness. It smooths out life's rough edges. But what begins as a coping mechanism can evolve into dependence. The shift can be subtle – a glass of wine after work, a beer with dinner – these habits are so culturally ingrained that they go unquestioned.

As a doctor, what strikes me most is how many of my patients remain in denial, not just about how much they drink, but about the ripple effects it has on their health. Alcohol is often there, in plain sight, quietly disrupting their well-being, relationships and long-term outlook, but the attitudes and expectations normalised in our society keep it concealed.

I'm not suggesting that everyone gives up alcohol altogether, but it's worth asking ourselves whether we truly need it as much as we think we do.

The myth of moderation

Matthew: When we say 'alcohol' what we're really talking about is ethanol, a substance that is essentially a toxin. When consumed, ethanol quickly enters the bloodstream and affects the brain by increasing levels of dopamine and GABA [gamma-aminobutyric acid is a neurotransmitter, a chemical messenger in your brain that calms you by blocking specific signals in your central nervous system], creating feelings of relaxation and euphoria.

This comes at a cost, however, as disrupting the delicate balance of neurotransmitters often leads, as many will know, to impaired judgement, slowed reactions and disrupted sleep. And over time, regular consumption of alcohol can damage multiple organs and systems, increasing the risk of developing serious health conditions. Even in smaller amounts, alcohol can contribute to them, especially as we age, making it crucial that we understand its impact on the body and approach it with caution.

You can learn more about Matthew and his work in the field of integrative and personalised medicine on his website www.myprivategp.co.uk.

Blood thirsty

As you can imagine, I have had a *lot* of blood taken for testing during my research for *Hack Yourself Healthy*. Pints and pints of the red stuff. (I'm surprised there's any left, to be honest, and you can see what I did with it all in the Appendix on Testing.) But why, you're wondering, am I raising this here? It's because from one of London's best-known phlebotomists, Julio de Oliveira, I learned something very specific about what alcohol does to your blood. It's so grim that it has stayed with me, and I'm going to tell you because it might make you think twice about that 'one for the road' glass.

'The blood from people who drink often has a distinct smell,' he tells me. 'If a sample spills, I can recognize the scent instantly, possibly due to the way alcohol affects red blood cells. Alcohol seems to make these cells more fragile, leading them to hemolyze (break down) faster. It stinks. Once you have smelled it, you never forget. The worst blood is that of alcoholic people, it smells of decay.'

When happy hour becomes unhappy

Now, let me introduce you to a woman who is, or rather was, the epitome of the hidden middle-class drinker: wife, mother and best-selling novelist, Clare Pooley. Clare is warm and funny, and extremely clever; she read economics at Cambridge and then spent the 1990s and the 2000s working in advertising for one of the world's best-known and most powerful marketing communications agencies, rising to become a managing partner. Like me, she could 'drink the boys under the table'. Also, like me, she once wore that as a badge of pride.

Until one day, at home with three small-ish children, she found herself pouring a glass of morning wine into a mug which read 'WORLD'S BEST MUM' and she realised that her drinking had crossed a line. She'd always loved wine, but now she couldn't function without it. She would give up, dealing with her addiction a day at a time, and sometimes on an hour-by-hour, or minute-by-minute, basis, processing her struggle by writing about it.

Her anonymous blog organically found a huge audience of women – and men – just like her, those middle-class drinkers in denial that Dr Matt Dennison speaks about. In 2017, it became a book, *The Sober Diaries*: one of the first and the finest pieces of what we now call 'quit-lit'. I wanted to talk to Clare because she speaks for many of us.

My name is Clare Pooley, and I'm an ex-wine addict

Clare: I grew up in the age of Bridget Jones and her Chardonnay, the girls from *Sex and the City* with their cosmopolitans, and the *Absolutely Fabulous* girls with their endless bottles of Bolly. It was the era of the ladette, when keeping up with the boys was seen as our duty as proud feminists. I was in advertising, and drinking was virtually compulsory. The office had a bar, and I had a huge expense account with which to take clients out for lunch, dinner and lots of drinks.

Then I had three children and totally bought into the cult of wine o'clock and me time. I was as likely to be offered a glass of wine on a playdate as a cup of tea. Wine was how we mothers coped with the crazy juggling of motherhood; it made us feel like we were still proper adults.

By the time I hit my mid-forties, however, I realised that alcohol had stopped being my friend. I was a terrible insomniac, anxious a lot of the time, two stone overweight and a terrible mother. I used to skip through bedroom stories as quickly as I could so that I could open a bottle of wine. And I'd often find myself, late at night, googling 'am

I an alcoholic' and doing one of those quizzes. 'Do you drink alone?', it would ask me. 'No,' I'd reply, because I was with the dog.

Nobody thought I had a problem or staged an intervention. From the outside, my life looked pretty perfect. Certainly nothing like the stereotypical 'alcoholic' pouring vodka on their cereal and collapsed on a park bench. I was nowhere near a rock bottom. But I knew that alcohol was making my life harder and harder.

At first, I tried to just drink less. You've been there, right? I set myself rules, like only drinking when out, or only at weekends, or only beer (because it didn't really count). But within weeks I'd have broken all my rules and was back to where I started. I discovered that I'm an all-or-nothing person. I just can't do anything by halves, not love, not crisps, not life, and not alcohol. It became clear that I had to quit altogether.

The final straw came the day after my forty-sixth birthday party, when I crossed one of my red lines. I poured some red wine into a mug (so that my kids wouldn't see) at 11.30am, to cure a hangover. I drank it, and it did help a little. But then I noticed that on the mug was printed 'THE WORLD'S BEST MUM'. That was the last drink I ever had.

I was too ashamed to tell anyone that I had stopped drinking. Not my family, nor my friends, not AA nor my GP. When I'd given up smoking, I told everyone and got endless pats on the back, but when you quit drinking, people find it difficult to know what so say, or do, around you. Alcohol is the only drug you have to make excuses for not taking.

Instead, by way of therapy, I started an anonymous blog called 'Mummy was a Secret Drinker' in which I wrote about what it felt like to go sober in a world where everyone drinks. All the ups and the downs, the triumphs and disasters. And I discovered that I wasn't alone. That blog went viral. Within the first year it had had over a million hits. Eventually, I published it as a memoir called *The Sober Diaries*.

Since then, I've had messages from thousands of people, from all over the world, telling me that my story is their story. We are the 'grey-area drinkers'. The people for whom alcohol is causing a problem, but who don't fit the outdated black-and-white stereotype of 'alcoholic'; the people who realise that waiting until you hit rock bottom to quit is a really, really stupid thing to do.

According to NHS England, in 2021, 21 per cent of adults drank to hazardous levels. And it's not the teenagers who are bolstering those statistics, it's actually the over fifty-fives. Twenty-eight per cent of 55 to 64-year-olds drink over the recommended limits. And the more well-educated and the more well-off you are, the more likely you are to drink too much.

When I first stopped drinking, I thought my life was pretty much over, that I'd never have fun again. In fact, my life was only just beginning. Quitting drinking (or cutting down, if you're the kind of person who's able to do that, in which case I salute you) is one of the most transformative things you can do with your life.

Sober is actually a super-power. You become less anxious, you sleep like a baby, you grow to adore the early mornings, your skin looks better, your eyes brighter, you have more energy, you lose weight, and you're much more able to deal with parenting and any lemons that life throws at you. Ditching the booze will help with any menopausal symptoms too. Drinking during the menopause is like throwing petrol on flames.

And going sober is really good for your health. The World Health Organization (WHO) say that alcohol is a group-1 human carcinogen. It causes seven types of cancer, including breast, mouth and bowel cancer. I had totally bought into the idea of moderate amounts of red wine being good for you. It's made of grapes! Part of a

Mediterranean diet! But the WHO insist that there is *no safe level* of alcohol consumption. According to breastcancer.org, just three drinks a week increases your risk of breast cancer by 15 per cent, and the more you drink, the higher the risk.

I am a part of these statistics. I was diagnosed with breast cancer just a few months after I quit drinking. Luckily, being sober I was able to deal with the diagnosis and the treatment without getting plastered and falling to pieces in front of the kids. And by not drinking, I have significantly reduced my risk of recurrence.

If you decide that alcohol isn't for you, you really won't be alone. More and more people are realising that going sober can be a positive lifestyle choice, and not just something you do because you have a 'disease' called alcoholism. Instagram is filled with people who are sober and shouting about it. Bookshops have shelves of 'quit-lit', and most of the big drinks brands, from Heineken to Guinness and Gordon's Gin have alcohol-free variants. About 30 per cent of young adults choose not to drink. At all. So you, my friend, will be surfing the zeitgeist!

Even if the sober life is one step too far for you, do try to drink mindfully. Make a note of how much you're drinking and think about why you reached for that drink. Is it just for social lubrication, or is it self-medication? Can you replace at least some of those glasses with something else? Your body and your mind will thank you for it.

Is your drinking a problem?

Clare used to do a multiplicity of quizzes online, mostly with a glass of wine in hand, trying to establish if she really did have a problem with alcohol. She has created a very simple one of her own, here, for readers of *Hack Yourself Healthy*. Answer it honestly, because Clare has been there, she knows what she's talking about and she's not judging you, she's asking you to judge yourself.

You probably know that drinking first thing in the morning, having blackouts, debilitating hangovers and physical withdrawal symptoms are signs that you're addicted to alcohol, but just because you don't tick those boxes, it doesn't mean that your drinking isn't becoming a problem. Here are some of the common early warning signs:

1 **Do you spend an awful lot of time** *thinking about drinking?* The truth is that people who don't have a problem with alcohol don't think about it. They don't plan it, feel guilty about it or try to stop doing it. It just isn't an issue.

2 **Have you ever googled:** *Am I an alcoholic?* It's another red flag. And, by the way, you're asking the wrong question. The questions you should ask are: *Is alcohol messing up my life?*, and: *Would I be better off without it?*

3 **Do you set rules** around your drinking? If you're always creating rules like 'I will only drink at weekends', or 'I'll only drink when I'm out', and you can't stick to them for long, then your drinking is a problem.

4 **Do you dislike yourself** when you've been drinking? Problem drinkers often wake up at 3am berating themselves for how much they've drunk, or something they've done or said or texted. (They also often take a while to remember how they got home, or where their handbag is.)

5 **Do you drink alone?** When we first start drinking, it's usually for social lubrication – to relax and have fun at a party. But over time it morphs into self-medication – we drink when we're feeling stressed or anxious, or bored or lonely. And that isn't healthy.

If you've answered 'yes' to two or more of these, it's a good idea to cut down on your drinking. And if you find that impossible, you really should quit altogether. The sooner you do it, the easier it is.

Clare navigated her own way to sobriety. You can find out more about how she did it at www.clarepooley.com or on Instagram @clare_pooley or on X @cpooleywriter. After *The Sober Diaries*, she wrote her first novel, *The Authenticity Project*, which was a Radio 2 Book Club pick and a *New York Times* bestseller and is published in 32 languages.

An alcohol exit plan

These days, almost a decade after the publishing phenomenon of *The Sober Diaries*, there's a lot more mainstream help for people wanting to quit or cut down as they seek to extend their healthspan. Here are Clare's personal top five tips:

1 **Find your tribe** They say that the opposite of addiction is connection, and it's true. It's hard to quit on your own, and you really don't have to. Instagram is filled with sober heroes. Check out @thisnakedmind, @sobergirlsociety, @soberandsocial_ @tribesober, @thriveacoholfree and @soberdave for starters. Or you can join an online group such as Kate Bee's The Sober School, Janet Gourand's Tribe Sober or Janey-Lee Grace's The Sober Club. If you'd rather meet sober friends in real life, you can find a local AA or SMART Recovery meeting.

2 **Read the 'quit-lit'** There are so many great books out there, filled with tips and inspiration. You could read *The Sober Diaries*, or try Annie Grace's *This Naked Mind*, Catherine Gray's *The Unexpected Joy of Being Sober* or Holly Whitaker's *Quit Like a Woman*.

3 **Create a personal toolkit** When the going gets tough, you need tools to help you ride through the cravings. Different things work for different people. My personal favourites are relaxing in

a hot bath with bubbles, going for a walk while listening to a great podcast, doing an exercise class or just losing myself in a good book or film. You have to find new ways of getting out of your head for a while.

4 Find something else to drink If you're used to pouring yourself a drink as a reward at the end of the day, you should still do that. Keep the ritual, change the ingredients. Try an alcohol-free beer or a super-healthy kombucha. Or an alcohol-free spirit. There are so many options now, and it'll stop you feeling that you're missing out.

5 Reward yourself You're doing an amazing thing – for you and the people who love you. And you're saving loads of money. Use some of it to reward yourself. Book a pedicure or a massage. Go away for a spa weekend. When I quit, I used some of the money I saved on a flower subscription. Every week a gorgeous bunch of flowers lands on my doorstep, and they always remind me what a wonderful thing I did.

And, finally, as Clare says, don't think about what you're giving up. You're giving up nothing but hangovers, bad health, insomnia, empty calories, guilt and regret. Think about what you're gaining – and the healthspan you're building.

Sipping pretty

There are many delicious ways to enjoy drinking with the low-alcohol and no-alcohol alternatives now appearing on the market. Here, I am turning to Helena Nicklin for advice. Helena is a freelance drinks writer and broadcaster, consultant, awards judge and co-founder of the HelenaSips Wine Academy.

She's a slender, glamorous honey-blonde, who's just launched an online wine academy with the aim of helping people to drink less but better. She's also applied her wine know-how to the no- and low-alcohol drinks space, seeking out the most delicious alternatives for those abstaining or wishing to moderate their consumption.

No/low wine

Helena says, 'The wine space has struggled the most when it comes to genuinely delicious, non-alcoholic drinks. This is because the alcohol removal process is so harsh that wine often ends up tasting cooked and un-fresh. The body it gets from alcohol also tends to be replaced by surprisingly high amounts of sugar, even if the wine doesn't taste officially sweet. The best bottles currently are as expensive as "real" wine and note that sparkling wines fare much better than still ones.'

No/low beer

Helena says, 'Ever since Lucky Saint gave us the first properly enjoyable non-alcoholic beer, more and more brands have popped up, giving us fantastic, booze-free IPAs, lagers and stouts. Today, even the big names are producing some fantastic versions – and on-tap too, which is a game changer in pubs. It's the non-alcoholic beers with benefits, however, that are really turning experts' heads, with artisanal brands producing refreshing, low-sugar beers that also include health-giving ingredients such as the fungi lion's mane and l-theanine (the amino acid you get in green and black tea) designed to improve cognition and mental aptitude, or guarana for a natural buzz.'

Spirits and liqueurs

Helena says: 'There's something a bit uncomfortable about non-alcoholic spirits and liqueurs, because what are these high alcohol tipples without the booze? Many can taste fairly flat; a bit like a slightly strange cordial and with a high price tag to boot.

Others, however, give you the right flavour hit with a kick on the finish that will just about fool your taste buds – especially if they are made to be mixed. These tipples also come in useful when you want a lower alcohol version of a regular cocktail or Aperol spritz-type drink. Using these means that you don't get the double hit of booze but you do get the desired blend of complex flavours in the glass – and some versions also include mood-boosting benefits.'

Delightfully different alcohol alternatives

Helena says, 'This relatively new drinks genre is growing exponentially – and for good reason. These drinks are not simply de-alcoholised and slightly disappointing versions of things we already know, or simple, sugar-filled soft drinks, but unique sippers in their own right. They can easily take the place of beers, wines and spirits, offering a delicious, complex drinking experience, often with natural flavours, no added sugar and, in some cases, extra health benefits. These 'functional' drinks, as they are known, use health-giving plant extracts that can also improve your mood, making you feel relaxed or more alert, as required. This is a space where there's something for everyone, and they're premium enough to feel like you're not missing out when at parties, the pub or just looking for an after-work treat. We're even seeing non-alcoholic beers and spirits using some of this 'functional' technology too.'

I have tried drinks containing a variety of plant compounds, including theobromine (found in cacao beans), caffeine and myrcene (found in hops and cannabis, and magnolia vines). Kombucha's tang – fruity and floral or spicy and herbal – and its bubbles make it a good alternative too.

So, cheers! Now you have no excuse. For more expert guidance, do have a look at helenasips.com or check out her new wine course at helenasipswinecourse.com and @HelenaSips on X and Insta.

One last sobering statistic, literally: the younger generation is drying out, unlike Gen Xers (that's my generation) and baby boomers. A YouGov poll from early 2025 showed that 39 per cent of Gen Z (18 to 24-year-olds) don't drink alcohol at all.

Happy hacks

- **If you're going to enjoy alcohol**, eat, sleep and exercise accordingly, and have plenty of water or an electrolyte drink too.
- **Don't feel the need to lubricate** every social situation with alcohol.
- **If you have any concerns about your consumption**, cut down. Being bothered is a big red flag.
- **Explore the lo- and no- market** – you'll be surprised by how much it has moved on in the last decade.
- **Find a non-alcoholic sipper** you love and make it your special drink – it's no more expensive than decent wine.

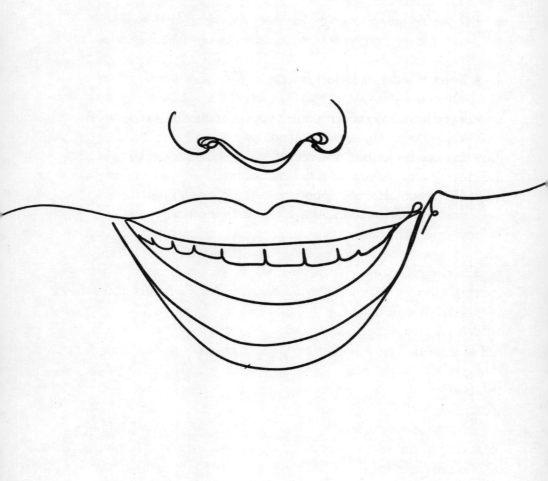

Chapter 5

Spit Happens

My children were given this strange game one Christmas that involves trying to talk with oversized mouthpieces. Plastic frames stretch the lips apart and expose the teeth, so it's impossible to look like anything other than a horse. The game is trying to say difficult words or sentences such as, 'He's my stealthy pet ferret named Garrett.'

Go on, try saying that with your mouth open.

Supine in a reclining chair peering up at functional dentist Victoria Sampson through pink-framed sunglasses, and wearing a similar type of mouthpiece, I was reminded of Garrett the pet ferret and looked, for sure, like Wallace from Wallace and Gromit.

'Ready?' Victoria asked.

'Wheeady!' I said, giving the thumbs up.

I was about to experience my first brush with guided biofilm therapy: the latest and apparently better way to clean teeth. (Biofilm is what we call plaque these days, in case you're wondering.)

I'm at a dental practice called The Health Society, which Victoria co-founded in the heart of Mayfair, central London. This is the future of dentistry and, like many pioneering propositions, it's exclusive and expensive-looking. Inside its great glass doors, Victoria polishes teeth using the latest oral tech, and she performs dental mini miracles to improve smiles. But there's a lot more to her work than that.

Just as the gut microbiome is revolutionising the way in which we look at health, the oral microbiome is also having a moment. At 28 'The queen of saliva' (as she was called on 'The Diary of a CEO' podcast) has invented a unique saliva test that not only measures the oral microbiome to test the virulence of certain bacteria in the mouth, but also takes into account genetic mutations that could play a role in identifying risks to your wider health. (Victoria is also a fully qualified dentist in the traditional sense, with a degree in dental surgery from Barts and the London School of Medicine and Dentistry.)

As you're about to learn, the health (or not) of the oral microbiome is increasingly thought to be linked to a host of diseases including heart conditions, rheumatoid arthritis, cancer, diabetes and pneumonia. It can also contribute to pre-term birth in mothers-to-be and impact erectile function in men. Staying on top of our oral hygiene could therefore be a heavy weapon in our defence against disease in multiple areas, not just our mouth. It plays a much more significant role in our healthspan and longevity than old-fashioned drill-and-fill dentistry once suggested.

(Find out more at https://www.thehealthsociety.co.uk/gum-treatment and follow Victoria @drvictoriasampson on Instagram.)

Lip service

Back in 490 BC, Hippocrates, the 'father of medicine', believed that dental pain and disorders might reflect imbalances in general health. He thought that by treating these dental issues, systemic health could be restored. He even apparently treated a woman's arthritis by pulling out an infected tooth. Now, fast forward to 1765, when the first ever school of medicine opened at the University of Pennsylvania, but dentistry was not on the syllabus. This was the beginning of the disconnect between the mouth and the rest of the body, which is just starting to be closed 250 years later.

If only we had stuck with Hippocrates.

Victoria Sampson talks about our oral eco system

Victoria: My professional journey began, like that of Hippocrates, with a patient suffering from rheumatoid arthritis.

For many years she had been unable to walk, hooked on steroids and painkillers to numb the pain. She had seen countless doctors and functional-medicine practitioners who attempted to reduce her inflammatory load with dietary changes and supplements. One day, her functional-medicine practitioner asked her about her teeth, and she told him that she'd had six extractions in the preceding year.

He referred her to me and we diagnosed severe gum disease. We did saliva testing that showed she had extremely high levels of inflammation, high levels of bad bacteria, and elevated collagen breakdown in her mouth. Rheumatoid arthritis is an inflammatory condition and, for it to improve, doctors need to have ruled out all sources of inflammation in the body – including the mouth.

After a few months of treatment, we re-tested her saliva and her rheumatoid factor. We found that not only had we improved her oral health significantly, but that this had a knock-on effect on her rheumatoid arthritis, allowing her to start enjoying her life again. This was my real Aha! moment.

Here at The Health Society we say that our work is about putting the mouth back into the body. And one way that we do this is by testing the oral microbiome.

So what exactly is the oral microbiome?

Scroll back to Holland in the 1670s when a man who was not a trained scientist – he had a fabric shop and sold ribbons and buttons for his living – got good at grinding lenses. He made himself an eye glass with 270-times magnification, ten times stronger than anything else then in existence. Using this magnificent homemade microscope, Antonie van Leeuwenhoek,[1] today known as 'the father of microbiology', made a series of sensational scientific findings, including the fact that a drop of water is teaming with bacteria.

In the spirit of discovery, he decided not to brush his teeth for a while to see what would happen. (People have been cleaning their teeth for millennia, although the first mass-produced toothbrush was not invented until 1780.) After a few days, a white film started to grow on his teeth and around his gums. He scraped it off and put it under his microscope. 'There were many very little living animalcules, very prettily a-moving. The biggest sort . . . had a very strong and swift motion and shot through the water (or spittle) like a pike does through the water. The second sort . . . oft-times spun round like a top . . . and these were far more in number', he wrote in delight to the Royal Society in London.

Today, we know a lot more about the oral microbiome, namely that it's the biggest in our body after the one in our gut, with 700 different strains of bacteria and a population of about 2 billion bacteria in everyone's mouth. We also understand that it is the gateway to the rest of the body; for example, a 2012 American Heart Association study suggested that gum disease could be as significant a risk factor for heart disease as high cholesterol.[2] Research has also shown that patients with periodontal disease are three times more likely to develop diabetes[3] and 70 per cent more likely to develop Alzheimer's disease.[4]

The great thing about the mouth is that oral diseases such as decay and gum disease are extremely easy (and cheap) to avoid. The WHO says that they're the most common non-communicable diseases in the world – and that they're entirely preventable. In the pursuit of more, better years of life, knowing how to care for your mouth, teeth and tongue is an easy win.[5]

Plaque to the future

As more evidence emerges about the importance of oral health as part of whole-body health, it's important to get young families to develop good oral habits. Brushing your teeth is one of the simplest biohacks we can all do – starting as soon as those baby teeth appear! Here are some brushing tips for all ages from specialist orthodontist, Dr Sarah Good.

- Electric toothbrush or manual? Either works, but electric brushes are generally recommended for older children and adults (and used more by dentists themselves). They can help you brush for the right amount of time (a minimum of 2 minutes, but if you or your child have wobbly baby teeth, replacement teeth or fixed braces, it will take longer. The genius of these toothbrushes is that they have inbuilt timers, and some have pressure sensors as well, which can stop you from damaging the delicate gum tissue by scrubbing.
- Timing is key. Find what works for you and your family. If bedtime brushing is rushed or skipped, consider adding brushing after dinner instead, as it tends to be a less tired/time pressured time of the day.
- Avoid acidic tooth wear. Don't brush for at least 30 minutes (ideally 45) after consuming food or drink, especially citrus juices or fizzy drinks. Regular water is fine any time.
- Savoury snacks are best. It takes about 45 minutes for your mouth to neutralise acids after a sugary snack of any size, so frequent 'sugar hits' throughout the day can cause serious damage.

Finally, both Victoria and Sarah agree you should test, test, test. Unfortunately, we cannot 'see' the oral microbiome, just the consequences of a balanced or imbalanced one. The only way to understand what bacteria you have, any genetic mutations that increase your risk of disease, and how inflamed you are, is by testing. In the Appendix, you can read my before-and-after results from The Health Society.

Happy hacks

- **Brush twice a day** and spit, don't rinse. It sounds simple, but this is the best way to maintain a good oral microbiome. When you don't brush, bacteria accumulate on your teeth and gums, which can cause dysbiosis (an imbalance of the gut microbiome, leading to health issues). Regular mechanical removal of the bacteria is key.
- **Floss daily** Nearly 30 per cent of the bacteria in your mouth is found in between your teeth and can only be removed by flossing.
- **Disclose your microbiome** Try using a disclosing tablet that dyes the bacteria in your mouth a different colour. This is a great visual tool to help train you and your family to remove it effectively. Brush first and then disclose to see the bits that you are missing.
- **Avoid aggressive mouthwashes** Unless recommended by your dentist, avoid strong antibacterial or alcohol-based mouthwashes. You are probably doing more harm than good. If you use a mouthwash (avoid those found in the supermarket) you should use it only for a prescribed period of no more than two weeks.
- **Avoid products that contain SLS** (sodium lauryl sulfate). SLS is a foaming agent that can disturb the soft tissues in your mouth and imbalance your oral microbiome. Many people are intolerant to SLS and may have sore gums or ulcers if they use it, and the same applies to whitening toothpastes.
- **Think about taking a probiotic** If you have no issues and just want to maintain a healthy, balanced oral microbiome, try supplementing it. Check out oral probiotics available online from companies such as Luv Biotics, Invivo and Healf.

- **Chew sugar-free and plastic-free gum** and/or mints to stimulate saliva production. Saliva is what makes the oral microbiome healthy and your bacteria happy. By chewing a mint or gum you stimulate saliva production, providing more food and nutrients for the good bacteria in your mouth.

- **Scrape your tongue** Use a copper tongue scraper a few times a week to gently lift the bacteria that live on there. It may help to reduce the build-up of the bacteria and fungi that can lead to oral infections such as gingivitis and thrush. It might also improve your sense of taste, which is nice. You can buy one cheaply from multiple online retailers or a good health and wellness store.

- **Eat well** Seems too simple, right? Just as you should try to eat well for your gut microbiome, eat well for your oral microbiome too. Try to have a diet rich in prebiotics such as fermented foods (see page 57) or kefir, and avoid processed foods and sugar (as discussed in Chapter 3). When you do eat them, chew some plastic-free gum afterwards to help with saliva production, as above. Enjoy foods high in flavonoids such as parsley, onions, blueberries, green tea and bananas.

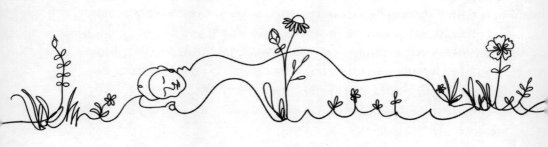

Chapter 6

Snooze or Lose

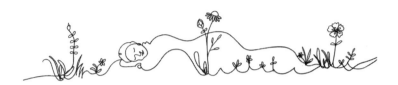

The reason we sleep is simple: our body needs that downtime to repair its cells, heal any injuries and rev up the immune system that keeps us safe. Our brain, freed from the burden of the body being awake, gets to do its filing and then puts the bins out. It has to be a critical function, because being asleep – which renders us unconscious and semi-paralysed – would have made our ancestors extraordinarily vulnerable to predators, both animal and human. We would have evolved very differently if it wasn't necessary for our health and longevity.

Physically, sleep allows you to conserve energy, grow and restore – it's especially important for the functioning of your cardiovascular system. Mentally, it helps with focus and concentration, and emotional regulation. It influences judgement and decision making – and there's truth in the old adage of sleeping on a problem: your brain loves to have a run at a knotty issue when the rest of the body is relatively quiet. Sleep is also when you lay down memories, the ones you want to keep forever, and the ones which help you learn how to go about your daily life: how to tie your shoelaces, for example.

Then there's what was discovered in 2013: that sleep helps detoxify the brain by flushing out the rubbish built up by a variety of metabolic functions during our waking hours. Waste chemicals drain from the brain along a series of channels surrounding our blood vessels. It's called the glymphatic system.

This breakthrough was made by a group led by Professor Maiken Nedergaard at the University of Rochester Medical Center in New York. She explains why the process (mostly) happens when we are asleep: 'You can think of it like having a house party. You can either entertain the guests or clean up the house, but you can't really do both at the same time.'[1]

(Among the waste products removed from brain tissue is a toxic protein called beta-amyloid, which is known to accumulate in the brains of people with Alzheimer's disease.)

So, given the amount of biology that happens when we are asleep, you can understand why we need it if we are to extend our healthspan. The Tudor dramatist Thomas Dekker wrote: 'Sleep is the golden chain that ties our health and our bodies together.' Queen Elizabeth I was on the throne at the time, and medical science was mostly herbal remedies and lucky charms, but he wasn't wrong.

Sleepy foods

- **Tart cherries** Admittedly, tart cherries are not that easy to get hold of, but there are supplements. They're a natural source of melatonin, which can help to regulate sleep patterns.
- **Kiwis** Another good source of melatonin, kiwi fruit can help you fall asleep faster and sleep more soundly.
- **Bananas** also contain melatonin, plus tryptophan (an amino acid that helps the body to release the happy hormone, serotonin), vitamin B6, and magnesium, which can all help you to sleep.
- **Oily fish** These offer vitamin D and omega-3 fatty acids, which can increase the production of serotonin.
- **Almonds** Good for magnesium, tryptophan, potassium and B vitamins.
- **Milk** Another source of tryptophan.
- **Chamomile tea** contains apigenin, an antioxidant that can promote sleepiness.

- **Rice** A carbohydrate that prompts the release of insulin, rice helps the brain's uptake of tryptophan. (Note: I have a genetic profile that suggests a reduced carbohydrate diet is more suitable for me and I should avoid starchy carbs at night. See Appendix.)

Pillow talk

Let's head to San Diego to talk to Satchin Panda, a professor at the Salk Institute of Biological Studies at the University of California. His lab is credited with some of the biggest break-throughs in what he calls the 'biology of time' in recent years. He's a world expert in circadian rhythms: that's your body clock, most notably its sleep–wake cycle.

The day he hops on to a Zoom with me he's newly back from China and suffering from the shift in time zones, just like the rest of us when we travel long haul. He's a big fan of having a nap, so he has a couch in his office. 'A couple of days ago, I still had jet lag, and I thought, okay, maybe a nap will help,' he laughs. 'I closed the office door, had 20 minutes and it was magical. For the next five, six hours, I was completely productive.'

I ask the professor to start by telling me about circadian rhythms as simply as he can.

Satchin Panda chats about circadian rhythms

Satchin: When we think of circadian rhythms, the first thing that comes into our brain is sleep. There are other rhythms, such as our feeding rhythm and our exercise rhythm, but sleep is the most profound. Broadly speaking, we have body clocks to anticipate time. It's very easy to explain. If your TV show, Julia, is at 6am, your body has to get ready from 4am onwards. Similarly, if your breakfast time is at 8am, your body is preparing you to eat from 7am onwards. When you go to sleep at 10pm, your body has been looking ahead to that from 7pm onwards. Just like in real life, if we don't anticipate and don't prepare ourselves, we don't get the best out of anything.

Our circadian rhythms also put together compatible processes in the body, so, for example, being awake and feeling hungry is a good thing, because you don't want to be hungry in the middle of the night. The reverse is also true, circadian rhythms separate incompatible processes.

Then there's what we call 'reset and rejuvenation'. Every organ, when it works, gets damaged, and must repair itself. Mitochondria [the powerhouses of every cell]: every day, they go through a repair process; our DNA repairs itself in the evening. When we are asleep our brain literally takes its own trash out. Much of this repair function happens while we are asleep. That's why we have a sleep–wake pattern.

Finally, our circadian rhythms help us to synchronise with our outside world. When we fly from one time zone to another, or work a night shift, or have an early start, our body is able to reset itself to anticipate what time we should be going to bed and what time we should be waking up.

Kitchen curfew: Satchin Panda's mealtime tips

'It's timing that makes food healthy or junk,' says the professor. 'Think of your best friend knocking on your door in the middle of the night for three nights. That won't make them your best friend any more. Even a healthy salad in the middle of the night, when your gut is not ready to digest, becomes junk. So, the question is, how do you figure out the optimum time window for eating?'

- When you wake up, wait for one to two hours before your first calorie, because that's when you have the maximum amount of the stress hormone cortisol in your body. We need a massive jolt of cortisol to drag us out of bed and start the day, but cortisol is not good for our digestion and nutrient absorption.

- At night, our sleep hormone, melatonin, prepares our brain for sleep, and slows down everything else too – including our metabolism. It reduces the rate at which insulin (the hormone we need for digestion and glucose absorption) is produced from the pancreas. It's like the changing of the guard in our body, and you don't want to eat when it's happening. Therefore, give yourself a three-hour break from eating *before* you go to sleep.

Ctrl+alt+snooze

Thanks to the professor's decades of work, we now understand far more, if not everything, about the mysteries of our circadian rhythms. As Satchin points out, we have lived with them for the last 200,000 years, but have only woken up to their importance in the last 25.

'The human brain is our own unique, expensive control system,' he reminds us. It is the only organ in our body that can be repaired by itself. It's not like a tooth or a cornea, or a heart or a liver, which can all be mended or even replaced, so it has become very important to figure out how it does what it needs to do. We know it cannot repair during the day. You have to put it in snooze mode.

'Think of it like this: your computer goes to sleep, and then it auto-updates its software, checks for viruses, and backs up all its files to the cloud. The brain does something similar. When we are asleep it updates itself, rids itself of toxins and stores information in its memory. And that is something we cannot abuse. We need to get the best sleep we can to let it work its nightly miracle.'

'Better sleep will give you a longer, healthier life, no question,' he says.

Here are Satchin's top ten rules for getting a good night's sleep:

1 **Eat at the right times** (see box above). The 'right time' to eat when travelling is going to have to be aligned to local/external clock time and *not* your body-clock time, but always remember to leave a three-hour gap between your last meal of the day and your local bedtime too.

2 **Avoid caffeine in the afternoon** Our body takes around six hours to break down half the coffee we drink, so that means no coffee after noon.

3 **Dim the lights** Enjoy a candlelit dinner – and don't go shopping in the evenings either. Supermarkets and pharmacies are extremely brightly lit and, although you might only stay 15 minutes, it's enough to slam the brakes on your melatonin production.

4 **Get outside into daylight** (as I am always telling you!). It doesn't have to be sunshine: daylight at any point will do. Even Satchin doesn't know exactly how this works, but daytime light exposure boosts the release of melatonin at night.

5 **Accept that psychology plays a role**, and it might impact your ability to fall asleep, especially in midlife, which can be an anxious or pressured time with its twin burdens of career and family. It is important to unwind for 30 minutes to an hour before sleep. Satchin, who was 53 at the time of writing, sometimes re-reads his daughter's old books. 'There's no drama or mystery, just a nice story with a happy ending. It works for me,' he says.

6 **Don't get sucked into a TV box set,** no matter how much you love it, because great television is the enemy of good sleep.

7 **Have a wash** Try washing your hands and feet before bed or having a shower. If you warm your extremities, it can help to regulate your body temperature, enabling you to drop off more easily.

8 **Try nose strips** If you sometimes wake up after 4–5 hours and struggle to get back to sleep, try a nose strip to keep

your nose open and increase the air flow. You may not have sleep apnoea (temporary pauses in breathing or reduced air flow during sleep), but your brain might still be grumbling that it's not getting enough oxygen. (I use nasal dilators from Oxygen Advantage throughout the day, sometimes while I'm exercising, to promote nasal breathing.)

9 **Never be afraid of having a nap**, because it's always good to catch up on sleep. Our sleep pressure (that is, the desire to sleep) rises at night, but in the middle of the day, six or seven hours after waking up, we have another moment of sleep pressure. It's not so strong that we can fall asleep for seven or eight hours as we do at night, but it might be strong enough to encourage you to take a nap.

10 **Don't lie in** It'll give you a kind of jet lag without having been anywhere. Get up, get on and have a nap later if you need to.

Snore and peace

Sometimes sleep just comes down to our age: as we get older, we wake earlier, like we used to when we were kids. It's partially to do with fluctuating sex hormones, which interact with our body clock to turn us into late risers as teenagers and young adults, only for us to be re-programmed by the menopause and falling testosterone levels in midlife.

Opening your eyes at 5am to 6am is normal for a woman my age, apparently, and it's started to happen to me involuntarily. Mostly, I can go back to sleep for another precious hour, but according to Satchin's research, that hour, which feels cherished to me, is not 'quality' sleep, as it disrupts my natural sleep cycle and could potentially throw off my body's internal clock. Consistency is best, going to sleep and waking up at the same time as often as possible.

The rule of thumb for working out what's optimal *for you* is to give up coffee ahead of a seven- to ten-day holiday (sorry!) and then monitoring how many hours per night you sleep without a coffee or an alarm clock. Then you can calculate your natural sleep requirement and try to implement it when you get home.

Sowing the seeds of sleep

I'm coming to the end of my time with the professor, but I want to know a little more about him and what inspired him to take this path.

It was nature.

Satchin is from the Indian province of Odisha on the Bay of Bengal. He went to one of India's Agricultural Universities, where he excelled in genetics and seriously considered becoming a plant breeder. 'The province where I grew up was a rice growing area,' he tells me. 'Rice flowers at four o'clock in the morning. It opens and then remains receptive to pollination, maybe for two hours. So that's when you have to go and tend to it. Wheat opens at six o'clock. Corn opens around 7–7.30am. They all have a precise time.

'I found it curious: how could a plant keep track of the length of the day or the length of the night and then decide what time to flower?'

Nature's timekeepers

As Satchin discovered, circadian rhythms are all around us in nature, they're found in animals and plants, fungi, and even blue-green algae. The name comes from the Latin 'circa', meaning 'around', and 'dies' meaning 'day'. They are simply cycles that repeat approximately every 24 hours.

The first circadian rhythm in nature known to have been recorded was in the 4th century BC when a ship's captain serving under Alexander the Great told the Ancient Greek philosopher and naturalist Theophrastus (a friend and follower of Aristotle), about 'a tree with many leaves like the rose, and that this closes at night, but opens at sunrise, and by noon is completely unfolded; and at evening again it closes by degrees and remains shut at night, and the natives say that it goes to sleep'.

It would eventually be identified as a tamarind tree, but it was the mimosa tree that finally proved the science behind this anecdotal observation.

If you've ever been lucky enough to touch a mimosa leaf (which I was in Mauritius on a mountain hike several years ago), you'll have witnessed the magic of their tiny bright-green fern-like leaves closing to protect themselves, like mini shutters when you stroke them. In 1729 French physicist and philosopher Jean-Jacques d'Ortous de Marian decided to investigate whether their ordinary daily opening and closing was due to sunlight. He stuck some specimens in perpetual dark and watched as they continued to open and close: their own internal clocks driving their leaf rhythms, rather than any external factor.

These master clocks are intimately connected with the life and health of all living things – us included.

Our sleep–wake cycle is critical to our physical and mental well-being, and therefore our predicted healthspan. Like many of us, I sometimes struggle to nod off or I wake up in the small hours. But I never consciously sabotage my sleep in the way that I used to before my cancer diagnosis, with an overnight drive, a last-minute work deadline or disastrously late meals in restaurants. I was careless with my sleep in my life before cancer, and I suspect it might have cost me dearly by making me more vulnerable to disease. These days, I am scrupulous about making deposits in my sleep bank, not withdrawals, viewing them as a nightly investment in my healthspan.

Sacred seasons

Kirsty Gallagher is the *Sunday Times* bestselling author of *Sacred Seasons*, a book of nature-inspired rituals designed to keep you in alignment with the rhythms of spring, summer, autumn and winter. Synchronicity with nature is a skill that many of us have forgotten or don't care about any more. Yet it is one of the loveliest and most important life hacks of them all.

Kirsty has created a simple reminder of nature's calendar. She writes: 'The turn of each season is marked by the solstices and the equinoxes, with cross-quarter festivals in between. These are wonderful opportunities to ask yourself where you are in your life, and whether it's where you want to be.

'Here are my suggestions for aligning yourself with them every year':

Spring equinox (approximately 21 March) This is the season of birth and growth where all that has been germinating beneath the surface begins to come to life, both in nature and in us. We take everything we learned from our winter hibernation and use it to determine what we want to create moving forwards. There is a feeling of hope, optimism and possibility in the air all around us as new life is emerging. Use this season to make positive change and to start something new – make things happen. This is also the beginning of the astrological year, so use this time to set some intentions and goals for your year ahead.

Summer solstice (approximately 21 June) This is the season of abundance and growth. Everything in nature is in full bloom and we can use this energy to grow our own desires and ideas, and expand beyond any limitations. This is the season to grow into all that you can be, to allow yourself to be seen and to shine, and to appreciate and enjoy all that you have nurtured in your life since the spring equinox. At this halfway point in the traditional year, check in with where you are: is it where you want to be? Make any necessary adjustments.

Autumn equinox (approximately 21 September) This is the season to gather in your harvest, feeling grateful for all that you have in your life and all that you have manifested, achieved and created during the spring and summer. As nature begins to transform, see that this is the season where we too begin to shed, to let go of all that we no longer need or want to take into winter with us. Nature is beginning to slow down and go inwards, and we are called to do the same, gathering our energy and withdrawing into our inner world to take care of, and nourish, ourselves.

Winter solstice (approximately 21 December) During the darkest and coldest time of year, nature draws into a deep hibernation, inspiring us to do the same. This is the season of introspection, rest and connecting with our inner worlds. It's in this quiet time of reflection that we get to learn the lessons from the year gone by, and make changes within, so that we are prepared for the traditional New Year and lighter days ahead. This is the perfect time to pause and reflect upon the past year and what it has brought you; a natural time to say goodbye to the old before welcoming in the new. It's an ending to create a new beginning.

Have a look at Kirsty's latest book *Your Cosmic Purpose* to find more of her wisdom, or go to kirstygallagher.com.

Happy hacks

- **Keep the lights dim** in the evening, to encourage sleep.
- **Try foods that aid sleep** one at a time and see what works best for you.
- **Be strict** with your sleep schedule.
- **Experiment with Satchin Panda's suggestion** of going without coffee and an alarm clock on holiday and let your body tell you how much sleep it really needs.
- **Go out into the daylight** early in the morning.
- **Have a nap** if you need one during the day.
- **Buy a beautiful journal** and write some reflections and intentions connected to the turning of the year, as suggested by Kirsty Gallagher.

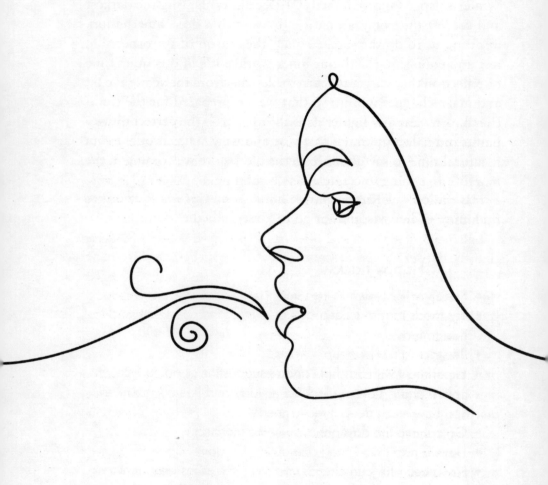

Chapter 7

Air Apparent

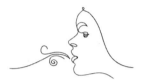

I've had to change things in my life to create better sleeping habits, improve my previously sugar-laden diet, and to exercise in a more deliberate way. I wrote about all of this in my last book *Walk Yourself Happy*. To me, these changes made sense, they're hardly rocket science, are they? (Unless you go deep, because then they really are a science.)

I also changed the way I breathe, although initially I found it slightly harder to justify the time for breathwork. Up until five years ago I had never given much thought to how I do it. Fast or slow? Deep or shallow? Through the nose or through the mouth? But breathwork, I now believe, is one of the most important and life-changing things that we can learn.

These days I do breathwork every morning when I wake up, practise different breath holds when I'm walking throughout the day, and include it as part of my night-time meditation. It's fascinating, gets easier over time and it's had a profound impact on my physical and emotional health.

Breathing is linked to brain function and multiple bodily processes, including heart and lung health, energy consumption, immunity, digestion and hormone release. It makes you feel stronger when you need to be, and calmer when you don't. I have come to depend on it as I seek to extend my healthspan.

If you read *Walk Yourself Happy*, you will already have 'met' my friend the breath expert Patrick McKeown, who has helped many people discover the power of breath, ranging from special-forces soldiers and elite athletes to children with asthma and teens with anxiety. Coldplay's Chris Martin, who is also a client, has recently helped put Patrick's book *The Oxygen Advantage* back into the bestseller charts.

I asked Patrick: 'What happens when we take a breath?'

A conversation with Patrick McKeown on breathing

Patrick: There's a common belief that breathing more air means more oxygen for the body. But that's not how it works. For example, when you hear people taking loud, deep breaths during a yoga practice, it may seem relaxing, but it can actually reduce oxygen delivery to the brain, muscles and vital organs. Breathing too heavily or too fast, especially through the mouth, causes too much carbon dioxide to be lost. This leads to blood vessel constriction and makes it harder for oxygen to move from the blood into the tissues. Feeling dizzy after deep breaths, or noticing cold hands or feet, or brain fog from breathing a little too much – minute after minute, hour after hour – is often a clear sign that your breathing is working against you.

Why is carbon dioxide essential?

Patrick: Once produced in the tissues, carbon dioxide is transported back to the lungs via the bloodstream. Although we exhale about 15 per cent of this carbon dioxide, the remaining 85 per cent is retained to perform crucial functions. Here's how it works: oxygen enters the lungs, moves into the blood, and binds to haemoglobin. But for oxygen to leave the blood and reach the tissues, we need carbon dioxide. This so-called waste gas helps in two vital ways: it dilates blood vessels to improve circulation and encourages haemoglobin to release oxygen where it's needed. So the key to using oxygen efficiently isn't more oxygen; it's maintaining the right level of carbon dioxide. Without enough of it, blood vessels narrow and oxygen stays trapped in the blood, unable to reach the brain, muscles and organs.

Can you explain how carbon dioxide unlocks oxygen?

Patrick: Beyond circulation, carbon dioxide plays a critical role in oxygen release. When carbon dioxide levels rise (for example, by Walking Yourself Happy with your mouth closed, or practising the 'breathe lightly' exercise described below), our blood pH drops slightly. This change causes haemoglobin to release oxygen more readily to the tissues. Given that the body can survive only few minutes without oxygen, this process is essential.

Can you change things for the better quickly by breathing properly?

Patrick: Yes. The empowering truth is that you can significantly influence your blood circulation and oxygen delivery simply by changing how you breathe. And here's the surprising part: it's not about taking big, deep breaths or breathing more air. Modern life often disrupts our natural breathing patterns, leading many of us to over-breathe. The real solution is to breathe less, to be slower and gentler. It's easy to overlook our breathing, yet it's one of our most reliable and supportive allies. By tuning into it – breathing gently in and out through the nose during rest, exercise and sleep, while softening our breath throughout the day – we can unlock profound benefits. There's no need for perfection or obsession; just dedicating five minutes here and there, six times a day, can make an incredible difference to how we feel. Think about it: we can not only improve the body's oxygen supply but also activate its relaxation response, fostering recovery and healing for both the body and mind.

The message in breathing

Breathing is more than a physical process, explains Patrick, it's a constant signal to your brain.

That message is either, 'We're safe, everything's okay,' or, 'We're under threat, time to gear up for survival!' Here's the big question: what is your body telling your brain right now?

The subtle signals in your breath:

When life gets stressful – whether it's work, family or not feeling well – your breathing changes. You might not even notice it. It's not like you're having a full-blown panic attack, but you might find yourself sighing more often, breathing a little faster, or feeling as if you're just not getting enough air. This kind of breathing isn't dramatic, but it's enough to signal to your brain that something's not right. Faster, harder breaths send a message, 'The body is under threat.' Your brain, being the overachiever that it is, takes this seriously. It cranks up the fight-or-flight response, pouring stress hormones into your system.

How to re-set the message: breathe lightly

The good news? You can take control of the message your body is sending your brain. Here's how:

1 Sit comfortably. Close your mouth and breathe gently in and out through your nose.
2 Focus on softening your breath. Take a very soft, gentle breath in through your nose, so light that it's almost imperceptible. Breathe in silently and lightly, then let your exhale be slow and relaxed.
3 Continue until you feel a slight air hunger. It's not uncomfortable, just enough to notice.

That slight feeling of air hunger is a sign that carbon dioxide levels are building slightly in your blood. This small increase helps to dilate your blood vessels, enhancing oxygen delivery to your brain and body. This gentle practice sends a powerful signal to your brain that the body is safe, triggering the rest-and-repair response.

Upgrade your airflow

It takes a while to get used to nasal breathing, and I still have to check myself throughout the day and give myself a nudge if I find I'm open mouthed. I tell my kids too, whenever I notice them sitting doing their homework with their mouths wide open, catching flies.

One little tip: when you practise, don't suck up violently through your nostrils as if you were breathing into the top of your head. Instead, breathe very gently as if you were aiming your breath at the back of your head, which is where your pipework leads anyway. And remember to expand your ribs and the area below them as you inhale.

If, like me, you struggle, you can try using a nasal dilator, as mentioned on page 97. I sometimes exercise wearing one, when I'm rebounding, or doing my fast Zone 2 (see page 295). I look like a surprised giraffe, but the occasional use of a dilator helps me to nasal-breathe comfortably the rest of the time.

To get an idea of how it works, place your thumb and your index finger on each side of your nostrils at the bottom of your nose. But instead of using them to block the airflow, use a gentle outward pressure to pull your nostrils apart. Essentially you're holding your nostrils open using your thumb and index finger. It should make your breathing feel easier and that's what a dilator does. Patrick advises, 'The key is to slow down the pace of whatever you are doing and focus on breathing comfortably in and out through your nose. It's not about forcing the air; it's about letting your body adapt naturally. Over a few weeks, as your body adjusts (and with the help of a nasal dilator), it becomes far easier to maintain nasal breathing during exercise.

Winning by a nose

- You'll need to breathe less air to sustain the same level of effort during exercise.
- Nasal breathing protects your airways by filtering, warming and humidifying the air entering your lungs.
- It improves oxygen delivery to your working muscles, helping them to recover faster after exercise.
- It slows your breathing, sending signals of relaxation to your brain.
- During sleep, nasal breathing promotes smoother airflow to and from your lungs, which can help keep snoring at bay.
- It helps engage your diaphragm – the key breathing muscle that powers movement, supports better posture, and boosts athletic performance.
- Your nasal passages produce nitric oxide, a gas that's drawn into your lungs with every breath. Nitric oxide is incredible: it opens up your airways, improves oxygen exchange, and it even helps your body to fight off airborne viruses.
- It's better for your dental health. Persistent mouth breathing can wreak havoc on your teeth and gums, contributing to gum disease, more cavities, and even bad breath.

Breathe (even) easier

Patrick's advice is free, but there are plenty of gizmos and gadgets that you can invest in, which will turbocharge your own efforts. To try some of them I turned to Anders Olsson, who discovered the power of breathing a little over 15 years ago. Back in 2009 he founded a company called Conscious Breathing. One person attended his first course and, er, two attended his second. He had to sell his house and live off his savings for six years, but he doggedly kept going until breathwork stopped sounding woo and found its place as a pillar of health and wellness.

Here are three things Anders makes to train the breath, which I've tested at home in London over the last year. I'm not suggesting you rush out and buy them, but I wanted to understand the lengths that practitioners are now going to. How we breathe plays such a critical part in healthspan, it's good to know that there are aids out there if you feel you need help. (Prices are correct at the time of going to print.)

1 **The Cardisuit** is a faff to get on (you're zipped in, a bit like putting on a scuba suit), but once you're cocooned, it does indeed calm you down. I first used it when I was filming an entertainment show for ITV called *The Real Full Monty*, to raise awareness of cancer. It was stressful and emotional sharing our personal cancer stories, so the soothing effect of the CO_2 on my near-naked body was welcome. Anders created the suit to help get your body and mind into a parasympathetic state (a resting state, as opposed to the fight-or-flight state). The CO_2 is absorbed through your skin, opening your blood vessels and airways, and leading to deep relaxation. You strip to your undies, and then get into the suit, which is inflated with CO_2 from a separate gas canister. I looked like a Teletubby, but once I managed to manoeuvre myself into a supine position on the sofa and close my eyes, a 20-minute session of mindfulness or meditation left me feeling utterly peaceful.
• Cardisuit: price: £1,700

2 **The CarboHaler,** on the other hand, energised me – but not to insane levels. It's a small black box with a face mask attached, intended to improve your body's oxygenation by adding a little extra CO_2 to inhaled air, for just a few minutes every day. It

certainly gives a boost to my mornings when I use it. I know that some people are ready to take on the world after a six-minute session – but I get an unhurried feel-good response that enables me to calmly and surely get on with my day. (Note: even if I'm using the CarboHaler, I still do my own breathwork exercises on my windowsill at dawn every morning.)
• CarboHaler: price: £600

3 **The Relaxator Breath Trainer** looks like a whistle. It's made using recycled plastic and non-toxic dye, and it is perfect to help you get into rhythmic, low, slower breathing cycles. It's good to remember that *inhaling* is activation and *exhaling* is relaxation, so you must ensure that your exhale is longer than your inhale. Because this little widget creates resistance when you breathe out (you can increase or decrease this with a simple twist), it prolongs the exhale, hence enhancing relaxation. I'm sitting in the back of a car now, on the way to film in Cornwall, using it. It's easy to forget to breathe properly when you're deep in thought, and this is a useful prompt.
• Relaxator Breath Trainer: price: £25

(The above products can be found on https://consciousbreathing.com/)

The wonder of the wanderer

Let's talk about the vagus nerve. 'Vagus' means 'wanderer' in Latin, and this nerve really does wander about from your brain down to your gut. It's hard to overstate its importance as the connector between your mind and your body – think of it as an information superhighway. The vagus nerve helps to activate the parasympathetic nervous system, the one that calms and relaxes you, as opposed to the fight-or-flight response of your sympathetic nervous system. There are multiple ways to stimulate it, the classics being breathwork, meditation and mindfulness, yoga and cold-water therapy. You can also buy specific devices to do the job, some costing many hundreds of pounds, but I want you to try humming. Because the nerve runs through your larynx (voice box) and your pharynx (your throat, or rather the passageway which connects your nose, mouth and throat), the vibration caused by humming can both soothe and tone it. It's very simple: just take a deep, belly breath in through your nose and hum gently on the exhale for as long as you feel comfortable. You don't have to perform Beethoven's *Symphony No. 5*, although you can if you want to. Three to five minutes of humming is a good start, but you might want to build up to ten, and you can do it as often as you like.

My top tips:

1 Sit comfortably, back straight, shoulders down – and you can also try shutting your eyes to see if you prefer it that way.
2 Keep your mouth softly closed, but not clenched.
3 Have your tongue resting gently on the roof of your mouth, if you want a visualisation, think about it being tucked behind your upper front teeth.
4 Make sure your throat feels open and soft. I don't play golf, but I was once told that you should imagine having a space about the size of a golf ball in there, and that works for me.
5 As you hum, try not to let your mind wander; instead, focus on your own 'wanderer' (your vagus nerve) by feeling the vibrations in your chest and head.
6 I'm a fan of the 'bee breath' or *bhramari pranayama*, which involves a humming sound too. I do a version of it sitting on a rolled yoga mat or cushion, knees drawn up in front of me, elbows resting on them, feet flat on the floor. I plug my ears with my thumbs, resting the other four fingers on either side my head (imagine sitting with your head in your hands). As I hum, I open and close my ears with my thumbs for a count of

five, then I repeat for about five to ten minutes. I find it truly calming.

How to hack this hack

Don't fancy humming, or you're short of time? Gargling with water will activate the muscles in the back of your throat, which are connected to the vagus nerve. Make sure you gargle at the back of your throat (without choking, of course) rather than in the front of your mouth. Thirty seconds to a minute should do it – and you can stack this hack by doing it when you brush your teeth.

Animal air-benders

As you know, I like to bring everything back to nature, and there are a number of animals that could teach us a thing or two about the benefits of reducing our intake of oxygen while upping our CO_2 levels. Thanks to some evolutionary acts of genius, they have mastered this, thereby increasing their longevity. It was Anders who first pointed them out to me – he talks about them in the lectures he now delivers to his clients around the globe.

- The long necks of giraffes act as large CO_2 reservoirs, enabling them to trap and recycle their own CO_2. Giraffes defend themselves against lions and other predators by headbutting. The force they generate with their heads is so powerful that a direct hit from an angry giraffe could be fatal to a human; however, thanks to their high CO_2 levels, giraffes maintain optimal blood flow to their own brains, protecting themselves from concussion. It's the same with bighorn sheep, but their CO_2 reservoirs are their horns. When their cranium is well-filled with blood, the brain is stabilised and doesn't slosh around inside the skull, hence they don't get concussed.

- The naked mole rat possesses remarkable features. It does not suffer from oxidative stress, never gets osteoporosis and is, broadly speaking, immune to cancer. It can live up to 30 years or more – ten to fifteen times longer than its closest relative, the mouse. How is this possible? Naked mole rats share labyrinthine underground colonies in an environment that is high in CO_2 and low in oxygen, with levels of up to 6 per cent CO_2 (150 times more than normal air) and 7 per cent oxygen (only a third of normal air).

- A bat can live up to 40 years which, again, is exceptionally long for such a small animal. One reason for this is that their caves contain up to 5 per cent CO_2. Imagine hundreds of thousands of bats roosting in a cave, exhaling warm, moist, carbon dioxide-rich air for 18 hours a day. This erodes calcium carbonate stalactites hanging from cave ceilings, while acidic bat urine erodes calcium carbonate stalagmites rising from cave floors. This erosion contributes to the formation of CO_2.

- We see something similar at work in the insect kingdom where science suggests queens who stay put in their nests – be they bees, ants or termites – benefit from higher levels of CO_2 than members of their colonies which go out and about. The queens live a lot longer as a result.

- But my favourite example is the woodpecker, which can hurl its head at a tree 100 times a minute without being hurt. That's perhaps 80 million times in its lifetime without getting concussed. There are two main reasons why, and one of them is its high tolerance to carbon dioxide. With higher CO_2 levels, blood flow to the brain is optimised, making the cranium full of enough liquid to withstand the knocking. And there's nothing bird-brained about that.

Heart rate variability . . .

. . . your heart's own Morse code.

One of the world walks I have always wanted to do is the Nakasendo Trail in Japan – specifically, I'd like to do it in cherry blossom season.

It was top of consultant cardiologist Dr Boon Lim's bucket list too, which is why he found himself in the ancient city of Kyoto with his family back in April 2024. He had spent five disappointing days in Tokyo without seeing a single bloom. Now, however, the blossom was cascading around him. He lay down sighing with delight, under the loveliest tree he could find. His breathing deepened and slowed, he felt resonance with this precious place he'd waited so long to visit, and the tug of emails and messages from London receded.

Of course, being one of Britain's top heart specialists, he recognised that this was his body shifting into an optimal heart rate variability (HRV) state. I'll explain what this is and why it's important in a moment, but the key thing here is that you can govern yours through your breath.

I asked Dr Lim to tell us about HRV; it's a bit of a tricky concept to grasp at first, but read on.

A conversation with Dr Boon Lim

What is HRV and why is it important?

Boon: The simplest definition is that HRV is a measure of the variability in time between heartbeats. The heart does not beat with metronomic regularity, and there are subtle variations in the time between successive heartbeats. This means that even if your heart rate is, on average, 60 beats a minute (bpm), the beat-to-beat variations might mean that your heart rate ranges between 58 to 62bpm (a low HRV), or 40 to 80bpm (a high HRV), but in both cases with the same average heart rate over a minute.

This variation is said to be a barometer of our overall health and longevity. It's different in all of us: normal HRV can range from below 20 to over 200 milliseconds depending on your age, sex, physical fitness and genetics. But broadly, the higher your HRV, the healthier you are, because the more adaptable and resilient your autonomic nervous system is showing itself to be.

You don't need to travel thousands of miles to Japan to achieve an optimal HRV. As Boon points out, we also have a 'Hanami' – a cherry blossom season – here in the UK. The difference? Full blooms in residential streets and in front of bus and train stations are overlooked in the daily hustle and bustle of the nine to five. The opportunity to experience the calm healing of nature often passes us by as we rush to be somewhere else. All it takes is a moment to pause and peacefully drink it in. And in that moment, which you might consider a waste of time, a deep physiological shift is occurring in your body as you move from a state of tension or chronic stress to one of relaxation.

DIY HRV

How to detect your own HRV:

1 Feel your pulse either in your neck or wrist (try two finger-widths below your wrist crease by the thumb).
2 Take a slow, deep breath in for six seconds and hold it. Then take a long slow exhale for six seconds and hold it. Observe the cadence of your heartbeat.
3 Put the book down – and try it now.
4 What did you observe? I hope most of you would see that on a long, slow inhale your heart rate increases slightly, and conversely, when you breathe out, your heart rate reduces. This is HRV in action!

The beat goes on

Boon says that there are two main ways to measure HRV properly, if you are interested in learning more about yours. You can get a wearable fitness tracker, a Garmin or a Whoop wrist band, or an Oura or Circular Ring, and they will give you an HRV value that is typically determined every night. It can be used to track changes in your stress response to things such as illness, exercise, diet, sleep, work-related stress, breathwork practice, alcohol and being outdoors in nature. Some wearables will also provide a 'readiness' or 'energy' score for the day ahead, considering your overnight HRV and other factors. You should always check these scores against how you feel when you wake up, but if you are feeling great, with a good score, you may have the confidence to try for a personal best in the gym, for example.

A better way to measure your HRV is to use an accurate heart rate monitor (such as the Polar H10 or Inner Balance) and to then export your data to some HRV software. If you do this, you'll have to measure your HRV in the same state and at the same time every morning, typically after having a wee. You will need to go back to bed, stay seated, and perform a one-minute breathing session (ideally six breaths in the minute) every day, or week, to track your changes.

A higher HRV usually means that your body can easily switch from one physiological state to another, which is a sign of good health, resilience to stress, and better fitness. Lower HRV can be a sign of stress, fatigue or poor health. HRV values are highly individualised, and we can't necessarily compare our stats to other people's. The most useful thing to do is to look at your own trends over time. Plus, HRV is very age-dependent, with younger people having naturally higher HRV than mid-lifers or older people.

Whatever your age, you can train yours using breathwork. Boon suggests many of the techniques you've just read about, including slowing down the breath and practising nasal breathing. He also recommends breathing in the present moment, which means: do not distract yourself with a to-do list or think-ing about what you're going to have for breakfast. Simply focus on the air flowing in and out of your lungs via your nostrils. Concentrate on following the route of the air with each breath.

HRV and me

In Boon's office at Hammersmith Hospital in West London, he hooks me up to a sensor that will measure responses through my ear, and sticks an electrocardiogram (ECG) on a chest band under my breast to listen to my noisy heart. As he instructs me to start breathing through my nose, I can hear it beating on his computer 'lub-dub lub-dub lub-dub', and I can see my HRV.

When I breathe in, my HRV speeds up, and the intervals between beats on the graph on the screen come closer together. When I breathe out, the beats slow down and the intervals get wider. I start breathing in for a count of six and out for a count of six, a long, linear breath. The graph tells me that my inhale is 65bpm and my exhale 50bpm. At this point something else comes into play, what's known as 'coherence value'. Anything above one is good, two is better and, within a minute, mine is four. It means that I am show-ing real consistency, that I am 'unencumbered' as Boon puts it, by performance pressure and all the instructions coming my way. I have used breathing to get control of my anxious heart.

'There was one hiccup: a moment where coherence value crashed,' he pointed out. 'It was when you were in the zone, your coherence shot up to 4.2, and I said "Julia, you're doing astonishingly well, keep it up!" Before then there had been no drama, but at that point you felt stressed that you had to perform.'

He was right. His words had been enough to engage the other side of my nervous system and his praise had, in this case, been a stressor. 'This demonstrates just how important the mind and our mental state is on our physiology,' he points out.

We went outside to re-run the experiment to see what the impact of nature would be. Together, we strolled to Wormwood Scrubs, a much-loved patch of green in west London. Initially, I concentrated on my breathing, but once I was in the flow, Boon asked me to feel the sun on my face and bask in the awe of nature. I closed my eyes, and then something extraordinary happened: my coherence score shot up to 8.7. My heartbeat was fluctuating between 58bpm and 75bpm and it was doing this in perfectly sequenced time, reflected in neat oscillations on Boon's graph.

'Phenomenal!' he said.

'Don't thank me, thank nature,' I grinned.

So the evidence is in: HRV is an important marker of our personal health, and we have an easy and impactful ability to change it using our breath. Aside from that, it was scientific proof of how profoundly important nature is in our lives. Awe, wonder, gratitude, some green grass and sunshine – they really do make our hearts sing.

Happy hacks

- **To improve the balance** between oxygen and carbon dioxide, try this: step out into nature, close your mouth and let your tongue rest on the roof of your mouth. (This signals to the brain that it can relax, try it right now.) Breathe in gently through your nose and proooolooooooooong your exhale, also through the nose. Extending exhalations beyond inhalations helps the body to shift towards the 'rest and digest' state, reducing stress, lowering blood pressure and promoting relaxation.

- **Familiarise yourself** with your own HRV, and use your breath to improve it, over time. My experience with Boon in a natural environment demonstrates how important mindset is. Be present in the moment and use your HRV monitoring time as another opportunity to calm your nervous system.

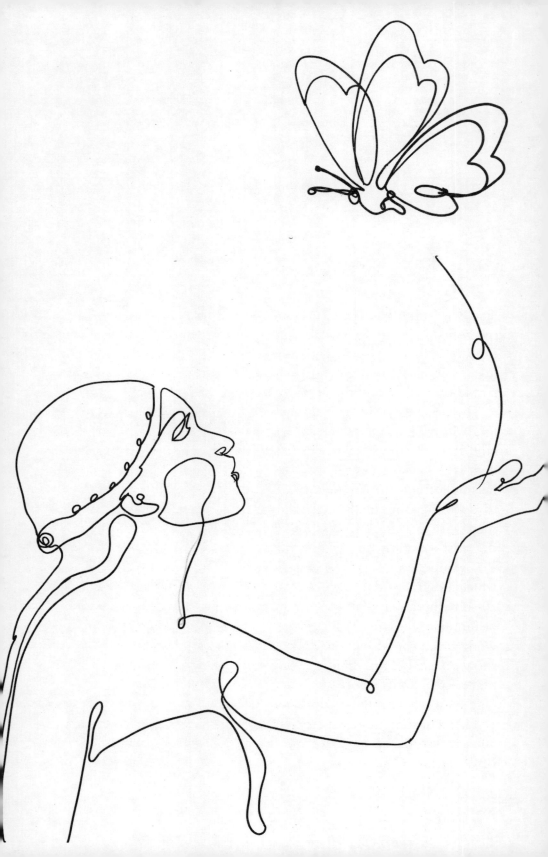

Chapter 8

Untamed: Rewilding People and the Planet

The Broughton Hall Estate near the market town of Skipton in the Yorkshire Dales has been in existence since 1097. That's not a typo, it really has been here since the 11th century. What's more, it's always been home to the same family, the Tempests: a golden strand of history running unbroken through 32 generations.

The Tempests are originally thought to have come over to England with William the Conqueror in 1066 and were gifted the land after his victory at the Battle of Hastings. The current custodian is Roger Tempest, a serial entrepreneur who has leveraged his intellectual curiosity, love of life and nature, and his courage, to do things differently at a 21st-century Broughton. He lives there with his wife, Paris, who shares his vision and commitment to transformation, and their small daughter, Aya.

If you've ever seen the cartoon strip 'Tottering-by-Gently', which has graced the pages of *Country Life* magazine for the last 20-something years (and I'll understand if you haven't), you will be familiar with Roger's big sister, Annie – the cartoonist – whose work was inspired by their early life in the hall: half-an-inch of snow on the billiard table, hip baths to catch the leaks and loos that needed antifreeze to keep them flushing in the winter.

It's not like that these days.

The 97-room honeyed-stone house has been subject to a 30-year restoration by Roger and has starred in series such as the BBC 1 hit *Gentleman Jack* (Suranne Jones as the first modern-day lesbian in Halifax) and movies such as *Wuthering Heights*, the one with Juliette Binoche and Ralph Fiennes. You can see it in *Made in Chelsea* and *All Creatures Great and Small* too.

Piggy in the middle

What's happened outside, on the 2,500 acres which surround Broughton, is where the real transformation has taken place, though. It's now home to a rewilding project, one of the most ambitious in the country. From being farmed to exhaustion (intensive sheep grazing, 6 per cent tree cover, limited wildlife), it's becoming a paradigm for change with more than 340,000 new broadleaf trees planted, Iron Age pigs truffling about, and a herd of Riggit Galloway Cattle.

The pigs are a cross between domestic pigs (think Peppa) and wild boar, bred to resemble the ancient pigs that once rooted the length and breadth of Europe. Their strong snouts with upturned ends turn over compacted soil, aerating it and making new microhabitats where seeds germinate and insects thrive. They are professional landscapers, the Monty Dons of the pig world. My children had a lovely piggy encounter when a young piglet lay down for them to stroke. From that point on they were nicknamed 'The Pig Whisperers'. (The appropriately named River, our nature guide, said he'd never seen the pigs so relaxed!)

The cows also roam free, pulling at vegetation with their tongues as they graze, enjoying a much (or should that be munch?) more diverse menu than the sheep ever used to. This results in a variety of vegetation heights and patterns, while their browsing, trampling, dunging and back-scratching against trees and shrubs is the equivalent of a gold-embossed invitation to a wide variety of flora and fauna. They mimic what bison and elk would have done 8,000 years ago.

As for the trees, there are 19 species from high-forest varieties including oak, beech and lime, to a patchwork of hazel and willows, down to shrubs such as hawthorn and elder. They've all been planted in the last three and a half years with the help of a landscape architect and a forest therapist.

Healthy land = healthy humans

It's worth highlighting that there is still farming at Broughton; Roger hasn't shirked the responsibility of feeding people, but it's that he's choosing to do it with a slow, sure shift to a regenerative agriculture.

Why am I telling you all this in a book about longevity? Because, as we're all beginning to realise (again), human health is linked to planetary health, and at Broughton, it's not just land that's being rewilded – it's people too.

What was Broughton Hall Estate has been renamed Broughton Sanctuary, and now has a healing and wellness centre called Avalon at its heart. There are woodland parties in a Cosmic Garden, music, dance and storytelling in a Fire Temple, a dark sky festival, a folk herbalist, wild swimming in the estate's own reservoir, tree nets for forest bathing, screaming fields (where you can go and release pent-up emotions by screaming) and a 16th-century Gothic-revival chapel for quiet prayer. There's even a new stone circle: a 33-stone helix built by Roger, and positioned by an earth shamen. That's a stone for every generation of Tempests, including the next, Aya, who'll be the first girl in 11 centuries to inherit.

The stone circle is where I began my exploration of Broughton, shoes off, barefoot on the damp August earth, encouraging my children to unlace their trainers and try it too. Afterwards I hiked back to the house and sat down to talk with Roger in his verdant walled garden about how he believes we can work in harmony with nature to extend human healthspan and happiness.

Tell me a bit about the history of Broughton:

Roger Tempest talks about Broughton

Roger: It's the social history of Britain, basically. Cromwell killed one of my ancestors on the lawn outside, and a priest from the estate gave the last rites to people on the Titanic as the ship went down. We've still got a mortgage document dating from 1326. In World War I the estate was paralysed, it lost many of its tradesmen – everyone from the gardeners to the stone masons. Post-World War II it was a struggle too – in the 1960s and 1970s it was all about 'killing the rich' politically, and we are still paying tax from that time. It took us to the edge of survival.

Today, from the air, you can look down on the UK and see solar farm, after wind farm, after road, after industrial estate, after over-farmed fields. There's no sense of wilderness anymore, and I am trying to change that, starting here in Broughton. This land was a monoculture of sheep, hormones, vaccinations, antibiotics, glyphosates . . . Now it's returning to a more natural state, a home for otters, storks and owls again – we have even got two beavers. The power of nature has been badly underestimated.

How does that relate to people?

Roger: We are trying to give people who come here the chance to align their inner nature with the outer nature we have been restoring. We're an experiment in the making. You don't have to agree with us, but I think we all know in our hearts that how we live today, shopping, the pub, polarised by social media, always on our devices, away from nature, that we've lost our way. Can our jewel of a house in Yorkshire be some kind of antidote to that?

The call of the wild

It's a tricky question. I mean, how do you replicate those lessons and those principles? How can you take the Broughton model of rewilding people and rewilding land and make it work for everyone? I don't know, but I do know that if Roger and Paris can take 1,000 years of history and make change for the better, it must be possible for us all.

Roger in particular has spent most of his life being defined by his stately home. (You're about to meet a key member of his team, Kelly Hollick, whose grandma was so flustered by his lineage that she curtseyed by mistake the first time they met. It's something they laugh about together now.) What he and Paris are doing today is brave and unconventional, a colossal commitment to the environment, and a bold statement that human health – our health – is dependent on that of our planet.

Finding your inner compass

Kelly Hollick's business title is nature recovery manager at Broughton Sanctuary. I think of her more as a nature crusader.

Kelly, 40, a mother of one, grew up in nature. She's originally from Yorkshire and spent her childhood planting and digging on the family allotment, summering under canvas and walking around the Yorkshire Dales every weekend. 'Come rain or shine', she smiles. I can relate. My childhood was spent hiking around the Peak District with my dad or pottering in the garden with my mum.

She gave me a tour, sharing both her practical work at Broughton and her deep, spiritual connection to place. After we were done, the mud knocked off our boots and our hands clasped around a welcome mug of tea, I asked her if she'd write me a guide to walking as she does – not about getting your steps in, but as a form of connection to your wilder self.

Kelly Hollick's walking guide

Kelly says, 'Energy flows where the intention goes – we are in relation to everything', so . . .

Go on an 'intuition walk' Leave the map at home and simply wander anywhere your intuition takes you. Be curious about everything you see, and look at nature as if it has signs and symbols to offer you. Tapping into your intuition quietens the voices of the world and awakens your heart's intelligence. In this heart space, you can hear your truth and listen to your callings.

Find a sit spot A great way to feel more connected to nature is to spend time sitting in silence and observing the wildlife around you. Find somewhere comfortable where you will be undisturbed and can spend at least 15 minutes sitting still and letting nature accept your presence. Learn to watch silently, patiently and with perseverance as you tune into the natural rhythms and movements of what's around you.

Take your shoes off Put your bare feet on the earth as often as you can. By kicking off our shoes, with their rubber or plastic soles, we connect with the earth's negatively charged electrons, which can neutralise those free radicals (unstable molecules that can damage cell structures). When we live in harmony with the earth's electrical charge, we recharge and restore balance to our bodies.

Enjoy a dawn walk Get out early into the morning sunlight to awaken your ancestral eye. When we align ourselves with the rhythms of the sun and the moon, we ensure that our circadian rhythms are working as they should.

Celebrate the changing of the seasons, and be outside in all weathers. When we align with the seasons, we ensure that we are using the same energies as the earth. By getting out into nature, whatever the weather, we can tap into these seasonal energies and find ways of living that are more in sync with the flow of nature and our natural way of being.

Mindful walking: hold in your heart your sense of co-existence
We are in relationship all the time with the rest of nature. We are
moulded every day by the microbiome we inhale, the sun-eating
plants we consume and the waves of gut biosis and dysbiosis
that influence how we think, behave and feel. While out walking,
whether that be in a green space or a busy urban area, cultivate
an awareness of yourself as an inter-being and consider the
many different interactions that are happening between your
body and other beings.

Mindful walking: be more animal We can easily get lost in the
busyness of being human, but underneath we are demonstrably
animal. While out walking, explore the similarities between
yourself and any other being that you meet along the way. You
have hair like a badger. You have teeth like a fox. You have eyes
like a fish. You think through the same filamentous connectivity
as the fungal networks within the soil. You have feet that can
stand on the ground like the roots of a tree. You are 'enmicrobed'
by the earth. It's a humbling feeling and deeply restorative.

Bringing Broughton home

A stay at Broughton Sanctuary might be out of your reach finan-
cially – not for nothing was it named as one of the 30 coolest
places in the *world* to visit in 2024 by *National Geographic*, but
if you are anywhere near Skipton, you have an open invitation to
the 30km track I hiked with my kids, the one where we met the
pigs. Access to the Odyssey Trail is free of charge. You can run,
walk or bike, stopping along the way to discover the essence of
the sanctuary. Even if you are not in North Yorkshire, you can go
for an 'intuition walk' and find a 'sit spot', as per Kelly's suggestion, wherever you are in the country.

Why don't you try it and let me know how you get on? To find
out more about Broughton Sanctuary go to:
www.broughtonsanctuary.co.uk.

Barefoot wisdom

You found me at the start of this chapter barefoot up a hill at
Broughton Sanctuary. I was 'earthing', wandering around a
stone circle in my bare feet absorbing nature's energy. (You might
also hear this referred to as 'grounding'.)

Here's the science: our earth is charged with negative electri-
city. If you wear rubber or plastic-soled shoes you're insulated
from it. It's just another facet of modern life – synthetic materials, electronic devices, and artificial environments – which separates us from nature. Grounding, or earthing, is about plugging
back in, making direct contact with the earth by walking barefoot on natural surfaces such as grass, soil and sand. (You can
also bathe in natural bodies of water.)

Earthing has a lot of celebrity fans. Gwyneth Paltrow[1] swears
by it and Naomie Harris[2] (007's Miss Moneypenny) uses it to
cure her jet lag. In the UK, the movement is headlined by a
woman called Jennifer Finlay who turned to it in desperation
after a decades-long battle with the autoimmune disease
Crohn's.

'There's no cure for it and the only treatment is a lifetime of
drugs,' she tells me. 'The drugs have side effects, and besides
they only treat the symptoms. Or you can have surgery, which
can be life-changing – it can leave you dependent on a colostomy
bag. Given this, I was hunting for a natural remedy as if it were
the Holy Grail itself. Boy, did I try everything!'

Her search led her to earthing, which she discovered during
the UK's second, long COVID lockdown in 2020. 'I was prepared
to try anything, and spare time was abundant, so I had the space
and the motivation to go on a fact-finding mission in my own
back garden. I started barefoot contact on the grass and on my
concrete patio, earthing every day, and the results were immediate and, for me, deep reaching.'

Jen is a super-groomed platinum blonde. She's just passed her
sixtieth birthday, but you wouldn't think so. It's hard to

reconcile her glamorous image and chatty warmth with the kind of physical and mental difficulties she's gone through – and that's down to earthing, she says. 'By reducing chronic inflammation in my body, I have completely transformed my health. I no longer suffer from anxiety, panic attacks, arthritic pain, poor sleep and low energy. There are no more nightly visits to the bathroom, and, most importantly, no more debilitating Crohn's flare-ups. It changed my life.

'Everyone needs to know about how our disconnect from Mother Earth has impacted on our overall health,' she says. 'I see it as the missing link, and believe it is as essential to us as good-quality water, oxygen and food. So, get earthing. Enjoy the miracle beneath your feet.'

(You can find out more about Jen and her work at: https://www.earthingrevolution.co.uk/)

You can earth using:

- Grass, sand and soil.
- Plants and living trees (especially those with wet bark).
- Gravel and rock (that is, touching the earth).
- Unsealed concrete (or coated with a water-based sealant).
- Unsealed brick (or coated with a water-based sealant).
- Bodies of water (such as oceans, lakes and streams).

What's the science? Is there any?

The science supporting earthing is small and often conducted by people with a vested interest in it – but that doesn't mean that it's wrong. More than a decade ago, America's *National Library of Medicine* published a paper entitled: 'Earthing: Health implications of reconnecting the human body to the earth's surface electrons'. Its purpose was to review existing earthing research and interrogate its potential.[3] It reminded us that: 'Chronic degenerative diseases have overcome infectious disease as the major causes of death in the 21st century, so an increase in human longevity will depend on finding an intervention that inhibits the development of these diseases and slows their progress.'

It went on to ask:

Could such an intervention be located right beneath our feet? Earthing research, observations, and related theories raise an intriguing possibility about the Earth's surface electrons as an untapped health resource – the Earth as a 'global treatment table.' Emerging evidence shows that contact with the Earth – whether being outside barefoot or indoors connected to grounded conductive systems – may be a simple, natural, and yet profoundly effective environmental strategy against chronic stress, ANS dysfunction, inflammation, pain, poor sleep, disturbed HRV, hyper-coagulable blood, and many common health disorders, including cardiovascular disease. The research done to date supports the concept that grounding or earthing the human body may be an essential element in the health equation along with sunshine, clean air and water, nutritious food, and physical activity.

Letting nature lead

We visited Broughton Sanctuary as a family in the summer of 2024 and had the most blissful screen-free four days. Martin Clarkson, the butler who has worked in the house for three years and has been a 'friend of the estate' for more than 30, looked after us. He's seen it all. From A-list actors to temperamental aristocrats, he's done everything from chopping their firewood to what you might call 'extreme shopping' in Skipton. (Oh wait, the kimchi was for me, because I'd forgotten my sauerkraut. Sorry, Martin.)

One evening we all tumbled into the back of a flat-bed truck heading uphill under a moody Yorkshire sky, the children bouncing around happily. Our destination was a small cold-water lake and a wood-fired sauna. I've managed to get all my kids and my partner to try a bit of hot–cold therapy over the years, and I'm proud to say that we all did it again that evening, with lots of screaming and yelping. I even got my friend, Sarah, to jump in with me and she does *not* do cold, but she does have a steely 'just get on with it' temperament, so she did.

Afterwards, we snuggled down by a campfire. I don't know when you last spent time sitting around a fire outdoors, but there's something magical about chatting together, looking into the flames. Historically, campfires were a central point for gathering and socialising, so sitting by one can promote a sense of community. The visual stimulation of the flickering flames on the mind reduces stress and yields a general sense of relaxation. Essentially, it triggers a primal sense of comfort and security, taking us back to our hunter-gatherer selves.

Studies show that it can exert a force powerful enough to reduce your blood pressure – just one more example of how being in nature has a measurable impact on our physical human health.

The Old English word for 'forest' is 'weald', but it can also mean 'power and authority'. There's some folklore that suggests this is because the wild has a will of its own – and what is rewilding but a return to the will of nature? As I say, it's only folklore, but I do believe in the broader, very real idea that we have to rewild bits of ourselves and our planet to ensure the health and longevity of both.

Happy hacks

- **Walk consciously**, as Kelly Hollick advises.
- **Take 15 minutes** just to sit and be in nature.
- **Walk** at sunrise.
- **Walk in the rain** instead of waiting for it to dry up.
- **Take your shoes off** and try earthing.

PS: here's a shaggy dog story. In Broughton, there's no shortage of well-behaved dogs enjoying the grounds with their humans. There has been a lot of research over the years that suggests having a dog is linked to a reduced risk of death, improved cardiovascular health, and – no surprise here – increased physical activity (which we know adds to our healthspan). There is also the companionship element, which can contribute to overall well-being. I will therefore always be personally grateful to the Tempests for introducing me to Show Cocker Spaniels, the breed we chose when we were getting our first dog as a family. It was Roger's sister, Annie, who extolled the virtues of show cockers, which she has herself, claiming them to be a top choice for children, since they are loving, loyal and trainable. Our beloved Zeus is all three.

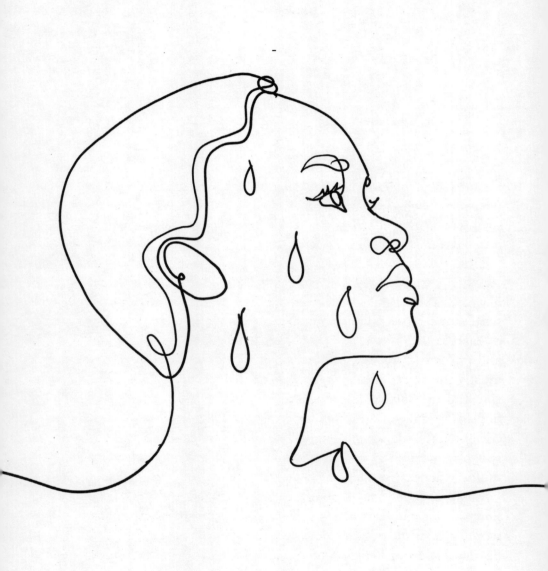

Chapter 9

Saunas – Sweat, Stretch, Chat

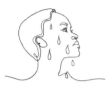

I want you to imagine for a moment a type of nematode worm (a tiny transparent worm that lives in the soil) and a fruit fly sitting in a tiny glass chamber where the temperature in the vial is equal to a sauna environment.

Hold that thought, and we'll get back to it shortly.

When I was filming across Ireland (where I was born) for a new TV series a couple of years ago, we stayed in some hotels with saunas. You might be picturing grand spa hotels with lots of marble and glass, but these were unflashy places with gyms and pools that looked like community sports centres. In fact, mostly they *were* community sports centres: big whiffs of chlorine and the sort of floors where it's wise to always wear flip-flops. The thing is, though, the saunas were always full and, curiously, the majority of the sweaty humans I encountered and spoke to were men, in various states of fitness, and spanning multiple generations.

I'd never pegged the Irish as big sauna users. That's the Finns: Finland has more saunas per capita than any country in the world. But from my anecdotal experience, it's a popular Irish pastime, and I had some interesting conversations in them there saunas, talking about everything from agricultural irrigation systems to dairy herds. And that's one of the many paybacks of sauna bathing: the social aspect. They're a phone-free environment where people go to sweat, stretch and chat.

Some like it hot

There's more, however, much more. I have been turned on to the numerous benefits of saunas for several years now, and this is where the nematode worm (*Caenorhabditis elegans*) and the fruit fly (*Drosophila melanogaster*) come in.

You see, a single brief heat exposure in these organisms has been shown to increase their lifespan by up to 15 per cent.[1,2] The mechanisms by which this happens relate to human longevity too and it has something to do with a family of proteins called 'heat shock proteins'. They're found in worms, flies, mice, monkeys and, you guessed it, us. Known as 'chaperone proteins', heat shock proteins (HSPs) are really important in maintaining our cells and helping them to function normally and protect them from stress.

They play a role in the immune system and DNA repair, aid the development of skeletal muscle and can also help to protect the brain. Our bodies generate HSPs when they detect exposure to short-term stress, such as the heat in a sauna (but also to cold-water swimming, fasting and exercise). We have evolved to handle this beneficial hermetic stress, and the more we're exposed to it the better we'll be at doing it again. If, like me, you switch the shower from hot to cold regularly, you'll notice that bearing the cold blasts gets easier – even though it's still hard to do!

Healthy people who sit in a dry sauna set to around 78°C for 30 minutes, increase their heat-shock proteins by 50 per cent, and once those levels are increased, they stay elevated for about 48 hours. This is much the same as forest bathing (the Japanese practice of immersing oneself in nature and especially wood-land), which has a lasting impact for several weeks after you've wandered through woods.

Uncontrolled chronic stress, on the other hand, affects our body differently, harming cells and promoting inflammation and disease. It's the difference between the *sympathetic* nervous system – the so-called fight-or-fight response – and the *para-sympathetic* system, which is our rest-and-digest mode.

It's easy to understand why being in fight-or-flight mode isn't healthy for us all the time. Stress hormones, such as cortisol, adrenaline and norepinephrine, course through our body to help us overcome a perceived danger, but it's not a state that we should be in for 24 hours a day. It's now widely understood that, unfortunately, we are frequently stuck there: our smart phones ping with alerts, emails drop into our inbox and sirens blast from the street as we walk to work, doomscrolling social media as we go. This barrage of information puts many of us on alert for much of the day – and this overall picture isn't forecast to get better soon.

It is estimated that 90 per cent of the world's data was generated in the last two years alone, says a Statista report from November 2024. Some studies suggest an average person living today processes as much as 74 gigabytes of information every 24 hours (the equivalent of 16 movies) via television, computers, smartphones, tablets, adverts and gadgets. Five hundred years ago, a highly educated person would have consumed just 74 gigabytes of information in their entire lifetime through books and storytelling.[3, 4, 5]

But what has this got to do with saunas and heat shock proteins?

Sweat it out

Well, it's essential to find as many ways as possible to introduce some calm into our lives and boost our body's defences against the 21st century. Our bodies need to feel the blissful, beneficial heat of the sauna, not the white-hot heat of technological advance.

Alongside the social benefits, and boosting lifespan via the production of HSPs, sauna bathing has been connected to a reduced risk of cardiovascular disease,[6] a reduction in blood pressure, the slowing down of muscle atrophy (muscle wastage, which happens as we get older – which is why it's important to build some resistance training into your weekly exercise, as explained in Chapter 14) and the lessening of inflammation.

Inflammation is a little like stress: short-term acute inflammation is a brilliant physiological response that helps the body to heal and defend itself, but it can become pathological or chronic when the body is exposed to a stressor that is too powerful or it doesn't end when it should – at which point you're in trouble.

The message of this chapter is that frequent sauna use helps to fix inflammation. In particular, it lowers a marker of inflammation called C-reactive protein (CRP) which is made by the liver. Elevated CRP levels are associated with cardiovascular conditions and the narrowing of your arteries. A study of 2,084 men found that the more frequently they used the sauna, the lower their CRP levels.[7]

I don't know if I'm fortunate enough to have something called the heat-shock protein 70 gene (HSP70), but one Danish study suggests that if you've got one copy of it, you can live a year longer than someone who is without it, and if you've got two copies, you get an extra two years. It's a genetic advantage, a lucky draw in life's lottery. But it can be echoed by using saunas, which boost HSP production and benefit your brain, heart and lung health. Doing exercise hard enough to raise your core temperature has the same effect, and so does a hot bath, although you'll need to be in the water up to your neck with your shoulders, arms and legs submerged. They're both genuinely great health hacks, but the sauna is the one you really want when you're working on your healthspan.

Off-grid heat

As a country, we're already on to this. Google searches for 'home sauna' rose by 84 per cent between January and March 2024 in the UK[8] and partly that's because of the work of journalist Emma O'Kelly.

Emma was sent on a writing assignment to an island off Finland back in 2016. (As I said, saunas are huge there: in 2019 Finnish sauna culture was added to UNESCO's list of Intangible Cultural Heritage.) After Emma had finished work for the day, she and her colleagues retired to the local sauna. They spent the evening plunging in and out of a cold lake, sweating and talking, and she was completely converted.

She published her first book *Sauna: The Power of Deep Heat* in 2023, and she's just written her second, *Wild Sauna: The Best Outdoor Saunas in Britain*. She tells me, 'When I started researching the UK guide in February 2024, I had 80 saunas on my list. By November this had stretched to almost 200, and new ones were popping up every day. Everywhere it's the same story: the passion and enthusiasm for sauna and the connection with nature, with people, the sense of community.

'These new "saunapreneurs" are fire starters. The wild-sauna scene feels like a movement, like the contemporary coffee-shop boom of the mid-1990s. And, like coffee shops, each sauna has its own atmosphere, its own culture and its own unique offering.'

Somewhere near you there will be a purpose-built hut in a forest, a modified horse box on a beach, a trailer in a clifftop car park, a tent sauna next to your municipal baths or a refurbished treasure at a local lido. Seriously, go and investigate – what have you got to lose other than most of your clothes and all your inhibitions?

Emma O'Kelly talks about the new sauna nomads

Emma: A huddle of horsebox saunas on a windswept beach is not the sort of place you expect to find an ambassador in his swimming trunks. Yet, one cold winter morning in 2022, the Estonian envoy to the UK pitched up in a chauffeur driven car, stripped off and settled into the steam at Beach Box in Brighton. Why? Because there's a sauna revolution sweeping the UK, thanks in part to Beach Box, and Estonia wants to be part of it – so does Finland, where a rich sauna tradition is being mined and made fashionable by a new generation, Lithuania, Norway and Latvia. Post-pandemic, legions of wild swimmers have taken to British beaches, and mobile saunas have followed, wrapping them up in a warm embrace.

But sauna is about more than just getting warm after a cold plunge; there are myriad proven health benefits too, as Julia mentions above. In addition, this 'heat therapy' can also help with fatigue and depression.[9] There's a reason why sauna-loving nations, such as Finland, Sweden and Norway, jostle for top position in the annual United Nations World Happiness Report. Yet the UK, cold and gloomy and prone to never-ending winters, has only now got hooked on heat. What has taken us so long?

Poorly ventilated, dingy gym saunas have, until now, been the only option for many of us, alongside too-pricey spas, where disposable slippers, fluffy robes and a bottle of prosecco are as central to the package as any sort of wellness.

Hot box

Emma: Beachside horseboxes, woodland trailers and bijou barrels therefore offer a third space that is simple, primal, intentional and often beautiful. There's something about sitting in a cosy wood-fired sauna, after being exposed to raw nature and unpredictable elements, that makes us feel safe, warm and connected.

In an attempt to document this fledgling sauna movement, I wrote a guide to the UK's wild saunas. I couldn't keep up: each time I boarded the train home from Cornwall, Wales or Scotland, another sauna would open behind me. Everywhere I went, I met bands of enthusiasts, heat evangelists eager to share the love. Menopausal mums, body-optimising athletes, people with Parkinson's, fibromyalgia and long-COVID, they all talked about how the sauna helps them to manage pain, inflammation, anxiety, depression and sleep.

Gen Z said that they loved sauna as a digital detox and enjoyed it as a real-time experience; ex-addicts explained how they craved the dopamine hit of hot and cold; retirees came for the company. As I washed the backs of strangers, had my body whisked with birch branches, was wrapped in honey and scrubbed with salt, I found a way to look after my health that is easy, cheap, accessible and fun.

I learned about the trees, herbs and seaweeds that grow on our islands and have been used as healing remedies for centuries. So too in the Nordics and Baltics where important rites of passage – birth, death, marriage – were held in the sauna, and spells were used to boost fertility, and to bring good luck and love. In Finland, the sauna was known as 'the poor man's pharmacy', and healers would travel from village to village curing the sick (they still do).

For *Sauna, The Power of Deep Heat*, I picked up cultural cues from Finnish community saunas, from the smoke saunas of Estonia and the floating saunas of Norway. Now, lots of them have landed here. We are tweaking and adapting the best bits from all these countries, and, like our cuisine, UK sauna culture is shaping up to be a rich melting pot of ideas and practices.

Archaeological evidence, however, suggests that our

ancestors had their own sweat-bathing traditions too. Bronze Age saunas and 'burnt mounds' – remnants of heat-shattered stones beside a rectangular water trough – have been found in Shetland, Orkney and Ireland. What exactly went on inside these dark, mysterious spaces is an increasingly hot topic on sauna benches. Were they similar to the Native American sweat lodge (*inípi*), the Mexican *temazcal*, the Celtic sweat lodge or the Korean *jjimjilbang*? In Ireland, more than 600 *teach allais* (sweat houses) have been unearthed, the last of which was in use until the 1930s. Those who were sick, in pain or needed a good scrub, went to the sweat house to be treated for everything from 'pains in the bones' to pleurisy, lumbago, sciatica, fever, pneumonia and influenza. Bathers would crawl, often naked with a pitcher of drinking water, through a tiny entrance and would sit on rush matting in the dark, often for many hours, before rinsing off in cold water.

Yo-yoing between hot and cold – or contrast therapy – is as old as time, and science can now tell us why it never goes away. It offers a thermoregulatory workout that boosts circulation, heart rate and blood flow. It creates hermetic stress – 'good stress' – and activates brown fat. (We are all born with brown fat, which helps to maintain our body temperature in cold conditions; it can help burn calories, enabling the body to lose weight [as explained in Chapter 1].)

Our ancestors didn't 'know' this, they just 'felt' it. The sauna offers us space and time to turn off and tune in to ourselves, so that we can feel it too.

Too hot to handle: sauna safety

Saunas are generally safe for most people, but there are some warnings and precautions to keep in mind:

Health conditions

It's best to avoid saunas if you have unstable angina, have had a heart attack, or you suffer with aortic stenosis (when the aortic valve narrows and stiffens, making it difficult for blood to flow from the heart to the body), or if you have any other heart or cardiovascular problems. You should also check with your doctor if you have uncontrolled high blood pressure. (Although some research suggests that regular sauna use might have a positive impact on lowering blood pressure, it is crucial you seek personal advice from your GP or specialist.)

Dehydration

Drink two to four glasses of cool water after each sauna session. Signs of dehydration include thirst, a dry or sticky mouth, not urinating much, and dark yellow urine. I also drink electrolytes.

Overheating

Limit your time in the sauna to around 20 minutes, and exit immediately if you feel nauseous, dizzy or sleepy.

Alcohol and medications

Avoid alcohol and medications that can impair sweating or cause overheating. Drinking alcohol in the sauna can increase the risk of hypotension, arrhythmia and sudden death.

Burns

Beware: the rocks and heaters in the sauna can get very hot.

Electronics

Annoyingly, some people at the sauna at my gym in London bring their phones into the sweat box, despite the signs. It just shows how addicted we have all become to our devices. If you choose to use electronics in the sauna, do so at your own risk. It might explode. (Or I might.)

Sperm count

It has been reported that frequent visits to the sauna might lower men's sperm count, although the effect appears to be temporary. In one study, sperm counts returned to normal after six months, but if you're trying to conceive, perhaps stay out of the heat – although the findings aren't conclusive enough to use this as a form of contraception.[10]

Exercise v. sauna

A study published in the *Complementary Therapies of Medicine* (June 2018) compared a 25-minute sauna session to a 25-minute session on an exercise bike doing about 100 watts[11] (that's a measure of how hard you are pushing or peddling). The effects on heart rate and blood pressure were identical. During the physical activity and the sauna session, both heart rate and blood pressure increased. Immediately after, both heart rate and blood pressure were lower than baseline levels. As well as lowering the heart rate, a 30-minute Finnish sauna session also increased heart rate variability (HRV), which is indicative of the heart's capacity to respond well under stressful conditions. Isn't that amazing?

Mighty mitochondria

Extremes of heat (and cold) help with the production and repair of our mitochondria, which are the source of our body's energy, although not the kind of energy you might be thinking about.

You know when people say, 'She's got such a nice/good/bad energy about her'? That's more of an aura-type of energy that I think emanates from the inside and is linked to personality. (People often comment on my energy, and I do feel something inside of me sometimes, a sort of verve.) Mitochondrial energy, however, is different. This is the physical energy created by our cells. In the biohacking and well-being world, people talk about mitochondria all the time, because they're important, which is why they're worth understanding.

I learned more about them than I ever expected to during my breast-cancer diagnosis when I discovered that I had 'reduced mitochondrial function'. Cancer cells often have fewer (and misshapen) mitochondria per cell, and mutations occur in something called 'the mitochondrial DNA' (mtDNA), which contributes to cancer development. Like most things in our bodies, they are also impacted by age, although there are things that we can do to help improve their function: heat is one and, guess what, walking is another.

As I said, it's complex, which is why I have asked Michael Ash, naturopath, osteopath, nutritional therapist and international educator, to explain it for us.

Our cellular powerhouses, by Michael Ash

Michael: As adults we are made up of some 37 trillion cells, and inside these are mitochondria, often called the 'powerhouses' of our cells. They are believed to have originated from ancient bacteria about 1.5 billion years ago. The hypothesis is that complex cells evolved after absorbing oxygen-using bacteria. These bacteria then transformed into mitochondria. This relationship was beneficial for both, with mitochondria providing energy from oxygen to the host cell and in return getting protection. This relationship marks the beginning of all living organisms, including plants.

Mitochondria (tiny, membrane-bound structures inside most human cells) are often in their thousands in each cell and are essential not just for making energy but also for balancing essential minerals such as iron and calcium, and for producing hormones such as melatonin. They interact with other cell parts, affect our body clocks, and connect with our gut bacteria and immune system, possibly serving as a key link in health and disease. Problems with mitochondria are associated with several common conditions, including metabolic syndrome, neurodegenerative diseases, cancer, heart problems, and inflammatory disorders.

Mitochondria are hard at work converting nutrients from food into ATP (adenosine triphosphate), which our bodies use as energy. ATP is the main energy carrier in cells, and it is crucial for maintaining metabolism, body temperature and essential functions such as digestion, circulation and excretion. ATP also acts as a signalling molecule that helps cells communicate and function properly. Essentially, ATP is the universal energy currency in cells, powering various biological reactions and sustaining life. Amazingly, an adult typically produces their body weight in ATP *every day*.

To understand mitochondrial function clearly, imagine the cell as a factory, where various processes come together to produce vital goods. In this cellular factory, mitochondria can be thought of as the dedicated workers, whose primary job is to produce energy and influence the essential services necessary for the factory to operate efficiently.

These mitochondrial workers need specific inputs to perform their jobs effectively. In this analogy, the inputs are the nutrients we consume: carbohydrates, fats, proteins and essential micronutrients, as well as specialised compounds from our food. Just as the quality of input materials in a factory affects the quality of the output, the quality of the food we consume directly impacts how efficiently our mitochondria can convert these inputs into energy. High-quality, nutrient-dense foods enhance mitochondrial function, promoting more robust and efficient energy production. Conversely, poor-quality inputs, such as ultra-processed foods high in sugars and unhealthy fats – for example, seed oils/chemically refined oils – can reduce mitochondrial efficiency and contribute to the production of less energy and disordered well-being.

As explained, the primary output of our mitochondrial workers is ATP. This energy allows the cell to perform vital functions such as growth, repair and maintenance; however, there is also a by-product of this energy production: oxidative stress. Think of this as smoke from the factory. Oxidative stress occurs when the energy-production process inevitably leads to the creation of free radicals, which are unstable molecules that can damage cell structures, including DNA, proteins and cell membranes.

Over time, like machinery that wears out, mitochondria can become damaged or old. When mitochondria are not functioning properly, or when they begin to degrade due to age or stress, they not only produce less energy but they also increase the production of harmful free radicals, and the 'smoke' can be blacker and thicker, indicating that the factory is not functioning well. This situation can escalate if the mitochondria are not properly fusing, dividing or being recycled by the cell, a process known as mitophagy (a way for cells to get rid of damaged or unnecessary mitochondria, preventing the build-up of dysfunctional organelles).

What happens when they power down?

Michael: Accumulation of damaged or old mitochondria can lead to another significant issue: sterile inflammation. This type of inflammation is not caused by pathogens, but rather by cellular debris and dysfunction. Damaged mitochondrial DNA and free radicals can activate a specific type of immune response through something known as the NLRP3 inflammasome. The NLRP3 inflammasome is a complex protein that plays a crucial role in the body's immune response, activating inflammatory processes when it detects cellular stress or damage.

This activation, if persistent, can lead to chronic inflammation, which is implicated in numerous diseases, including metabolic disorders such as diabetes, cardiovascular diseases, and age-related conditions. Therefore, maintaining mitochondrial health is critical for efficient ATP production via oxidative phosphorylation, as well as supporting immune function, regulating apoptosis, sustaining metabolic processes and stabilising intracellular calcium levels. Optimal mitochondrial function is essential to mitigate oxidative stress and prevent inflammatory conditions that accelerate healthspan compression and age-related pathologies driven by mitochondrial dysfunction.

In summary, just as the efficiency and well-being of a factory depend on the health and productivity of its workers, so too does the health of our cells rely on the robust functioning of mitochondria – and by extension our entire body.

Your mitochondrial health

Michael explains that mitochondrial quality control is key to keeping mitochondria healthy, and it involves removing damaged mitochondria, recycling mitochondria and creating new ones.

The chemical processes by which this is achieved in the body can be helped in a number of ways to which we can contribute ourselves, namely exercise, diet and specific supplements.

Quality control: exercise

Physical activity is a basic human trait that's built into our genes. Nowadays, many people think of exercise as something special or extra, because we have become used to being less active; however, being active is our natural state, and not moving around much is really the change from what's ancestrally normal. Inadequate physical activity can cause problems with our mitochondria, and this lack of movement is a common reason for many of the chronic diseases we see in modern societies. It's why walking has so many benefits – from the molecular to the macro.

Quality control: phospholipids

Phospholipids are the main structural components of cell membranes. To understand their importance, consider them as the bricks and mortar of the mitochondrial walls. When these components are fresh and intact, they help to maintain the optimal function of mitochondria, including the vital process of energy production; however, like any structural component, phospholipids can wear out or get damaged. If they are not adequately replaced, the integrity of the mitochondrial membrane suffers, leading to a decrease in mitochondrial effectiveness. If your diet lacks sufficient phospholipids, or if your body simply does not produce enough of them, supplementation might be necessary to avoid mitochondrial degradation. This is where specialised phospholipid supplements come into play. (I have recommended NTFactor to my patients. It's a patented formula that claims to support the restoration of membrane potential and the overall health of the cells.) The idea is to replace damaged phospholipids in mitochondrial membranes to improve cellular function and energy production.

Help on a plate

To replace phospholipids naturally, focus on foods rich in lecithin, which includes egg yolks, soya beans and fish. Organ meats, lean meats, shellfish and cereal grains also contain phospholipids. Polyphenols, compounds found in fruits and vegetables, have antioxidant and anti-inflammatory properties that can support mitochondrial health. (I drink a shot of polyphenol-rich cold-pressed extra virgin olive oil most mornings.)

Some help from vitamin Zing!

Here are some of the most common supplements prescribed to support mitochondrial function, energy production and antioxidant protection. As supplement quality can vary, I do not recommend that you purchase these without consulting a professional nutritionist, as detailed in 'Supplement sleuthing' below.

- **Essential fatty acids** Omega-3 fatty acids, particularly EPA and DHA, have been shown to improve mitochondrial function and membrane quality.
- **Coenzyme Q10 (CoQ10)** A powerful antioxidant, CoQ10 is crucial for energy production within mitochondria, but its levels decline with age.
- **B vitamins (B1, B2, B3, B5)** These vitamins are essential for energy production in the mitochondria.
- **Creatine** Although primarily known for muscle building, creatine also plays a role in energy production within the mitochondria, particularly during high-intensity activities.
- **Nicotinamide adenine dinucleotide (NAD+)** NAD+ is a coenzyme that is involved in many metabolic processes, including energy production in the mitochondria.

Supplement sleuthing

In the supplement world, words like 'promising', and phrases such as 'may contribute to healthy heart function/cognitive ability/improved sleep', and so on, are often used, so approach a professional rather than trying to prescribe for yourself. Qualified nutritionists have preferred suppliers, and they should have sourced the cleanest and most reliable formulas. I don't advise taking supplements willy-nilly – don't order from unknown brands off the Internet, for example – and it's advisable to work with a professional in the first instance to assess your personal needs. Sometimes, a couple of consultations is all that is needed to get you on the right road.

One of your biggest clues

General fatigue is a common symptom that can indicate mitochondrial dysfunction; however, it is essential to note that it can have multiple causes, and you'll need a proper diagnosis to determine the underlying cause. There are more than a few ways to assess mitochondrial function including: high resolution respirometry, HRR (a technique that precisely measures the oxygen consumption by cells or tissues), MRI scans, genetic testing and cheek swab tests. These would all need to be done under the guidance of a specialist. I have been genetically tested (see Appendix) and I have several 'unhelpful' genes that might contribute to poor cardiovascular health. Mitochondrial dysfunction is increasingly recognised as a contributor to cardiovascular diseases such as heart failure, heart disease, hypertension and cardiomyopathy, so this is an area of focus for me.

Happy hacks

- **Investigate budget sauna** options near you.
- **Sauna blankets or tents** can be a good at-home option.
- **Arrange to go to a sauna with family** or friends to increase the social benefits.
- **Invest in a bath thermometer** (from as little as £4) and take hot baths. Most scientific studies suggest temperatures in a range of 38–41°C as therapeutic. Add essential oils or Epsom salts to avoid drying the skin out.
- **For mitochondrial health**, try a shot of high-polyphenol extra-virgin olive oil every morning, or drizzle it on your veg if drinking it is too much. My kids and I glug it down, but it might be a half-Greek thing!

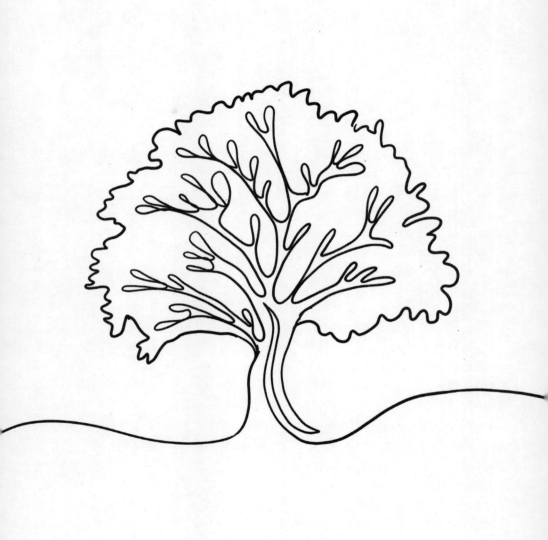

Chapter 10

Fifty Shades of Green

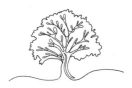

It's February 2025, and outside the prevailing south-westerly wind is whipping huge grey waves all the way up Gyllyngvase Beach in Falmouth, Cornwall. Gyllyngvase is from the Cornish *an gilen vas*, which means 'shallow inlet', although everyone here just calls it Gylly. Usually, it's a year-round swim spot, a wide, soft half-moon of pale sand protected from the Atlantic by the Lizard Peninsula. Today? Not even the hardiest of souls are venturing in. It's cold, blowy and wet. As for me, I'm snug underground in an old wine cellar at the St Michaels Resort, Falmouth.

Down here, it's warm, calm and there's coffee on call. It's tastefully done: grey flagstones, dark wood and old brick with vintage leather club chairs draped in sheepskin rugs that look perfect for slumping in later. Around me the walls are decorated with empty magnums of Veuve Clicquot champagne. It would be a great place for a party, I think, as the rain howls down.

Not that I can see much of the weather. The only natural light is from the floor-to-ceiling glass doors, which look out over a little patio and up a flight of stone steps. My only glimpse of nature is electronic: a glorious screen saver projected on to a big screen that slides around the world, from Lake Bled in Slovenia to the palm-fringed shores of the Caribbean.

And that is kind of the point, because today is the day I meet a team of academics whose work I have long admired – and about which I talk frequently. I have become the subject of one of their famous experiments: trying to quantify the beneficial impact of nature on the human body and healthspan. I've been purposefully kept inside, busy and a bit stressed, so they can measure the restorative qualities of the natural world when I get back out into it.

Natural lab

The academics are from the European Centre for Environment and Human Health (ECEHH) based at the University of Exeter. It's a globally recognised centre of excellence in this field and is responsible for one of my favourite facts (and one of the centre's most frequently cited statistics): that spending two hours in nature every week significantly boosts human health and well-being. They demonstrated this in 2019, discovering that it didn't matter if the 120 minutes were spent in a single visit or spread over several shorter visits; it worked for men and women, across all age groups, and for different ethnic and economic groups; and it worked for able-bodied people and for people living with disabilities.

It just works.

I am with Ben Wheeler (who's a professor in environment, health and inequalities), Dr Lewis Elliott (an environmental psychologist), and Dr Becca Lovell (an expert in the links between nature and health) who, like me, adores trees. She started her career as an apprentice forester with the National Trust in Cambridgeshire and then moved into Forest Research, part of the Forestry Commission, studying the social values of trees, woods and forests to people, communities and society. Later, she tells me that she has her chainsaw licence as well as her PhD.

Since they need a 'control', someone to measure me against, I've brought along my big sister Gina. She's such a whirlwind of activity that we call her 'Zanussi' – because she's permanently on a human spin cycle. She helps me run my work and my family life and 'The Outdoor Guide', the website we set up to showcase the best walks in Britain. The experiment isn't tricky – but it is important. It goes to the very heart of what I believe and have been telling people my whole career: being outside is good for you, your body and brain. Now my big sis is going to help me to show it.

Lewis is going to give us a series of online tasks designed to suck up our full attention; we need to be fast and accurate in the face of challenges designed to make us err.

Afterwards, I get to lace up my boots and swaddle myself in my coat and tramp along the coastal path from Gylly Beach to Swanpool, the next cove along. I can't go with anyone or take my phone; I'm not allowed to think about work, just the horizon, the wide-open sea, and the abundance of marine life here: at low tide the rock pools fill with shrimps, crabs and squat lobsters. Seals, and even whales, can be spotted from the shore, if you're lucky.

Gina, in contrast, gets another cappuccino and an hour to power through her emails in the cellar.

After I get back, we will rerun the experiment to see who's got faster or more accurate, and who has slowed down, or got sloppier. What's interesting, Lewis tells me, is that the fine focus demanded by the test is the same as what's needed by those of us who live in an urban environment, because people and traffic and the busyness of city life means that we are always 'switched on'.

I'm feeling confident, because this isn't an academic challenge (under which I shrivel) and I think my response time is quick; however, I have noticed over the last few years that it has become easier for my attention to wander. I'm blaming social media and the doomscrolling phenomenon. Now, when I'm working or writing at my desk, I make sure that my phone is out of sight, because my natural instinct is to pick it up and check for updates, about *anything*, even though my notifications are switched off.

It's a thing. A 2017 study found that the mere presence of your phone, even if it's turned off, reduces available cognitive capacity. The authors of the study called this 'brain drain'.[1]

Gina is very quick off the mark and definitely a nimbler typist than me, so this will be interesting. Phones safely away, minds set to focus, my big sis and I are crouched over our keyboards ready to jump like grasshoppers.

When we finish the tests, which are pretty horrible, I zip up my new parka (I get through quite a few in my job) and step outside. The wind is blowy enough to lean into, and as the fresh sea air hits my nostrils, I feel the instant relief that comes with a sniff of nature. I make a concerted effort to look outwards and wide. The theory is that this helps our attention recover because there are fewer threats and distractions that we need to effortfully attend to. It's called 'horizon gazing' (and regularly focusing on distant objects can be beneficial to your vision too). I think about how grateful I am to be here, immersed in the beautiful scenery, nodding smiling hellos to passers-by to boost my social fitness along the way. 'We're always very jealous of your job!' some fellow walkers call out.

'Yes,' I respond smiling, 'I'm very lucky, and I'm even "working" today.'

Just under an hour later, I am back in the cellar re-running the tests with Gina.

An explanation by Dr Lewis Elliott

Can you describe the 50-minute fix

Lewis: This first experiment was designed to illustrate attention restoration theory (as per Kaplan & Kaplan, 1989).[2] This theory posits that for most people, everyday life and its demands deplete our directed attention, which is needed for tasks requiring focus and cognitive control. However, engagement with a 'restorative' environment

– that is, one that permits distancing from stressors and promotes a sense of immersion, 'soft' fascination (effortless attention capture), and compatibility (alignment with needs and preference) – can restore directed attention. It is thought that these properties are more often experienced in natural, as opposed to urban or indoor, environments. Short-term effects of restored directed attention can lead to immediate potential well-being benefits, such as reduced stress, improved mood and enhanced cognitive function generally. More importantly though, an accumulation of restorative experiences could play a role in mitigating age-related cognitive decline.[3]

To test this theory with Julia, we designed an experiment to see whether a coastal walk would better restore attentional capacity than not doing this walk. We asked Julia and Gina to firstly perform a cognitively demanding test that requires them to inhibit the automatic response to read the *name* of a colour printed on a screen, and instead to respond by saying the *colour* of that word instead. Secondly, to measure their directed attention capacity following this, Julia and Gina completed a task which asked them to press a spacebar for every number seen, apart from the number 3. We recorded the number of errors Julia and Gina made, along with their reaction times.

After this, Julia was instructed to take a coastal walk and focus on the extent and sense of immersion she felt in her environment. Gina continued her laptop work requiring effortful attention. Combined, these simulate a typical 'intervention' and 'control' group respectively; the kind you would see in a psychological experiment testing attention-restoration theory.

Following this, both Julia and Gina were re-tested. The aim was to see if the coastal walk had benefited Julia's capacity for direct attention compared with Gina. Although a similar number of errors were made, Julia's reaction times were 20 per cent *quicker* than they had been, whereas Gina's reaction times were 14 per cent *slower*. These results suggest that the coastal walk had improved Julia's directed attention capacity, whereas the continuation of work for Gina had actually reduced hers.

Reaction times are the most sensitive measure in this kind of experiment; it's not how many things you get right or wrong, it's about how long it takes you to respond. Gina and I both improved our error rate to pretty much the same extent, but my walk made me significantly faster, and my big sister's strong coffee and assault on her inbox in the comfort of the wine cellar made her slower. If ever there was an argument for regular nature snacks, as I call them, to boost productivity, surely this is it.

Billion-dollar baby

Later that afternoon we head up to join Ben, Lewis and Becca at the ECEHH on the University of Exeter's Penryn Campus. It's a 70-acre site on a blustery hill above Falmouth, and by the time we get there the winter sky is a grumpy grey, hanging so low it's scraping the St Austell hills on the horizon. Inside, the centre practises what it preaches with a mass of pot plants thriving amid the books and mugs and clutter of academic life. I find a large spider crawling over my chest, which Becca rescues and pops back onto a leaf.

My next challenge is to work through my week in 'outside minutes', as Lewis taps furiously on his laptop beside me. These minutes must be spent in a green space with fresh air – birds and wildlife are considered a bonus! (Technically this shouldn't be your garden or private space, it should be publicly accessible, as the point is to quantify the value of nature to the population as a whole.) I'm very glad to have Zeus, my dog, and his need for frequent walks boosting my total because, ironically, writing a book about health and wellness does tend to keep you at your desk. At the end, after a bit of working out, Lewis gives me a score, which astounds me, and it should make you sit up and listen too, because what he shows is that I am a billion-dollar baby.

Lewis's survey exercise – the green dividend

Lewis: The European Centre for Environment and Human Health (ECEHH) has long harnessed the power of large-scale datasets to answer questions about people's interactions with nature, and what they mean for public health and well-being. A good example of this kind of data is Natural England's Monitor of Engagement with the Natural Environment survey (Natural England, 2019) and its follow-on, the People and Nature Survey (Natural England, 2023). These essentially query people's recent leisure visits to natural environments, what they do there, and their perceptions and attitudes around nature more generally. The ECEHH has used these data to uncover a raft of findings including:

- Uplands and coastal margins are perceived as the most restorative of all natural environments in England.
- The more visits we make to nature, and the more 'connected' to nature we feel, the more meaning we find in our lives, and the more likely we are to act pro-environmentally.
- Spending 120 minutes in nature a week is associated with greater well-being for a host of demographic groups.

We asked Julia to complete an excerpt of the original Natural England survey and found that she had recorded 12 visits to publicly accessible natural spaces in the last week. Using an accepted formula, we converted these visits into a standardised unit of energy cost (called a metabolic equivalence of task – MET), which can be applied to any type of activity from sleeping and sitting, to cycling and surfing and everything in between. For example, walking with a dog requires about three times greater energy expenditure than being seated at rest.

The next step was to turn Julia's MET score into an estimate of how many quality-adjusted life years (QALYs) were associated with this level of activity. Using another accepted formula, we determined that the physical activity in nature Julia probably undertakes each year is equivalent to around 32 days lived in full health.

We calculate that this is worth £1,732 per year to the NHS in terms of costs saved. But, of course, Julia is just one individual. If we imagine that Julia's activity was representative of the whole adult population of England (which it is not – Julia spends considerably more time in nature or viewing it, according to our own research than most people do), this figure would reach a whopping £81 billion.

In reality, we found that recreation in publicly accessible natural environments in England was worth around £2.2 billion in adult health cost savings every year. This underscores nature's public health dividend, but also shows how much room there is for improvement if more people could visit these spaces more often for active leisure.

The free pharmacy

It's been a revelatory day with Ben and his team, seeing at first-hand the provable health benefits of being out in nature. But there's still one more astonishing natural health hack to come – and that's discovering that nature can be a painkiller too.

For this we need to head to the University of Vienna where you'll find the legendary Professor Mathew White. He was a key member of the team at the University of Exeter until he moved to Vienna in 2020, and I have followed his work for years. It was through him that I was introduced to PhD student Maximilian Steininger, who's been working on the links between exposure to nature and a reduction in acute pain.[4] I asked him to tell me more.

A conversation with Maximilian Steininger

How birdsong can dull pain

Maximilian: It's 5.30 in the morning. My 18-month-old daughter has woken up crying because she is struggling with her digestion. Over the last couple of days, this has caused her a lot of pain. I take her in my arms and carry her into our kitchen. From here, we can see the green courtyard behind the building we live in. The sun is just rising, and we hear sparrows chirping as they hop around the lime tree outside our window. I try to get my daughter to notice the rustling of the leaves in the breeze and the shadows they cast on our windowsill. For a few fleeting moments, it seems as if she's forgotten about her tummy troubles and the pain they bring. In these moments, I experience first-hand what studies, including our own, have shown time and again: nature can help us ease our pain.

It all started with an article from 1984 that reported that patients looking at trees as compared to a brick wall from their hospital bed needed less pain medication and were sent home earlier by the medical staff. Since then, many researchers have found a similar result: when people are in pain, being in contact with nature tends to help them. In a systematic effort to summarise the available studies on the topic, our research team looked at more than 60 papers and found that contact with nature, on average, lowered the subjective burden of pain. Even though the results did not match up in all studies, in most cases, nature helped to reduce pain. Listening to the sound of water, immersing oneself in a virtual natural scene, or repotting plants, all led to lower pain ratings. But how?

Pain is complicated and can be affected in many ways. Scientists piece the complex experience together like a puzzle using small, understandable parts. Different areas of our brain are specialised to handle these parts separately, and do so fairly piecemeal. If we cut our finger chopping vegetables, special sensory neurons in our hand, called 'nociceptors', send a signal through our spine up to our brain. One of the first things our brain figures out is where (in our finger) the pain is and how intense (based on the cut) it is. Then, a series of complex processes happen that not only tell us where and how bad the cut is, but they also control our feelings towards the pain and our motivation to do something about it.

How we feel pain can be influenced by changes in one, two, or more of these parts of the experience; for example, when we rub our elbow after hitting it on something, the pain reduces because our brain gets less information about where or how intense the pain is. Taking a sugar pill, thinking it's a potent pain reliever, on the other hand, makes our brains care less about the injury from an emotional point of view.

How, then, does nature do it? To answer this question, our research team studied how the brain reacts to pain while people experience nature. We recorded their brain activity while they received electrical shocks while also watching videos of either natural, urban or indoor scenes. Not only did we find that people reported pain as less intense and unpleasant when viewing nature, but also that the brain areas that inform us where and how strong the pain is were less active during these videos. Unlike placebos, the early information tied to the bodily experience changed and not the emotional reaction to pain. It was as if looking at nature had turned the participant's focus away from the early pain signals of the body and towards nature, much like the little sparrows and the rustling of the leaves that distracted my daughter from her pain that morning.

Happy hacks

- **Remember that taking a break in nature** will restore your ability to focus, not reduce it further. As I say time and time again to my friends and in talks: tell your boss that you're going to be more productive if you take regular nature breaks. And you can cite my experiment!
- **Any time in nature** – even walking along a tree-lined street if that's all you've got – is beneficial. Looking at nature, as I do every morning when I do my breathwork, also counts. Time spent in hills, in woodland and on the coast gets you extra brownie points.
- **One-hundred and twenty minutes a week** – not necessarily spent consecutively – is the golden number for a cascade of physical and mental benefits.
- **Pain can be less intense** and less scary if you are immersed or exposed to nature. Exercise can seem less strenuous too.

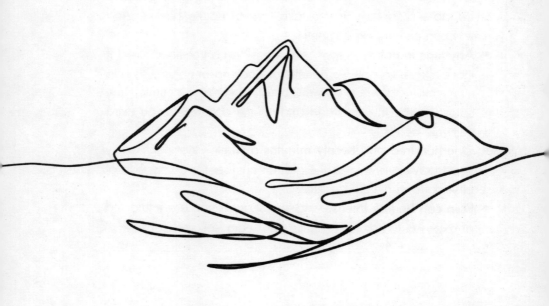

Chapter 11

Ananda: The Healing Himalayas

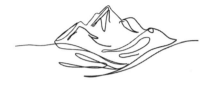

Driving up through the lower Himalayas, you get your first glimpse of Ananda from the Ganges valley. Mostly, you see the dense green of the sal forests (the *Sharia robusta*, a tree native to India), the grey slabs of mountain, and the crimson sky of northern India. But every now and again, the sunlight flickers onto a lemony building held aloft by a great Himalayan crag. You climb and climb until your ears pop and the bends in the road become proper hairpins, and then you see it in all its loveliness.

We are heading for one of the world's leading Ayurvedic clinics, Ananda, where the ancient Indian medical system is used for 21st-century healing. The sanctuary is in the foothills of the Himalayas, located in two historic palaces, the oldest was built for a maharaja, the other was built by him to accommodate a viceroy during the days of empire.

It is 100 acres of idyllic surroundings: dense vegetation and beautifully manicured gardens; monkeys potter along the walls; deer come to drink from the water that surrounds a white marble music temple; and a colony of bees makes honey from the sal blossom, wild curry leaf and wild basil. At night, I would walk through the grounds in wonder, absorbing the multitude of smells and sounds, reflecting on our symbiotic existence with nature. Our own health and planetary health are so intricately linked, and abundantly green, nature-rich places amplify this.

I haven't come for the views, however (well, maybe a little), or the wildlife, or even the honey, although it is remarkable (curry leaf doesn't taste of curry, by the way: it has a musky citrus flavour). I'm not even here for the oldest billiards table in India, or to see a laughing thrush, which sings like someone laughing, and looks like Rod Stewart. I'm here because Ananda is a place of pilgrimage, healing, learning and wellness, that draws everyone from British royals and Hollywood A-listers to scholars and yogis.

Ayurvedic medicine is a very different discipline from Western medicine and, as I recover from cancer and work out how to be the healthiest I can be, I want to know what lessons there are for me here.

Ayurveda is about cleansing, rejuvenating and revitalising for health, healthspan and longevity, and it's been successfully practised for the last 10,000 years. What interests me more than anything is that it considers mental well-being as important as physical health: the two are totally entwined. Whereas I have worked hard to rebuild my body following my mastectomy and breast reconstruction, I am coming to understand that my emotional health is another story.

I will be in the care of Dr Sreelal Sankar, Ananda's head of Ayurveda, and it's going to be an intense seven days of treatments. I will eat a diet prescribed according to my body type, or *dosha*, and follow Ayurvedic principles of sleep, sunshine and exercise. I will deepen my yoga practice and understanding of breathwork and study a little *vedanta*, an ancient Indian philosophy, which teaches students how to live a life of both mental peace and dynamic action. (*Vedanta* is a Sanskrit word meaning 'end of knowledge', though this is a very literal translation. Think of the word 'end' more in terms of 'fulfilment', and you'll get the idea.)

Finally, I will also go on one of the hikes of my life, climbing a modest mountain from where I can gaze on the sacred beauty of the snow-capped high Himalaya, and the gateway to Tibet.

The basics of Ayurveda

According to Ayurveda, the universe is made of five primordial elements: earth, air, fire, water and ether. These elements individually are inanimate but, in combination, they give rise to three different biological forces in the human body. They are called '*doshas*' and, although every human being has a different balance of elements, one *dosha* is typically predominant in each of us and it dictates both our character and our constitution.

Me, myself, and *vata*

Dr Naresh Perumbuduri is a senior physician at Ananda, a fourth-generation Ayurveda medic from a family in southern India. I meet him in a wood-panelled consulting room where his aura of calm well-being highlights my un-calmness. I am talking to Dr Naresh about *vata*, my own *dosha* (my body type) and he's giving me the skinny on the other two: *pitta* and *kapha*.

We're born with a unique combination of three 'bio-energies', and although we all have one predominant *dosha*, everyone has a little of the other two. Dr Naresh likes to explain the characteristics of each *dosha* with metaphors from the animal kingdom. 'No person is 100 per cent *vata*, *pitta* or *kapha*,' he points out. 'If they were 100 per cent *vata* they would be like a monkey: quick and fickle, both physically and mentally. Someone who was 100 per cent *pitta* would be like a ferocious animal: a tiger, if they were to get angry. If 100 per cent *kapha*, that would be like an elephant: slow, in a good way, not over-stimulated and rarely provoked.'

He describes the different *doshas* as follows:

Dr Naresh Perumbuduri talks about the *doshas*

Vata

Naresh: *Vata* people are often dark complexioned, they can be tall or short, but their hands and feet will be always cold. They don't like extreme weather, not too much cold, not too much heat, they want to be in a mid-zone all the time. Often they have dry skin. Simple dietary changes give them constipation, they have an irregular appetite and digestion, sometimes a very good appetite, sometimes very poor which makes them feel either light and well, or bloated; it's fluctuating and unpredictable.

About 70 per cent of this chimes with me. I always have a good appetite; I do have a sensitive stomach, but I like it both very hot and very cold, which reflects another *dosha*.

Naresh: Mentally, *vata* are very energetic, eccentric, enthusiastic, multitasking, creative, talkative, hyperactive, jolly, friendly people; they forgive and forget very fast. They need others around them, or they go crazy. If there is any imbalance in *vata*, it is that simple things make them nervous unnecessarily. They start worrying about something that might happen or might not, and too many things buzz around in their head. It's difficult to shut down their mind. Although they want to focus on certain things, they keep shifting their attention and end up doing something else – and that's where they create stress and anxiety-related issues for themselves and end up losing sleep. They are very light sleepers. When they're lying in bed, they sometimes remember irrelevant things, and then struggle to fall back to sleep. Ayurveda divides the night into *vata*, *pitta* and *kapha*; 2am to 6am is a *vata* time. Those who have a *vata* imbalance always end up getting disturbed after 2am or 3am.

Yes, yes, yes! (Apart from the forgiveness bit. I'm working on that.)

Pitta

Naresh: The *pitta* person is moderately built, often fair of complexion and can suffer from premature greying of the hair, they can lose their hair earlier too. Their hands and feet will be always warm – they like cold weather and hate humid, sweaty conditions, which make them irritable. They have sensitive skin. *Pitta* people have a very good appetite, digestion and metabolism. They don't gain weight quickly until and unless they completely deviate from their lifestyle.

Mentally, they're very organised. They always live by a plan (whether they follow it or not, that's different), but they need some structure to go forward. They set rules in their life and never cross them. They have a typical routine, and they don't alter it often. They expect others to follow some routine in their life too – if they don't, then a *pitta* person will get agitated. 'Why don't you follow this? It makes your life easy,' that's what they keep telling other people. It can make them aggressive by nature, although they don't react to every situation. They are very analytical, trying to understand people, tasks and situations, which means that they can handle life very well. They're good at handling one task at a time; however, they can also multitask when required. In fact, they work efficiently under stressful conditions: it motivates their personality, plus they have good concentration. They always care about quality and will not jump on to a second thing without finishing the primary one. They always prioritise.

They have a good but selective memory. If they feel something is relevant, they remember it forever. They're very, very picky with people, brands, possessions, restaurants, foods – if they like it, they will go to the same restaurant again and again. If they don't, however, it's gone, and they never think about it again. Usually, they're highly goal-oriented: they go aggressively and forgo anything to achieve their goals. When you have a mild imbalance of *pitta*, you will become more instructive, giving instructions to people: try to do this, try to do that, in the home or outside. Where there is a drastic imbalance of *pitta*, they always end up having inflammatory conditions like soft-tissue disorders such as tonsillitis, polyps and piles, digestive disorders, skin issues, etc.

Kapha

Naresh: The *kapha* personality is very hefty; they have good stamina, radiant skin, and they like things a little on the cooler side. They have a good appetite, but slow digestion and a very slow metabolism, so they gain weight quickly, and it's very difficult for them to lose it, even after doing an intense workout and following strict dietary guidelines. They're very slow and methodical, they take their own time to understand things. They need time to execute any task, and they need their own space too. They don't like too many people around their introverted, reserved personalities, and they don't often get angry, because they don't want to be involved in any troublesome situations.

If they see trouble, they just walk away from it. Polite, loving, compassionate and sensitive, they get attached to people, places and pets. They are very consultative, they always take the opinions of others. *Kapha* people have good memories. They're stable mentally and physically, but if there is any imbalance in *kapha*, they will become lazy and lethargic, even calling someone to fetch the TV remote for them or to bring them a glass of water when there is one within reach. If there is an imbalance of *kapha*, most people end up having a metabolic disorder that results in obesity, diabetes and high cholesterol, and they are prone to depression. They're so sensitive and emotional that if something happens to people they love, they truly feel lost. Even if it is a pet, they feel that their pet is for their lifetime and they will never have the same connection, never be able to give the same kind of a love and affection to another animal. They can be opinionated, and if you don't share their opinions, they don't trust you, but if they connect with you, they will be loyal – there's no grey area.

I know a few *kaphas*, but I won't call them an elephant to their face.

What *dosha* are you? You can find out through various online questionnaires, but obviously, seeing your own Ayurvedic doctor or healer is the best way to explore your Ayurvedic type.

My *dosha* decoded

I am a *vata* with a *pitta*, apparently. At Ananda everything I eat, every treatment I have, and every moment of my daily routine – starting with which tea I am allowed to drink with my breakfast – is prescribed for my *dosha*. I was scrubbed, touched, massaged and moved in ways I never thought possible, taking me to a place of deep union between my body and my mind.

The one I'll remember with a smile was an extraordinary movement treatment. I was lying on my back on top of a young, supremely cheerful therapist. As she lay underneath me, her arms were hooked under my armpits and her legs wrapped around my thighs, stretching me firmly in opposite directions. Then she rolled me over and started prising my legs apart using her heels while tugging my arms the other way. 'How old are you?' she enquired.

'Fifty-four,' I replied.

She looked surprised. 'You are the same age as my mother, but very flexible!'

Afterwards, I felt like a rusty lock that had been unpicked and re-oiled.

The one I won't be rushing back to do was a nasal detox. Warm, medicated oil is dropped into both nostrils, you inhale gustily and then attempt to cough it out. You follow the oil with rasping smoke. I'm sure it's beneficial, but I have two words for you: curried tonsils.

I wish I had enjoyed it more because *nasyam*, as it is called, is a pillar of Ayurvedic therapy, designed to remove toxins from the head and neck area. It reduces inflammation and clears the nasal passages, relieves headaches and sinusitis, and balances the three *doshas* (*vata*, *pitta* and *kapha*).

The very efficient enema My *sneha vasti* oil enema wasn't uncomfortable, just a little awkward – having your rear end pipe-cleaned is bound to be. Once the medicated pippalyadi oil had been gently inserted with a plastic funnel, my legs were pumped like a baby's, so that it could take full effect. And it did. For some days afterwards, including up a mountain with no en suite. Like *nasyam*, the nasal detox, *sneha vasti* is a core Ayurvedic technique prescribed to balance the vata and flush out toxins at a cellular level.

The thing I brought home Days at Ananda start in the garden, chanting. I now chant most mornings at home too, having adopted a new mantra *sadhana* I learned there. Chanting isn't about religion for me, it's about sound-energy vibrations. It was a nice mental challenge to learn some Sanskrit verse, and I find the rhythmic pattern of the words soothing and calming. The well-established benefits include better cognitive function, improved mood and reduced fatigue and anxiety (very similar to walking). It's also said to improve one's focus and concentration, and it helps us balance our emotions. Importantly, it's another free thing that we can all do. (Calling it a hack somehow sounds wrong.)

My morning (and sometimes night-time) chant is a Vedic chant dedicated to Lord Shiva and known for its protective and healing powers. The mantra is believed to grant liberation from death and promote spiritual growth. Its chanting evokes divine energy, fostering peace and well-being – and who doesn't need a bit of that?

Pyjama party

The reconciliation of a peaceful mind and a healthy body begins at check-in at Ananda when you're given a pair of dazzlingly white *kurta* pyjamas to wear for the duration of your stay. Most guests wear nothing else, even at dinner. When I sent a picture home, a friend joked that we looked like we'd joined a cult, in our matching outfits with our long strings of *rudraksha* seed necklaces swishing about. But here's the thing: the PJs are comfortable and simple, and they take away a superfluous layer of thought and decision making. It's a tiny tweak which puts a huge distance between the external you with your 'floordrobe' at home and your inner self.

That's the space I was in when I met Blossom Furtado, Ananda's emotional wellness consultant, who does for the mind what Dr Naresh and Dr Sreelal do for the body. She wore a warm, cheerful smile and the eyes looking at me through gold-rimmed glasses were just as kindly. But I guessed, rightly as it turned out, that this was going to go deep.

Full blossom

Before taking me through a visualisation journey, Blossom explained a few home truths. Our 40 trillion cells soak up every bit of trauma, all the emotions, good and bad, that we experience in our lifetimes. We have approximately 60,000 thoughts per day, and because of our negative bias, a large majority, up to 80 per cent, tend to be negative. A significant portion are repetitive too. This constant barrage of negative and repetitive thoughts can significantly impact our mental health, happiness and overall quality of life. Very few of us make a conscious effort to switch off from this, even for a few minutes.

Yet, if we all put aside just ten minutes a day for mindfulness or meditation that would equal just 0.69 per cent of our 24 hours.

We've become human doings, not human beings. Add to this the traumas and challenges that we all encounter in our lives and then consider this: how does this constant onslaught affect us? How does our nervous system cope? These are things that I have only just started thinking about and trying to address in my own life post-cancer as I look ahead to my healthspan and longevity.

I told Blossom my worries about handling my diagnosis, feeling short of time, my family issues, some concerns for my children, and an ugly work situation.

'The mind, body and soul is a divine trinity,' she told me. 'Awareness, acceptance, action, that's the AAA framework and it can help you work through change and tackle negative thought patterns. But it requires time, and space and some reflection. Can you give yourself that gift, Julia?'

I wasn't sure, but I knew I'd like to try.

The essence of AAA is that you can't create change without awareness. Understanding your situation, feeling it and approaching it with curiosity and openness, is the first step. It's only when you can accept who you are in the moment, and don't resist, that you can move forward. Acceptance doesn't mean agreement, but resistance indicates an absence of alignment between your mind, body and emotions. Action can only follow acceptance.

I have now started to ask myself questions when I'm facing a challenge, and these include:

- What am I really feeling right now?
- What is this situation or person telling me about myself?
- What is good about this situation that I'm not yet understanding?
- What is the next logical step and the path of least resistance?

Next, Blossom led me through a guided visualisation in which I ended up sitting on an imaginary white bench talking to people I chose to sit with me. I was asking for their help, sharing emotions and off-loading my thoughts. Tears streamed down my face, even though I didn't feel sad; it was an eruption of emotions I had clearly been holding on to.

It was as if many of the emotional cuts and bruises I'd gathered in half a lifetime had been released in one satisfying emotional burp. I would go on to spend more hours with Blossom, in her room with its picture windows and glorious Himalayan garden view, and I believe that they have helped me build greater healthspan for myself.

If you want the science-based explanation: it's impossible to stay healthy if your body and mind are in a constant state of 'fight or flight'. This doesn't have to mean running from the proverbial tiger, it could be a moment of road rage, a nasty text, a new deadline from the boss, a stroppy child, or just a massive pile of PE kit to launder for tomorrow. Genuine physical changes occur when we're in this state. Adrenaline increases the heart rate and blood pressure, increasing blood flow to the muscles and brain (to help us run). The neurotransmitter and hormone responsible for our flight-or-fight response, noradrenaline, has similar functions, and cortisol (the primary stress hormone) increases blood sugar levels and the availability of substances that repair tissues. They're brilliant physiological responses to stress and danger, but they're a disaster if you live mostly in this state. Your body and your emotions literally get worn down by them all.

I am now ready to accept what I struggled to before: that you can love your life, your family and your work, but even when everything is running smoothly, you're not impervious to their jolts and stresses.

Physical and emotional recovery from a mild stressor, such as road rage or cross words with a colleague or loved one, can take anything from a few minutes to a few hours. It's wise to remember that these smaller events can impact your entire day

> unless you learn some coping mechanisms. Breathwork, move-ment, cold water and rest, can all help. If someone cuts me up when I'm driving or queue jumps, I take a couple of calming breaths and don't let it ruin my day.
>
> So my answer to Blossom's question is: yes.
>
> Yes, I can gift myself 0.69 per cent of my own day. Maybe even a little more.

Stillness and serenity

I have a few new habits about which I can now say, 'I do this every day.' Meditation is one of them. I'm not professing to be a guru, but I put aside 10 to 15 minutes every night to meditate. Which means that I lie down, legs up against the wall (to help ease anxiety and relieve the pressure of the day) and I do a guided meditation or I 'go within', as author and guru Deepak Chopra teaches. At the very least I'm creating 'quiet', which I didn't give myself before, and every time I swipe away a thought and try to get back to my mantra or sound, I feel a sense of achievement. I'm choosing to do this over something less productive, such as watching Netflix, because I know it will aid my sleep, improve my mental health and help me to be still.

I don't think of meditation as an escape from the spinning world but an invitation to step inwards, into the rhythms of my own being – to listen, reflect and discover what lies beneath the surface of my mind. Meditation is not about banishing thoughts but observing them, to try to become more aware of their tapestry. Through medi-tation, we can learn to sit with our emotions and impulses and, over time, we become more skilled at reading these inner patterns. It's no coincidence that rivers and water metaphors are widely used in mindfulness and meditation guides. It makes sense to me, because when I meditate I really do feel like an observer watching the currents of a river, without judgement or resistance.

I have been meditating with more intent since 2021. I probably commit a little more than 0.69 per cent of my day as prescribed by Blossom, because I try to do something every morning and then always before bedtime to anchor myself. During daytime meditation, I generally sit in the traditional cross-legged lotus position with my hands in Chin Mudra: folded index fingers touching the inside base of the thumbs, the other three fingers straight, palms facing upwards. This mudra is believed to enhance concentration, memory and mental clarity. I have added some things that Blossom taught me, and I am following the teachings of Malati Mehrish, Ananda's head of yoga and meditation expert. Here is her beginner's guide to meditation, written specially for *Hack Yourself Healthy*.

Meditation: a journey within

Malati explains how meditation reaches a deeper part of yourself.

Imagine yourself as a swimmer who has spent your life on the surface of the ocean, only to discover that there's an entire world of wonder that lies beneath the waves. Meditation offers a way to dive deep beneath physical experiences into the depths of consciousness itself. Think of it as a powerful path that allows you to go beyond the limitations of your identifications in life and connects you to something deeper.

What is meditation?

In the yogic tradition, meditation is known as 'dhyana': a state of complete awareness, attention and absorption. The winds of life blow into the mind through the windows of the senses. There is a constant stream of information flowing in from the outside world. Meditation begins with gently closing these windows and turning your attention inwards. You turn away from the sensory inputs — not to escape them, but to discover what lies beyond them. It's important to know that meditation isn't about controlling your mind, but it is about bringing together its wandering tendencies. The mind, like a scattered beam of light, gets transformed into a laser – it is the same energy, but concentrated and infinitely more powerful.

Being the witness

One of the most essential aspects of meditation is learning to separate yourself from your experiences. Like a viewer watching a movie, you might get completely absorbed in the story, but you know that these are actors on the screen. Similarly, meditation teaches us that we are not our thoughts, sensations or experiences – we are the witness that observes it all. When we turn inward, we begin to see our own thoughts, memories, dreams, and moods – like watching a private screening of our internal world. In the state of *dhyana* (true meditation), we go beyond both of these states, to a point where both inner and outer projections cease.

Evolution of consciousness

When you're not meditating, you are like a traveller lost in a bustling marketplace, distracted by countless sights, sounds and sensations. Meditation is your compass pointing homeward: it brings you closer to your true self. It is a communion with your inner being. Meditation isn't about shutting down the mind, but of transforming it into something greater. Just as a caterpillar transforms into a butterfly, regular meditation practice can help your mind to evolve into what ancient yogis called a 'super mind': a higher state of consciousness and awareness. Through regular meditation practice, we make a profound discovery: the source of our problems and unhappiness isn't in the external world – it's internal. Meditation teaches us to dive beneath the surface turbulence to find the inherent stillness that was always there. Meditation invites us to return to our essential nature: the simple truth of who we really are beyond all our experiences and perceptions.

Brain box

You can see, I hope, why meeting Malati had such an influence on my own practice. Meditation might seem difficult to access in the beginning, but I have found it worth pursuing. Additionally, brain scans have shown that long-term meditators tend to have increased grey-matter density in regions of the brain, including the hippocampus, which is important for memory and emotional regulation, and the prefrontal cortex, which is responsible for executive function.[1] Studies have also found a decrease in the volume of the amygdala, the brain region associated with processing emotions such as fear and anxiety. Perhaps this is another reason why people like Oprah Winfrey, Ariana Huffington, tennis player Naomi Osaka, and LinkedIn founder Jeff Weiner all meditate.

One hill closer to heaven: my Himalayan walk

O dear Himalaya . . . why are you so amazing, can I kiss your peak or can I just let your silence speak . . . O dear Himalaya . . . (Santosh Kalwar)

Dawn is breaking as we roll out of bed and start the drive into the Shivalik Range (the name means 'tresses of Shiva'). We pass through snoozing villages and up, up onto forested slopes. Mostly, it's a forest of Himalayan oaks. Water washed through their roots is said to aid digestion, making the natural springs around here very popular. (I don't think the locals call this 'biohacking', but it kinda is.) Among the oaks are hundreds and hundreds of elegant pines, their tops fluffy post-monsoon, as if they've had a bouncy blow-dry.

This is the road to Tibet, just 200 miles away. At 1,800m (metres) we stop and tuck into breakfast, eating while our guide, Manish, tells us about the mountain opposite, which was once home to seven sister fairies who may or may not have made a flute player disappear. The Himalayas is that sort of place.

We lace up, and turn and climb, quickly leaving the road behind us and walking onto the mountainside, tussocky and steep, and looking, it has to be said, a lot like Switzerland at its picture-postcard best. Huge rhododendron trees cling to the slopes, with junipers dotted here and there. Iridescent-feathered pheasants whirr from the ground in front of us at almost every step, crying out in surprise, for the trail we are on is little known, and little used, other than by local people walking from one village to another.

We walk and talk, and climb and pause to look, and then, just as we start to summit, Manish runs ahead of us. 'Give me a minute,' he cries and disappears. We gratefully take a break until we hear his voice summoning us from the cool grey mist ahead. A moment or two later we join him. 'I wanted to check . . .', he says and gets no further before we turn to see what he's pointing at. And there they are: the snow-capped peaks of the upper Himalayas, as fierce, as white, a awe-inspiring, and as breath-taking as you could ever imagine, standing sentinel over us.

It feels surreal basking in the sunshine – and technically we are in someone's back garden – looking at this. I feel blessed and deeply lucky, for these early days post-monsoon have remained hazy this year and a clear view is vanishingly rare. About the back garden: we aren't trespassing; the family who live up here with their cow and their bean patch have invited us in so that we can see better. This view is theirs every day.

We take some pictures, but I know that there's nothing I can film on my phone that will do justice to this, and that when I want to remember it, I'll be looking at it in my mind's eye, not on my camera roll. An hour later, we hike another 250m up to what is technically the top, and begin our descent, plunging down a pebbly path through a forest of highly scented deodor cedars. They're named after the Sanskrit term 'devadāru' which means 'wood of the gods', a blend of deva (god) and dāru (wood and tree).

Back at the bottom, I crank the handle of a well, pump out some ice-cold water with which to wash my dusty hands, and then go to hug the biggest pine I can find. He is huge. I wrap my arms around him and cuddle my face into his rough red bark. The friend I was with took a picture of us embracing. If it looked like a real love story, then yes, it was, between me and my mountain and the trees.

Feed well, live long

Diet is a huge part of Ayurvedic medicine. The basic Ayurvedic food principles are set out below, although they may well look familiar to you, as they share many Western principles of healthy eating. I loved everything I ate at Ananda, with the exception of the morning I was given vegetable porridge. Broccoli, yes, oats, yes, just not in the same bowl.

- Eat fresh, whole fruits, vegetables, grains, legumes (peas, beans and lentils), nuts, seeds and herbs.
- Minimise processed foods, which are often high in calories, fat, salt and sugar.
- Eat warm, cooked foods, which are easier to digest than raw.
- Pay attention to the taste, smell and texture of your food, and eat in a calm place without distractions.
- Eat seasonally and focus on foods to match your state. In Ayurvedic medicine foods are referred to as 'heating' or 'cooling'. Certain foods are recommended depending on the time of year, your Ayurvedic constitution and your current state of imbalance. See theayurvedacentre.com/cooling-and-heating-foods/ for a list of foods, and search www.anandaspa.com (Wellbeing Blog / Healthy Cuisine) for articles on Ananda's *Ayurveda*-based cuisine.
- Eat three meals a day at fixed times, ideally without snacking in between.

Before I got to Ananda, I underwent a purifying process called *ama-pachana*, which is intended to clear toxins and kindle your digestive fire. I'm reproducing it here because it's easy to do and I found it beneficial.

Morning elixir Start your day with a morning elixir of cinnamon, cumin and ginger tea. Put a small piece of cinnamon stick, a small piece of peeled fresh ginger and ⅓ teaspoon cumin seeds in a saucepan, and add a glass of water. Boil for 2 minutes, filter and drink warm.

Cleansing herbal water Drink plenty of warm water or this cleansing herbal water throughout the day to flush toxins out of the body through the urine. Put 3 thin slices of peeled fresh ginger, ¼ teaspoon ground cumin, ½ teaspoon fennel seeds and 2 black peppercorns in a saucepan and add 1.5 litres water. Boil for 2 minutes, then add 2 leaves of fresh mint and let it steep for 3–5 minutes. Pour it into a vacuum flask and sip it throughout the day.

The medicine chest in the garden

I meet chef Diwaker Balodi not in the restaurant at Ananda or even in the kitchen, but in his herb garden. We wander between *kalmegh* (a leaf more bitter than quinine, with multiple medicinal uses), snakeroot (good for blood pressure), *partharchatta* (helps with kidney stones), *brahmi* (for the memory) and *nagar-motha* (for gargling away a sore throat). You get the picture: it's like walking through a pharmacy. There's a lot more besides, including an insulin plant, which is related to ginger, and is believed to help control glucose levels.

Together we pick turmeric, carom and clove leaf, which we crush and turn into tea when we get back to his kitchen. As we chat, Diwaker rolls up the sleeves of his whites and starts to demonstrate some of his skills. His menus for Ananda are elaborate and delicious but feature very little added sugar (usually just dates, prunes, figs and honey) and no beef or pork; lamb occasionally and a little chicken and fish.

Watching him work is fascinating, because so much of what he makes is fat-free, gluten-free and not overly sweet and, erm, it's all incredibly moreish. For example, he's experimenting with mung beans – a high source of nutrients including manganese, potassium, magnesium, folate, zinc and essential B vitamins – plus they're full of protein and dietary fibre. Diwaker uses them for muffins to make his version of an eggs Benedict (served with mushrooms and an eggless hollandaise) but is planning to try them in a high tea as scones and as a dessert, in place of profiteroles.

'You eat 21 meals in a week. If you eat red meat and sugar in two or three of them, that's fine,' he says. 'But they're ingredients you should keep in a cupboard marked "rare". We eat for more than for health, it has to be a joy, but the smartest thing to do is to associate joy with healthy eating.'

One of the things we made together was Date, Fig and Lemon Ladoo. We loved them so much that Diwaker made another batch as a goodbye gift, which we discovered only when we opened our packed dinner in the airport at Dehradun on our way home.

Diwaker's Date, Fig and Lemon Ladoo

Serves 7
5g ground ginger
5g ground cinnamon
zest of 1 lemon
zest of 1 orange
1g salt
150g dried figs
150g dried dates
60g porridge oats
a few lemon basil leaves, or camphor basil or lemon balm, or
    a mixture of all three

1 Put all the ingredients in a blender and whiz to combine.
2 Make small hand-rolled balls from the mixture and leave to air-dry until firm.
3 Store in an airtight jar in the fridge.

Thank you, Diwaker.

Ananda. The word itself means 'happiness' or 'bliss state' in Sanskrit. Was I happy there? Yes. Deeply. Seven days was not enough to change the habits of a lifetime (some people move in for a month), but it served as an introduction to a way of life that deeply resonated within me. I left with as many questions as I had when I arrived, but feeling calm, enthused and inspired. Almost a year on, to borrow a Himalayan analogy, I'm still in the foothills of my learning, but I'm climbing with energy, purpose and confidence.

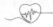

Happy hacks

(The first three come with my thanks to UK Ayurvedic practitioner Dr Sam Watts.

- **Embrace your circadian rhythms** Ayurveda has an entire discipline devoted to this, called *'dinacharya'*. The simplest way to train our circadian rhythms is to maintain consistent waking, eating and sleeping times, and also to get out into natural light within 90 minutes of sunrise (see also Chapter 6). The 21st-century addition to *dinacharya* is blue-light-blocking glasses to reduce the impact of screens and indoor lighting, things that we didn't have to deal with until relatively recently.
- **Experiment with self-*abhyanga*/massage** In Ayurveda, a daily self-massage is a cornerstone of self-care, said to boost immunity, reduce inflammation, reduce stress and increase the secretion of feel-good hormones. Simply warm a few tablespoons of

a pure oil, such as almond or sesame, and gently massage your whole body (or at least your feet) in a slow, rhythmic and mindful way for five minutes each morning.

- **Use detoxifying spices** Add ginger, turmeric, coriander, fennel and fenugreek to your meals. In Ayurvedic medicine, these spices are believed to support the flow of toxins from the skin, urinary tract, colon and liver.
- **Always leave a quarter of your tummy empty** after meals to give your digestion the space it needs to do its job.
- **Practise meditation** for just ten minutes a day – give yourself the gift of time, as suggested by Blossom.
- **Breath, bend, believe**: a yoga hack. I did some wonderful yoga with Malati at Ananda, and it's worth adding that the origins of yoga in Rishikesh (the nearest town) are deeply rooted in spiritual practice, not fitness. Rishikesh itself has been a hub of spiritual learning and yoga practice for centuries. The physical postures we now associate with yoga (*asanas*) were originally minimal and designed not for exercise but to strengthen the spine, calm the nervous system and prepare the body for long periods of seated meditation (often in lotus pose under austere conditions). Only a few poses were emphasised, and they were typically static and grounding. The evolution of yoga, influenced by Western ideals and a growing wellness industry, has seen a big shift from a spiritual path to a workout routine. I have practised yoga for most of my adult life, but what I learned at Ananda has changed what I do, and how I do it, and it might be helpful for you too. I focus on the slower, purposeful, more mindful Hatha yoga, which is taught at Ananda. I also learned a technique that finally helped me to make a connection between my mind and body. When I move into each *asana*, I do it first with my eyes open, and then a second time with them closed. On my third go, I visualise myself in the pose, seeing myself in my mind's eye. It makes such a difference.

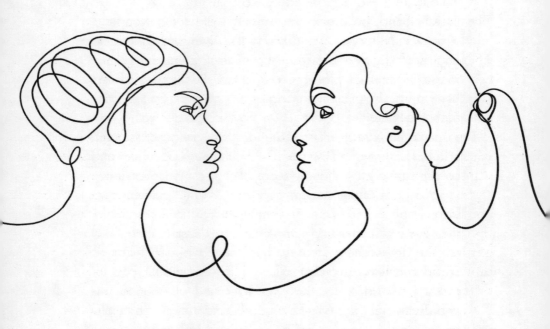

Chapter 12

The Two-Way Street: Mind–Body Health

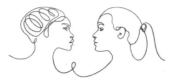

The armchair is made from velvet, the colour of a wild damson. 'Hello Julia, sit down,' says Dr Gabor Maté, scrutinising me. There's a fierce intelligence in his eyes, hooded beneath a bird's nest of tousled grey hair. His agile, rail-thin frame is so comfortably settled in the chair opposite me that it's impossible to believe that he's 80.

I'm on stage in front of an audience with him at a conference where he's speaking. It's not a scheduled appointment, but he wanted a volunteer and here I am.

'So, tell me about your happy childhood,' he encourages, and I do. I share with him memories of my past, describing the old rectory in an idyllic village, the apple trees in the garden, the veg in the plot that made their way to our kitchen table, and the love and care of my parents who loved each other too.

'Overwhelming' is a word that comes out of my mouth unbidden, and he probes the consequences of having to maintain this sense of perfection. 'Were you bullied?'

'Yes, I was.'

'When?'

'Between the ages of 14 and 16.'

'Did you tell your parents?'

'No.'

'Why not?'

'Because, because . . .', my mind reaches back 40 years, 'because I didn't want to bring my problems to them. I was afraid of their reaction.'

He asks how it made me feel, and in that instant, the misery and the loneliness of being the talkative girl with no one to talk to, flooded my body. The unhappiness and confusion of being accepted into the 'cool girl gang' one week, and given the silent treatment the next, came rushing back; as does being mocked for my Greekness at a school in Sheffield, and belittled for my career ambitions. My heart races, I can feel a cascade of stress hormones hurrying my heart and my breathing. I feel safe with him, held by the other people in the room, but physically, it might as well be yesterday. That's the power of trauma and stress.

'It was isolating and scary, and sad inducing,' I admit.

'Isolating and scary and sad inducing', he lets the words settle. 'By the time you were 14 *you* had learned that *you* were, in this sense, alone; that there was no one there for *you*. It's no accident that you were bullied; bullies exploit someone else's vulnerability for their own aggrandisement, you were not bullied by accident: the abuser always has a laser sense of who to choose. So, there's your happy childhood, Julia. Fair enough?' Then he says something that both fascinates and terrifies me.

'Your breast cancer had everything to do with what we are talking about here. This pattern of self-repression and the abandonment you felt but did not acknowledge.'

We sit and regard each other for a moment. The audience is still, quiet and attentive. I have taken the microphone thousands of times in my career, but never like this, never to be put 'on the couch' in a room full of strangers.

'You may be right,' I say, holding my lips together in a smile.

'Of course I am,' he laughs.

Sad, tired and wired

It is March 2024 and we are on the fourth floor of London's County Hall with a spectacular view of the capital. Outside, it's a speedwell-blue day, and the late-spring sun is shining on the Houses of Parliament just across the grey-green of the Thames. Gabor Maté has flown in from Canada to talk about how our bodies hold on to mental and emotional trauma. Although this does not directly cause disease or chronic health conditions, Dr Maté believes they create the conditions in which illness can take hold.

Gabor Maté is a world expert in the impact of trauma and stress on our health. His 2019 book *When the Body Says No: The Cost of Hidden Stress* examines the mind–body links to arthritis, diabetes, heart disease, irritable bowel disease and multiple sclerosis, as well as cancer. Basically, his argument is this: some diseases are genetic, but having the genes which predispose you to developing them is not a pre-determinant, and, inversely, you can develop illnesses to which you are not genetically predisposed as a legacy of early trauma or unrelenting stress.

He cites examples of like-minded physicians such as Sir William Osler (1849–1919), the first doctor to suggest that rheumatoid arthritis might be linked to stress, and Soma Weiss, Hersey professor of the theory and practice of physic at Harvard Medical School until his premature death aged 44 in 1942. Weiss would tell his students that 'social and psychic factors play a role in every disease, but in many conditions, they represent dominant influences' and that 'mental factors represent as active a force in the treatment of patients as chemical and physical agents'.

Of particular personal interest to me was a 2019 study by researchers at the Harvard School of Public Health and Moffitt Cancer Center, which found that women with six or more symptoms of post-traumatic stress disorder (PTSD) had double the risk of developing ovarian cancer, the most deadly of all gynae-cological cancers.[1]

How often do we say, 'Aargh! The stress is killing me!' when we're in a sticky situation?

Well, it really might be. Consider these statistics:

- The American Heart Association says that people with high levels of stress and anxiety have a 48 per cent higher risk of developing heart disease compared to those who don't.[2] Chronic unhappiness can increase blood pressure, raise cholesterol levels, and contribute to plaque build-up in the arteries.[3]
- Researchers at the Carnegie Mellon University found that people with stress are up to three times more likely to catch a cold, because it impairs the immune system.[4]
- Studies from the American College of Gastroenterology show that people with high levels of stress are twice as likely to develop irritable bowel syndrome (IBS) and other gastrointestinal disorders because of the disruption to the gut–brain axis.[5]
- Research published in *Proceedings of the National Academy of Sciences* found that unhappy people have higher levels of inflammation markers, increasing their risk of diabetes, auto-immune conditions and cancer.[6]

All this means that if we are to live longer, healthier lives, we are going to have to deal with our sh*t.

A kitchen disco could save your life

There's growing evidence that dancing is good for the mind–body connection. Here Dr Indika Gunaratne, a former GP who posts on Instagram as the joyfuldancingdoctor, explains why:

1 **It rewires your brain** Dancing doesn't just move your body, it rewires your brain. A study shows that it improves mental sharpness by up to 76 per cent[7] while also balancing the two hemispheres of the brain. This harmony connects logical thinking with creativity, helping you to solve problems and approach challenges with fresh ideas. If you've been stuck in overthinking, dancing can shift you into clarity and creativity.

2 **You can achieve a meditative state** – without sitting still. Listening to rhythmic beats for just 13–15 minutes can shift your brain into theta[8] state – a meditative state where stress dissolves and your mind naturally processes emotions.

3 **It helps with emotional release** We all carry emotional weight: stress, trauma, frustration. These emotions often get stored in the body, creating physical tension. This can dysregulate the nervous system and cause changes in your connective tissue (fascia), leading to pain and fatigue.[9] Dancing is an effective way to release tension, promoting both physical and emotional healing. Research suggests that it has more therapeutic benefits than antidepressants or cognitive behavioural therapy (CBT).[10]

4 **It will regulate your nervous system, joyfully** Dancing aligns with the Polyvagal Theory,[11] which explains how your nervous system shifts between fight or flight and connection and safety. Rhythmic movement and music stimulate the vagus nerve, which helps the latter.

5 **You can use it to reclaim your relationship with your body** Programmes such as 'Move Dance Feel',[12] which supports women recovering from cancer, show how dancing rebuilds trust with your body. Results include:
- 96 per cent improved mood.
- 86 per cent reduced stress and anxiety.
- 63 per cent greater body appreciation.

For more dancing inspiration, go to: www.drindika.com/dance

> **Dance it out like the trees are watching:**
> I would add that doing this outside in nature adds an extra dimension of freedom. There's nothing quite like dancing away to a good tune under the trees.

Sorry, not sorry

One of the common stressors in our lives, thinks Dr Maté, is not living in a way that is true to 'you'. We withhold our expression of emotions or validly held opinions for fear of offending others, of being unpopular, of compromising our personal relationships or our working lives. Sometimes we just don't want to hurt or worry the people we care about, which is why I didn't tell my parents that I was being bullied.

Another stressor is being unable to say no. 'Nobody is born not knowing how to say no,' he says. 'That's something we learn over time. Ask yourselves: "What is the hidden story behind my inability to say no? What is the belief there? That someone won't like me? I will feel guilty? I am only valuable if I am serviceable to other people? I am unkind, unloveable?" Who would you be if you *didn't* believe these stories? Who would you be if you could say no?'

It's a great question. You can see pretty much everyone in the audience thinking about it. But I already have. A lot of women who've had breast cancer do. Protecting your mind–body health by learning how to say no, is really, really hard at first. Women are particularly prone to prioritising everyone else when they should be making time for themselves – and that, says Gabor Maté, can have a cascade of health consequences.

So how do you do it?

If you read my last book, *Walk Yourself Happy*, you'll remember that I spoke to Oliver Burkeman, the best-selling author of *Four Thousand Weeks: Time and How to Use it*. (Four thousand weeks is how many you'll get to enjoy if you live to be 80, which should give you pause for thought.) His most recent book, *Meditations for Mortals*, is a four-week guide to making time for what matters to you – and that definitely means having to say no to other people and other things.

Oliver Burkeman on the unapologetic no

Oliver: The secret to making time for yourself, and specifically for healthy and life-affirming habits, begins with facing an annoying truth: strictly speaking, you *can't* make time for yourself. You can't 'make time' at all. You will always have the same 24 hours in a day as everyone else – 16 really, if you're going to get serious about the foundational healthy habit of sleep. Besides, it's highly likely you feel that your hours are already extremely full of important or unavoidable things. It follows from this that if you're going to claim time in your week for yourself, something else is going to have to receive *less* of your time.

There's no avoiding this fact. It's just maths. The good news is that when you stop avoiding it, you become empowered to make wiser and more fulfilling choices, because you get to give up the futile quest to fit absolutely everything in (which was never going to happen in the first place). Instead, you begin to see that using your time in any way at all requires *some* kind of sacrifice – the sacrifice of all the other things you could have done with that time – and your only challenge is to decide which sacrifice you'd like to make.

The trade-off might be an easy one: if you spend eight hours a week watching streamed TV dramas that you barely even enjoy, consciously cutting that back to six hours at first will surely be the way to go (baby steps!). But it's far more likely that making time for exercise, journaling, meditation or anything else will mean spending a bit less time on something that feels genuinely important, even obligatory.

It might mean spending a bit less time keeping the house in perfect condition, which could feel like letting your family down; or it might mean spending fewer hours with an elderly relative who truly cherishes your attention; it might mean not volunteering for quite so many school fairs or neighbourhood events. The crucial thing to remember is that by consciously pulling back from one or two of these activities, you're not declaring that they aren't worthwhile; you're simply acknowledging that there are many more worthwhile things on which you could, theoretically, spend your time than you'll ever actually have time for. You're also saying that although many things you are doing are valuable and valued, perhaps you can also do a bit less of them and think a little more about yourself – it's absolutely appropriate that some proportion of your time should be spent on nurturing yourself. In the long run, your household, elderly relative or local community will almost certainly benefit from that choice.

Don't forget the deep truth that in some sense you don't need to change at all. It would be *nice* to do so, certainly. But your self-worth, your basic adequacy, your right to occupy space on the planet – none of these depend on your making any great transformation in your life. In the strongest sense of the word 'need', you don't really *need* to become more focused, or fitter, or more patient with your kids.

The ironic truth here is the one identified by the psychotherapist Carl Rogers: 'The curious paradox is that when I accept myself just as I am, then I can change.' Realising that you don't *need* to change makes it easier to do so. You're fine as you are – *and* you have the chance to get better. So why not try? On the days when I'm successful at seeing things from this angle, making a little time for myself stops seeming like a heavy, difficult, forbidding and intransigent sort of problem. Instead, it becomes a prospect too tempting to resist.

Chronically bad

Stress, trauma and emotional issues can manifest themselves physically, as we have seen – in fact it can be a circular route. They can bring on chronic pain or ailments, then that chronic pain prevents us from living our life fully.

According to the World Health Organization (WHO), 619 million people were affected by lower back pain in 2020. It's the leading cause of disability worldwide, and the hardest hit is the 50–54 age group. Frozen shoulder is another significant issue, estimated to affect 2–5 per cent of the general population. That's huge. The cost burden? An estimated US$3 billion in the US alone.

I met Boniface Verney-Carron at a wellness event last year. He's an engagingly passionate Frenchman and a functional osteopath. Banish your ideas about osteopathy: he does so much more than 'crack your back' (that sound, by the way, isn't a crack; it's the rapid release of gas bubbles within the joint fluid, and not the bones cracking. I hope that makes you feel better).

'Whether it's a frozen shoulder or chronic lower back pain, it's not just a physical sensation. It's an interruption, a signal, a call to attention,' he told me. 'Pain is not a flaw in the system. Nature created it as a brilliant biological alert system – designed to protect, guide and communicate. It's the body's intelligent way of saying, 'Something here needs care.'

In acute situations, pain keeps us safe from further harm. But when pain becomes chronic, it shifts into a different kind of language: one that speaks of imbalance, overload, or unprocessed emotional weight.'

A conversation with Boniface Verney-Carron

Why does pain exist?

Boniface: Pain is the body's messenger. Pain isn't your enemy – it's information. It's the voice of a body that has been holding more than it can carry, often silently, often for years.

What is frozen shoulder?

Boniface: In conventional medicine, frozen shoulder is frequently labelled 'idiopathic': a word that means we don't know why it happens. However, we often see it appear after trauma: physical (such as a car accident, surgery or illness) or emotional (such as a loss, a divorce or a major life upheaval). The link between emotional shock and musculoskeletal tension is well known in somatic therapy (where treatment focuses on the body and its link to the emotions).

Symbolically, the shoulder represents a bridge between responsibility and expression, power and burden. A frozen shoulder might reflect repressed emotion, fear or a loss of control. The body, in an attempt to protect or contain something unprocessed, locks down.

At home, gentle rhythmic shoulder circles, within a pain-free range, can help to reintroduce movement. But this must be paired with internal work: visualising the area, connecting to it, and restoring agency. It's not about forcing movement; it's about inviting reconnection.

What is the cause of chronic lower back pain?

Boniface: From a symbolic perspective, the lower back represents support, stability and survival. It's our foundation, from which we hold ourselves upright in the world. Pain here often reflects a deep lack of support, either externally from others, or internally from the way we treat ourselves. It can stem from financial stress, social insecurity or the burden of long-held emotional weight.

This is where our 'comfort crisis' comes in. We've designed lives that minimise movement and insulate us from natural discomfort. But comfort becomes numbness, and the body eventually speaks.

Emotionally, the lower back might hold unspoken anger, grief or family pressure. It's not unusual for people to feel disconnected from the area. Disowning a part of oneself is common in chronic pain.

The antidote is reconnection, not just through major movements, but through small, conscious ones. Practices such as the Alexander Technique, somatic Pilates (where mindful body awareness is combined with mindful movement rather than strict form), or slow, breath-led floor work help to rewire the nervous system. It's better to do ten minutes a day than one big session a week – consistency helps to re-establish trust within the body.

On a biochemical level, chronic pain is also linked to inflammation. Breathwork and anti-inflammatory foods support a healing terrain. If you want one simple, powerful habit, create three small moments in your day – just seven minutes each – to concentrate on your breath, have an awareness of your body and perform some small movements to wake up and stretch your body. I would suggest arching your back upwards and then downwards when on all fours (the cat stretch), or lying on your back with knees bent and tipping up and lifting your pelvis to strengthen your core.

You're training your system to remember: I am here; I can feel; I can heal.

I find it fascinating, and alarming, that two of our most common physical complaints today – a bad back and a frozen shoulder – can be directly linked to stress and emotional trauma. As I said earlier in this chapter, you really do have to deal with your sh*t.

Being more Marcus

In the Appendix, you'll read that I'm genetically wired for stress, which means that I have to work hard to maintain my equilibrium. Being in nature, walking, and mini-breathwork routines all work – and so does my newfound ability to say no.

I have also embraced the idea that things can and do go wrong in life, but it's how you respond to them that matters. This, of course, is the philosophy of the Stoics who lived around 2000 years ago – Marcus Aurelius, Seneca and Epictetus. I was reacquainted with it through the work of writer and 21st-century stoic, Brigid Delaney.

Brigid embraces the belief that a lot of life is simply out of our control: that it's the journey not the end that counts; that happiness is a side effect of living well rather than a goal in itself; and that you should measure success by who you are, not by how others see you. If they all sound relevant to our lives today, that's because stoics lived in a world that looked and felt a lot like ours, says Brigid.

> They also dealt with chaos, war, plagues, treachery, corruption, anxiety, overindulgence and the fear of a climate apocalypse. And just like us they strove to live well in the time that they had. They also longed to find meaning and connection, to feel whole and tranquil, to love and be loved, to have a harmonious family life, fulfilling and meaningful work, intimate and nourishing friendships, a sense of community and a wonder at the natural world.[13]

You can read a lot more about this in her charming and clever 2022 book, *Reasons Not to Worry: How to be Stoic in Chaotic Times*.

Brigid Delaney – ancient resilience for modern life

Brigid: If you want to approach life more stoically, the first thing to do is to learn and apply the following test:

A cornerstone of stoicism is the 'control test', as found in a collection of teachings by Roman stoic Epictetus. It's properly known as the *Enchiridion*. Epictetus – whose handbook was published *c.*125 CE – wrote: 'Within our power are opinion, motivation, desire, aversion, and, in a word, whatever is of our own doing; not within our power are our body, our property, reputation, office, and, in a word, whatever is not of our own doing.'

Essentially, he's saying that our field of control consists of our own actions and reactions, our desires, our character and how we treat others. The rest – including our bodies, the actions of others, our reputation and our fortunes (personal and financial) – are out of our control.

As responses are *within* our control, it is worth considering how you respond to things, particularly setbacks. It's also good to keep in mind that often our responses are the result of our judgements. We make judgements quickly, often without adequate information, and sometimes when no judgement is needed at all. So much of what we label 'good' or 'bad' is actually neutral, it's our judgements that are powerful and they dictate to a large extent what we do next.

If we were to treat most events in a neutral way, we would be less likely to get upset by them. Being indifferent to things outside our control means that we are more likely to maintain our tranquillity.

The state of *ataraxia*, the Greek word for tranquillity, is a key element of stoic philosophy. It's about being serenely calm, unperturbed and undisturbed. I think my Greek heritage is more on the fiery side – *anatarachi*, which means 'disturbance or agitation'. I know I must be more of the former, and less of the latter, so I've had to learn to let go, say no and build a bulwark of time for myself.

Happy hacks

- **Practise the skill of remaining calm** wherever possible. A study in the *Journal of Behavioural Medicine* showed that when sensations of stress or anger become persistent, our immune system weakens. People who are less able to control their anger response were shown to heal significantly slower than subjects who were better at dealing with stress.[14]
- **Laughter has been reported to have a beneficial effect** on the immune system. Studies have demonstrated that showing people funny films up-regulates the expression of genes involved in the natural killer-cell immune response (essential for fighting viral infections), so store some amusing films on your tablet or laptop for emergencies.
- **Have a kitchen disco** Make a playlist, grab some speakers and just dance, and/or join a dance fitness class to have fun dancing with others as well.
- **Be brave enough** to say no.
- **If you have physical pain**, ask yourself what message it's sending, and whether there's an emotional issue that needs your time, care and attention.
- **Next time you're in a jam**, apply the stoics' control test and see if your challenging situation is something you can control – or whether the only thing you have any jurisdiction over is how you respond to it.

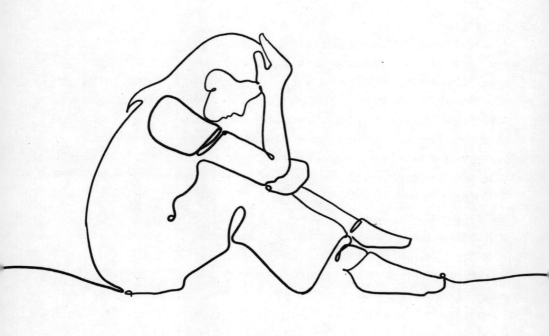

Chapter 13

Emotional Adulting

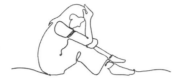

The silver one-shoulder jumpsuit looked fantastic. It had been a gift from my fashion-designer friend, Melissa Odabash, sent on spec because she thought I'd like it. She was right: I loved it. I was already in a taxi by the time I realised that the revealing top was cut diagonally on the same side as my newly diagnosed breast cancer. I looked down and understood that this was the last time I would be red-carpet-ready in my old body.

It was September 2021 and I was heading to the National Television Awards, but I wouldn't be able to tell any of my telly mates about my cancer or the fact that I had a mastectomy coming up in a fortnight's time.

It was a complicated night.

The paparazzi were out in force, flashbulbs popping, the champagne was flowing and the whole TV industry was partying as only it knows how. I wasn't drinking and was perhaps a little subdued compared to my usual fondness for a good night out.

My friend Ben Shephard, now presenting *This Morning* with Cat Deeley, asked, 'You OK Jools? No bubbles tonight?'

There weren't. In fact, it would be a while before I had anything to celebrate again. Yet, for all that I was going through, and the surgery I was about to endure, looking back I can honestly say that there would – in time – be many positives too. For one thing, a cancer diagnosis would force me to focus on my emotional health.

Having previously neglected this part of my life, I have had to learn how to love and believe in myself, not in an egotistical, narcissistic way, but with softness in my heart. Compassion, grace and gratitude have slowly become part of my vernacular. My body is battle worn, but I have gathered new skills that enable me to look at myself in the mirror, with my odd-shaped prosthetic left breast and all the other scars that I've collected along the way, and say, very quietly to my reflection, 'I love you. Even now. Especially now. I love you.'

It's about being resilient, not hiding from challenging things, but considering them, getting them in perspective and then stepping up. And this is not just about managing life – it has a very real impact on your physical health too. The following list comes courtesy of psychotherapist, author and broadcaster, Anna Mathur.

Anna Mathur – stress fracture

Anna: Below are some of the ways our emotional health impacts our physical health:

Pain sensitivity When someone is emotionally distressed, their tolerance for physical pain is decreased. People who experience chronic health or autoimmune conditions such as migraine, back pain, muscle aches or skin complaints, often see a direct correlation between the experience of stress and an increase in discomfort and symptoms.

The immune system When we experience emotions such as grief, anger or anxiety, our bodies release cortisol and adrenaline. These stress hormones put our body on high alert and in survival mode. This is intended to last for short periods of time, yet so many people are living much of their lives in this heightened, inflammatory, energy-draining state.

As the body is focused on momentary survival, the immune system is robbed of resources, and therefore we become less able to fight off illnesses or to heal. Instead, with the resulting increased levels of physical inflammation, the risk of related diseases such as cancer, arthritis and diabetes is heightened.

The heart When someone feels stressed, depressed or anxious, a higher blood pressure and heart rate is evident. This increases the risk of cardiac disease. (Amazingly, when people feel connected to others – safe, secure and calm – all these risk factors drop, showing a strong link to emotional and physical health.)

The gut Just as excitement and trepidation lead to a very physical experience of 'butterflies in the stomach', and anxiety can find the stomach literally churning, our emotional health impacts our gut health. The gut–brain axis is the channel through which our brain and gut communicate with one another. The gut is often termed 'the second brain' and the vast majority of the so-called 'happy hormone', serotonin, is actually produced in the gut. Therefore, when our stomachs are churning with anxiety, or our gut feels punched with grief, there are chemical and hormonal changes occurring. Those people experiencing irritable bowel syndrome, reflux or other digestive issues, often notice a link between increased stress and their symptoms, and when the stress levels are reduced, the gastrointestinal tract tends to become calmer and more predictable.

Quality of sleep Anxiety, grief and rumination can disrupt our sleep. When we're tired, we're low in energy and resources. Chronically disturbed sleep impacts every system in the body, from the immune system to how we metabolise food.

In short, those who are bottling things up or struggling emotionally are more vulnerable to physical disease than those who have better emotional health.

The wilderness cure

Emotional health is about how we handle life's ups and downs, how we express ourselves and connect to others. We will all experience setbacks, but even these can be beneficial experiences, if we know how to frame them. Nature can help us with that – and you won't be surprised to learn that I leaned on it a lot as I mourned the loss of my old body and came to appreciate my new one.

Spend a day outside, underneath the big sky (in contrast to a low ceiling of energy-sapping LED lights indoors). This can evoke feelings of awe and gratitude, and a connection to your deeper self. These aren't just fleeting feelings: they nurture our emotional reservoir. Humans are 'set to negative' to help protect ourselves. Our negativity bias has a value in keeping us safe, but we need to bolster our positivity reserves. We can do that by acknowledging and absorbing the little wins we have throughout the day. Hugging that tree, hearing those birds, gratefully acknowledging the time that you have given yourself in nature – they are all natural curatives.

I met Anna Mathur on a fitness retreat in Spain, where the first thing I noticed was that she had the most incredible selection of onesies. On this retreat, the group took turns to tell after-dinner stories. Anna told one story about an afternoon wading through a massive pile of laundry for her family – a tiresome chore. It was pissing her off until she stopped and reframed the situation, 'I'm so lucky to have a family to do this for, I have a washing machine and a lovely home. I can wear clean clothes.' Bloody hell, we all thought. She's only gone and turned the washing into a gratitude practice!

For *Hack Yourself Healthy*, I asked her to offer her expertise on emotional health (not laundry), what it is, how to find it, how to keep it, and what to do when your emotions feel fragile or uncomfortable.

Feel it to heal it

Anna explains:

Emotional health is the ability to process, understand and express our feelings in a way that supports overall well-being. It's not about feeling happy all the time but learning instead to navigate the full range of emotions with self-compassion, balance and resilience. Emotional health means being responsive to our feelings rather than reactive, it means we feel safe within ourselves and don't immediately tip into a state of stress or overwhelm when faced with a challenge.

Ten golden rules for nurturing your emotional health

1 **Movement** Move your body in a way that serves you according to the energy levels you have that day. Whether you opt for some high-intensity cardio or a walk round the block, movement is a powerful way to improve your emotional health. Moving your body and raising your heart rate triggers the release of happy hormones, such as endorphins, which help to boost and regulate mood.

2 **Journaling** Writing your feelings down is a way of externally processing and releasing stress and emotion. People often report feeling a reduction in stress, and increased self-awareness. Memory, communication ability and cognitive function are also enhanced when we take time to articulate our thoughts, set goals and organise our thinking. All these benefits work to support physical health by improving immune function, and can even increase sleep quality when journaling is done before bed!

3 **Joy and gratitude** Consider something you are grateful for in this moment, or take a couple of minutes writing a gratitude list. Even if your list is full of tiny things you tend to overlook, it is a powerful way to shift your focus from the negative to the positive. It's not a denial or avoidance of tough things happening, but the recognition that good and beautiful things are *also* happening in your life alongside them. Gratitude can reduce levels of depression and anxiety, and halt rumination, when we can't stop thinking over and over about something that is troubling us. Gratitude is also known to improve sleep quality due to reducing our focus on sleep-disrupting negative thoughts.

4 **Rest** When life feels busy, rest is often overlooked, yet rest is the true antidote to burnout! The more we do in life, the more rest we need. Choose to not overlook an opportunity to slow down and rest, but see it as a chance to process what you've been through and refuel yourself for the hours ahead. When we're tired, our ability to navigate stressors is impacted. Rest reduces physical anxiety and moves our body into a state of refuelling and processing. It increases mental clarity, mood, self-control, focus, memory and emotional resilience.

5 **Talking** to someone you trust about how you're feeling enables you to feel supported, heard and validated. This meets a deep human need, and it helps to quash feelings of loneliness and improves connectedness to others. As we talk through feelings, we are able to understand ourselves a bit more, gain fresh insight and resolutions, and release emotional (and therefore physical) tension.

6 **Reshape your critical inner dialogue** The conversation you have in the quiet of your mind is the single most important dialogue of your life. If your internal dialogue is critical or bullying, it will directly impact your anxiety and stress levels. Begin to introduce to yourself a kinder, more compassion-

ate voice, even if it feels clunky and tiring at first. When you begin to replace criticism with kindness, you nurture a healthier, more supportive relationship with yourself. This helps you to navigate stress more effectively, as you are more likely to coach and guide yourself through it rather than criticise yourself for each perceived failing or weakness. This improved self-relationship boosts physical health by reducing stress hormones (cortisol) and, in turn, improves your immune system and general sense of well-being.

7 **Get out in nature** There are so many things that you can do to support yourself, but getting out in nature has to be one of the most cost-effective and accessible. Nature has a calming impact on your stress levels and it reduces anxiety and depression. Recognise how you feel before and after taking a walk, or even hugging a tree. Nature prompts mindfulness and offers space for reflection. The profound impact on reducing blood pressure and heart rate are a testament to the power of nature on our minds and bodies. Make a pledge to interact with nature more often, be it standing at your window and breathing in some fresh air, or leaving ten minutes early for your commute so that you can get off a stop earlier and walk the last part of the journey. Even if you work in a town, you may be able to spend that walking time enjoying the exercise, and hopefully there will also be some trees or greenery along your route.

8 **Wild swimming and cold-water therapy** There's solid reasoning behind the fact that so many people rave about the transformative benefits of spending time in water. Whether you opt to join a wild-swimming group or turn your shower on to the coldest setting for a moment in the morning, the benefits are undeniable. The cold water stimulates the parasympathetic, the calming, stress-reducing arm of your

nervous system. It also triggers an influx of mood-lifting happy hormones (endorphins). Plus, as you emerge from the water, the sense of pride and well-being boosts your mental resilience and increases your tolerance to stress. Not to mention the physical benefits of improved circulation, metabolism, immune system and recovery! (Note: if you feel uncomfortable rather than energised after your cold swim/soak, it might be that your body is not able to benefit from it and it is therefore unsuitable for you. See the Outdoor Swimming Society's website for more on this: https://www.outdoorswimmingsociety.com/risks-cold-water/. Also be aware that women can respond differently from men, because of hormonal and physiological differences. Women, for example, have a higher density of cold receptors in their skin, potentially making them more sensitive to temperature changes.)

9 **Gardening** Whether you are nurturing a plant in your kitchen, cutting a lawn, working on an allotment or planting a window box, tending to nature offers powerful benefits to your emotional and physical health. Seeing the direct impact of your time and energy through growth and flowering is really empowering. Enjoy the mood-improving, heart-rate slowing benefits of these pursuits as you get your hands dirty.

10 **Helping others** There is something incredible about seeing people thrive and change because of the impact you are having on them. Helping others also benefits one's emotional and physical health, because it meets the human need to feel that we matter to others. Whether you engage in a small act of kindness, invest in a relationship in which you support someone else, or support a charity or a campaign, contributing to someone else's well-being improves your mood and sense of connection, belonging, fulfilment and purpose.

Feeling fragile

As you know, I've been working hard on my physical fitness at the Hooke Clinic in London. But what was also clinically measured at Hooke was my emotional health, my resilience. And, friends, some of my scores were low. Very low. I wasn't surprised, as this came after a long period of challenge and change: my breast cancer, some family issues and, obviously, I work in the media, which is fast evolving too. A triple whammy.

I was examined by Aneta Tunariu, a professor of applied psychology and a chartered psychologist with the British Psychological Society, who has taught and practised in Britain for decades. She is originally from the city of Brasov in Romania, where her work with young people in an orphanage would later inspire her career in mental health.

Aneta places existential philosophy at the heart of her approach. She tells me: 'In a nutshell, existentialism is a philosophical line of questioning that nudges us to ask "what is a life worth living to me?", and to remain mindful of our freedom to choose our responses, and to be able to talk honestly to ourselves in a responsible and empowering way. Existential lenses as ways of seeing are not dogmatic nor imposing,' she says, 'but designed to help the client [in this case, me] towards a mindset that allows healing, insight and graceful defiance.'

Questions on the couch

Aneta has given me a list of questions to gently interrogate myself with while I buttress my emotional health as part of my pursuit of healthspan. They're general, rather than related specifically to me, so you can try them too:

1 What makes me smile? How do I participate in a way that will generate more of this?

2 Whose company tends to bring out the best of me? How can I keep company with these people?

3 When do I feel most lovable? Are these times related to both 'being me' and doing things? If not, where do I strike a harmony between those two ideas?

4 When do I feel most deserving? Is this good for me? Or do my choices set a conditional, transactional self-regard? For example, 'I must do X to be worthy of love and happiness?'

5 Is there another way of looking at things? What am I not seeing?

6 What have I achieved today in spite of any difficulties?

7 When I am lost or overwhelmed, I can ask myself, 'What do I know for sure?'

- My values (these delineate me and require that I honour them in action and talk).
- My embodied breath (this feels like me).
- The things that I am grateful for (I am more than this unpleasant predicament).
- My hopes (I am the boundaries of the emerging me).

Be a tree: when it's stormy, bend don't break

Aneta has also created a special *Hack Yourself Healthy* seven-point plan designed to help build resilience as we navigate our way through life's personal and professional challenges. Holding and understanding emotions just long enough to make sense of them, and possibly reframe them, is hard and takes practice. After my sessions with Aneta, I often recall the phrase, 'I am my choices.'

1 **Normalise** Emotions are the flavour of our every moment and experience. They give us insights as well as fuelling the orientation of our actions. Normalise emotions and build awareness of their presence. Remember, we cannot help

feelings or emotions rising inside us; however, we can help how we make sense of them, what we learn from them, and how we respond to them.

2 **Mindset** Step back and take a bird's-eye view of the emotion or emotional behaviour you are examining. Choose self-compassion. See what you encounter for what it is, and accept it without judgement or an ego-led reaction (such as reacting with rejection, or a sense that it is unfair).

3 **Name it** Name the emotion as accurately and objectively as possible (including having at hand a good vocabulary of emotional nuances). This will help you disentangle its message and its significance.

4 **Feel it** Stay with this emotion; stay with the feeling of this experience for a minimum of two minutes. Tolerate this discomfort, because the emotion is a source of learning. Tolerating it is a way of accepting its reality.

5 **Acceptance** Resist the temptation to leap ahead. Engage in internal dialogue and tell yourself, 'I am not this emotion. This is a passing moment that carries insights. Once it passes, I will still be standing and I will be wiser for it. What am I not seeing? What would be good for me to learn? What else should I know?' In this way, we refocus our attention and diminish the risk of reaction, and thereby we increase the possibility of insight.

6 **Integration** Let go without forsaking your experiences. By processing things that matter, we become grounded; we come to a deliberate choice rather than following our normal or familiar patterns of action. With repetition, choice becomes our new normality.

7 **Claim the outcome** Welcome change with grit and self-accountability. This will help you to recover faster from falls, mistakes and failure, and to become more able to grow through adversity and challenges. We come to see how peak performance is not merely about time or effort spent, but rather about how awareness and energy are invested.

Lonely in a crowd

Right now, my partner and I are fully immersed in parenting young children and running our respective businesses. Both require a lot of time and energy; there's not a lot left for socialising. The fall-back is old friends who we feel happy and secure with and newer school-gate mates. A decade ago, we were out and about all the time with all kinds of people in all kinds of places: nourished, inspired, educated, as curious about them as they were about us. Now, a night in, cooking with family, is my ideal, but I'm aware that we're not nurturing new friendships with all the freshness and energy that they bring to our lives.

Like many people, I'm just not as socially fit as I was. For me, that's a combination of work, parenting and having cancer. For others it might be the legacy of lockdowns, moving to a new city, divorce, redundancy, retirement, or splintering from an old friendship group. In many cases, it's just the age we live in: our digital life persuading us to bury ourselves in our screens in lieu of connecting with other human beings.

Yet, strong social connections are so critical to physical wellness and healthspan that in 2023 the World Health Organisation launched a special commission to try to publicise what they call this 'global threat to public health'. 'High rates of social isolation and loneliness around the world have serious consequences for health and well-being. People without enough strong social connections are at higher risk of stroke, anxiety, dementia, depression, suicide and more,' said WHO Director-General Dr Tedros Adhanom Ghebreyesus.

According to the WHO, a lack of social connection carries an equivalent, or even greater, risk of early death as other better-known risk factors – such as smoking, excessive drinking, physical inactivity, obesity and air pollution. Social isolation also has a serious impact on physical and mental health; studies show that it has been linked to anxiety and depression and can increase the risk of cardiovascular disease by 30 per cent. It's a known risk factor for Alzheimer's disease too.

It's one of the easiest things to fix, however. A quick chat to the barrista as you buy a coffee, a hi to someone else walking their dog, a cheerful interaction with the person standing behind you in the supermarket queue – they all count as flexing your social muscles.

The royal seal of approval

I'm not saying that book clubs are booming, but the number of book club listings on the global event booking platform Eventbrite rose by 350 per cent between 2019 and 2023, with eight out of ten clubs meeting face to face as opposed to online. Queen Camilla has her own: it's called The Queen's Reading Room.

Book clubs are a fantastic way to increase your social fitness, because you are meeting other people who you automatically have something in common with – reading – and you automatically have something to discuss: your book.

Reading can also be a good 'stacking hack', because it doesn't just make you more socially fit. In 2024 The Queen's Reading Room unveiled positive research about the benefits of reading:

'Just as we always suspected, books are good for us – and now the science is proving us right,' said Queen Camilla at the time. 'In addition to our five a day and our 10,000 steps, we should all be aiming for at least five minutes of reading every day for invaluable benefits for brain health and mental well-being. Literature, quite simply, makes life better.'

Five minutes of being lost in a story was sufficient to reduce stress by nearly 20 per cent and to improve concentration and focus by as much as 11 per cent. Additionally, The Reading Room showed that picking up a book earlier in the day helped people feel more connected to others and ready to tackle challenges. Reading fiction significantly reduced feelings of loneliness, helping to combat the social isolation we know is linked to an increased risk of developing different dementias.[1]

I would add that it's also a great way to help you to go off to sleep at night. Sleep experts suggest nothing too exciting or gory (suggestions on a postcard please), but the real pages of a book are much kinder to our circadian rhythms than blue screens.

Socially fit, not socially feral

We know that being connected to people, having genuine bonds and friendships, and even casual interactions in the street, add to our healthspan. To find out more I spoke to David Robson, an award-winning science writer whose 2024 book *The Laws of Connection* has gained a huge following for its practical science-based strategies to improve your social fitness. (Ironically, I didn't get to meet him; we hopped on Zoom to speak from our respective homes.)

David grappled with shyness and social anxiety growing up in a little village near York. A slight speech impediment did nothing for his confidence. 'I struggled to say my Rs, which is tricky given that my name is Robson,' he smiles, relaxed about it now. Despite his shyness, he followed his dream of becoming a journalist, and ended up with the BBC.

'You know what they say – research is often me-search,' he laughs. (Yep, that's why I'm writing this book.) 'Becoming a journalist was a kind of informal exposure therapy for me, and the result was me wanting to write the book I would have liked to have given my 15-year-old self.'

A question-and-answer session with David Robson

What exactly is social fitness?

David: Social fitness is feeling equipped to have the social life you personally desire. It's not about the number of connections you have, your tally of Facebook friends or Instagram followers, but about getting to a place where you feel loved, supported and truly understood by others. It's perfectly possible to feel lonely even when you are a popular person, and that's just as damaging as being physically isolated.

How can someone improve their social fitness if they're naturally shy?

David: Start small by practising regular interactions. Push yourself out of your comfort zone gradually. Treat it like any form of exercise: repetition builds confidence and skill.

Tell me about weak ties?

David: Weak ties, brief interactions with strangers or acquaintances, provide significant mental-health benefits. They help to train your social muscles and can lead to unexpected connections and personal growth, so they are a crucial part of building a stronger social network overall.

What's the biggest barrier to making social connections?

David: This is the 'liking gap' where people consistently underestimate how much others like them. It's been proven in lots of experiments that when you introduce two people who didn't know each other beforehand, but who get on, each person goes away thinking that they liked the other person more than the other person liked them. That can be a major barrier to social connection, because if you don't have faith that the other person reciprocated your feelings, you're less likely to suggest meeting up again. Try to really emphasise how much you appreciated them, don't just take it for granted that they will know, because they probably won't. Just telling them that you would like to meet up again is so powerful. When you start doing this, you'll be surprised at how warmly those overtures are received.

How can we start to improve our social fitness?

David: Reconnect with an old friend. Send a message expressing how much they mean to you. Research shows that people are often much more receptive and appreciative than we expect them to be.

What are your top social-connection hacks?

David: Listen carefully. If someone's coming to you, especially with something that's upset them, don't jump in and talk about your own experiences, because it's as if you're grabbing the microphone and making it all about you. Once someone has told you, you can share because you're validating what they're saying, letting them know that they're not alone. We often feel we're weird and a failure because of something that's happened. Actually knowing that someone else has had similar difficulties can be very reassuring. The research shows that when we're willing to share our true selves – our hopes, fears and passions – that's when we really start to establish a sense of shared reality and intimacy with others.

The friendship formula

I really enjoyed my conversation with David. I like the idea that a warm and interesting encounter with a stranger makes a difference. I make an effort to smile and say hello to people when I am on the bus or the tube – it makes you feel buoyed and happy. Another interesting fact that David shared is that the average person has 150 meaningful acquaintances, and then successively smaller layers of people that matter, down to a core of five or fewer people they love and need.

That's definitely true for me. Is it true for you?

Making a porpoiseful connection

As ever, we can look to nature to see how social fitness should be done. Gregarious dolphins are the masters of this art, the creators of complex social networks, pods within pods, if you like, to build alliances and friendships. They communicate with each other through whistles and clicks, often just to strengthen their social bonds but also to synchronise their movements as they swim and play with other dolphins they like. Their friendly characters and behavioural patterns stay with them for life, suggesting that their social fitness plays a significant role in their development and survival.

Tapping into the inner me

Hands up if you've heard of the Emotional Freedom Technique, EFT for short. It's a gentle type of therapy that combines cognitive behavioural therapy (CBT) and acupressure, and which includes body tapping. It's been shown to have beneficial effects on specific markers such as HRV (heart rate variability), RHR (resting heart rate) and blood pressure. Even depression and

PTSD (post-traumatic stress disorder) have been improved through EFT therapy.

Working with a therapist is great, but it isn't something we can all access regularly. The body tapping bit of EFT, however, is something we can do safely at home on our own, and it can be really effective. I've been experimenting with tapping for the past six months and using it to help a member of my family who suffers from anxiety.

This is how it works:

- Discomfort (such as a headache or a racing heart) can be significantly reduced, or even completely alleviated, quickly, when you practise tapping while simply focusing on the part of your body that feels anxious or is in pain.
- Tapping can reduce cortisol (one of our stress hormones) and can stimulate the body to release beneficial chemicals. It can help to reduce pain (as we have seen above), and there's a suggestion that it can even create epigenetic changes in our genes, linked to stress. (See Chapter 3 where Dr Kara Fitzgerald explains epigenetics. Although we can't change our genes, we can influence how they express themselves.)
- Like breathwork and forest bathing, tapping has a long-lasting impact on our physiology that reaches beyond the actual time spent practising it; even if you're not feeling anxious or stressed, but you have a history of those feelings, tapping can be used as a preventative measure, and doing it regularly can restore your body to a calmer baseline.

EFT therapist Dafni Serdari, from the Forbes Clinic of Integrative Medicine in London, has created this guide for you to try when tapping in your daily life.

The three stages of tapping self-help

Dafni's method, as developed by the founder of EFT, Gary Craig, is easy to follow and to benefit from.

1 First, decide on the problem you want to solve; for example, 'I'm stressed because I'm running late', 'I'm angry at my partner for making that comment', 'I'm so frustrated by the tight deadlines at work'.
2 Now, tap on the side of either palm (the fleshy part), using the tips of four fingers, while stating the problem in the following way: 'Even though I [enter problem], I deeply and completely accept myself.' For example: 'Even though I'm stressed because I have a book deadline/I have exams/I'm awake when I want to be asleep, I deeply and completely accept myself.'
3 Next, tap on the following eight points of the body while repeating the *negative* emotion; for example, 'I'm stressed.'

The eight points:
- Top of the head with the five fingers of either hand.
- Beginning of the eyebrow with two fingers (right or left).
- At the side of the eye with two fingers (right or left).
- Below the eye with two fingers (right or left).
- Above the top lip with two fingers.
- Below the top lip with two fingers.
- Between the collar bone with a fist.
- At the side of your torso, about the height of your bra-line/nipple with four fingers.

At the end of the tapping round, you should feel better. And you can go for as many rounds as you like, because tapping is a safe process.

If you are into positive affirmations (which I am), tapping can also be used when you say them out loud to super-charge the feeling. You might have heard about neuroplasticity: the ability to retrain the brain and learn new responses. This is one way to try to access that superpower.

Something I've started doing is tapping to reconnect with the calmness I feel when I'm out in nature; nature makes me feel happy, so if I'm feeling stressed and I can't get outside, I use tapping to take me back to the level of ease and happiness that I experience when I'm under the trees.

If you had told me ten or fifteen years ago that I would be meditating, doing breathwork daily and trying out new techniques, such as tapping and chanting, I would have laughed in your face – I didn't think that I had a problem with stress. How wrong I was. Now I accept that things can and do go wrong, and it's how you respond to them that matters. Learning how to hack my own emotional health, as well as gathering knowledge from experts, has been unbelievably helpful to me. People always talk about learning a lesson from cancer, and this was mine.

Happy hacks

- **Re-read Anna Mathur's ten golden rules** on page 209 and ask yourself which ones work best for you.
- **When something bad happens**, ask yourself what it's taught you and what you can use going forward.
- **Flex your social fitness muscles** at every opportunity.
- **Remember that nature** will always give you a sense of perspective.
- **Tap into your problems** to relieve anxiety.

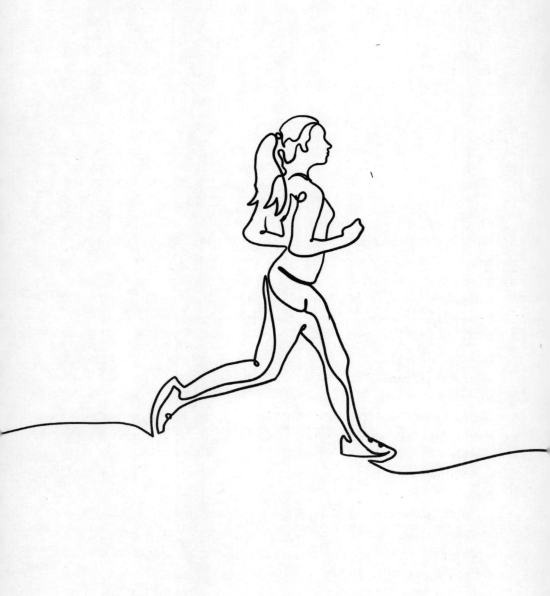

Chapter 14

Flex Appeal

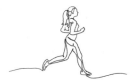

There was a point in my life that I had never expected to experience at the age of 50: I could not lie flat on the floor and put my arms above my head. It was after my mastectomy, and I'd been sent home from hospital with a list of exercises that were so simple they made me cry. They weren't tears of joy because they were easy, however, quite the opposite. I was desperately sad because they were so straightforward and yet they were still beyond me.

At that stage of my recovery, I could not even get my left hand to do a spider crawl up the door of the cupboard in my bedroom, never mind get my arms over my head. Those bleak memories will always be with me, and if ever I am tempted to skip an exercise session, I only have to think back to the days when my big sister Gina had to come round and dry my hair for me.

I will forever be grateful for the range of movements I now have.

At the age of 54, I'd argue that I am fitter, more flexible and stronger than I was before I was diagnosed with cancer – I'm probably in the best shape of my life. For me, healthspan means being able to continue doing all the things I enjoy as I creep (or should that be creak?) into older age: cooking for my family, driving myself from A to B, walking the dog, or carrying suitcases.

I don't want to wait for the day when I can't pick up a heavy casserole or reach behind me for my seatbelt, or bend down far enough to clip on Zeus's leash.

They are all actions that we barely register, doing them almost unconsciously – until we can't. I've been there, and it's awful.

Try this:

Pick a joint of your body and hold it stiff, eliminating movement completely, and see what effect it has on you; for example, try going about life holding one ankle completely rigid for five minutes. Do you find it difficult, uncomfortable, does it add stiffness to other parts of your body? Yes. Eye-opening, isn't it?

Let's try not to seize up but to keep moving, literally, throughout our lives. In my first book *Walk Yourself Happy* we met Hannah Beadle, the CEO and head coach of Wildfitness, whose brand of green exercise – moving in nature while being at one with it – sees her running transformative fitness retreats around the UK and Europe.

She is returning to *Hack Yourself Healthy* with a set of positions (designed specially by Wildfitness) to assess the varying ranges of motion that we're all going to need to lead a free and fulfilling life well into older age. What Hannah is talking about here is not the kind of exercise I did at Hooke: measuring and maintaining a healthy VO2 max, doing Zone 2 work (see page 295), or resistance training to maintain muscle mass. It's about specific movement patterns that unlock myriad health benefits in terms of healthspan and longevity.

They're what we all need to do, every day, simply to ensure that we can go on doing them. I don't count my regular walking, stretching and rebounding as part of my exercise regime; they are simply essential to keep the Bradbury wheels oiled. These other ranges of motion come under the same heading. In time they'll allow me to get up off the floor, climb steep stairs and give my grandchildren piggy-backs (if I am lucky enough to have any).

Hannah Beadle – moving to make life easier

Hannah: Your body is the vessel through which you experience every element of life and the world around you. The limits of your body will set the limits of your life in all respects: mentally, physically and emotionally. As human beings, we are adaptive organisms. Our bodies listen. For better or for worse, the way in which we move (or don't) every day is what gives us our potential and sets our limits.

The positions below are a self-check-in, highlighting the key patterns we need in order to lead a free and functioning life. If these ranges are limited, we'll notice the knock-on effects. Our knees will start to hurt, our back begin to ache, and moving about will become just that little bit more difficult. Practising these positions regularly and making them part of your daily routine, on the other hand, will give your body positive stimuli to which it can adapt, bringing forth forgotten ranges of motion while reinforcing and strengthening the ones you already have.

Being able to do these things is going to make ageing easier.

Hannah's tests

(The tests are the property of Wildfitness Ltd.)

Scoring

1 How to score your movement: each movement is scored on a scale of 0 to 5.
2 A score of 0 indicates pain and an inability to complete the movement to the basic level. The top end of the scale represents the movement being done perfectly, and it lets you know that you're ready to progress further, as discussed at the end of this chapter. In the case of movements that require a score on both sides of your body, take note of

each, but unless you have a specific injury, use the lower of the two scores as your true mark.

3 You will find it easier to visualise the positions if you check the accompanying illustrations and read the score chart before you begin each one. You may also find it best to have props such as yoga blocks, a pillow, and a rolled-up blanket or towel to hand too.

The movements: bend it like Bradbury

Knee to wall

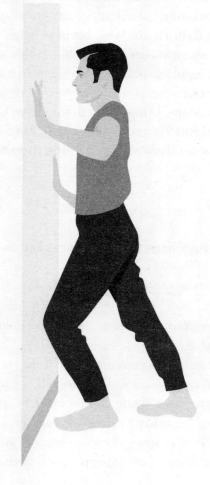

1 Knee to wall

Stand close to a wall, with one foot against it, as illustrated, and your hands on the wall. Now tap your knee against the wall.

What does this assess? Ankle flexion.

What are you looking for? How far away is your foot when you tap your knee to the wall?

Your everyday benefit Being part of your base, ankle flexion is involved to a certain extent whenever your foot moves, whether that's walking, going down a flight of stairs or bending over to pick something up.

Coaching points:
1 Test one side at a time.
2 Shoes off.
3 Knee tracking over the toes.
4 No heel elevation – the last point before your heel lifts is your score.

Scores for knee to wall

0	Pain
1	Toes touching the wall, knee touching the wall
2	Toes 2.5cm (1in) from the wall, knee touching the wall
3	Toes 5cm (2in) from the wall, knee touching the wall
4	Toes 7.5cm (3in) from the wall, knee touching the wall
5	Toes 10cm (4in) from the wall, knee touching the wall – no asymmetries present (both sides are balanced)

Kneeling toe test (parts I and II)

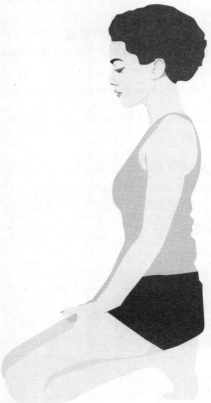

2 Kneeling toe test (part I)

Kneel as the illustration, with your toes tucked underneath your bottom and your knees on the floor.

What does this assess? Knee flexion.

What are you looking for? Can you sit comfortably with your bottom on your heels in this kneeling position?

Your everyday benefit From going up and down stairs to lifting, gardening, driving, sitting down, standing back up, putting your shoes on, or bending to put your dinner in the oven, the simplest of tasks will be affected if your knee flexion is limited.

Coaching points:

1 Consider your knee flexion, and support yourself with yoga blocks, a stack of books or any hard/stable surface under your hands if needed.

2 You should be completely comfortable with your bottom resting on your heels and able to sit there for a few minutes without pain.

3 Ensure your knees, feet and heels are together.

Scores for kneeling toe test (part I)

0	Pain
1	Knees becoming immovable early after beginning knee flexion
2	Large pillow or two required as prop between the bottom and heels
3	Small pillow/towel required as prop between the bottom and heels
4	Bottom to heels with some sign of discomfort, or no sign of discomfort but a small gap still present
5	Bottom to heels, no daylight, no signs of discomfort at all – no asymmetries present (both sides are balanced)

3 Kneeling toe test (part II)

Kneel as the illustration for part I, with your toes tucked underneath your bottom and your knees on the floor.

What does this assess? Big toe flexion.

What are you looking for? What is the angle in the big toes when sitting in a toes-tucked-under kneeling position?

Your everyday benefit Did you know that most of the control in the foot comes from big toe flexion? If your big toe does not flex, your gait and balance will be compromised. You may also experience pain in the foot itself and further up your body.

Coaching points:

1 To ensure that you have no knee pain, which might limit the test, ensure that you have props to hand as in the previous test (yoga blocks, a stack of books or anything hard/stable).

2 You should be completely comfortable with the ball of your foot resting on the floor.

3 Keep your torso upright.

Scores for kneeling toe test (part II)

0	Pain
1	Big toe almost completely straight/unable to bend
2	Large pillow or two required as prop between the bottom and heels
3	Small pillow/towel required as prop between the bottom and heels
4	Ball of foot to floor but some sign of discomfort/no sign of discomfort but small gap between bottom and heel (with no prop)
5	Foot at full 90 degrees, weight on ball of foot pressing into the floor, no sign of discomfort – no asymmetries present (both sides are balanced)

Kneeling ankle test

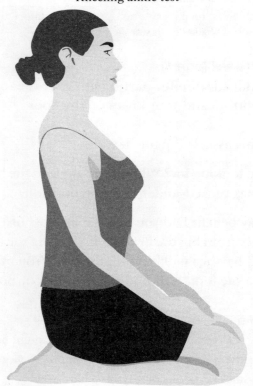

4 Kneeling ankle test

Kneel, this time with your foot flat, as the illustration.

What does this assess? Ankle flexion.

What are you looking for? Can you sit comfortably with your bottom on your heels in a toes-pointed kneeling position?

Your everyday benefit Stability, balance, walking, running and jumping.

Coaching points:

1 Check your knees, and grab yoga blocks or a cushion/ large pillow, a small pillow or a towel to put between your bottom and your heels if you need one, as per tests 2 and 3.
2 Aim to be completely comfortable with the top of your foot resting on the floor – there should not be daylight between them.
3 Ensure your feet are straight and your heels are not flopping out to the sides.

Scores for kneeling ankle test

0	Pain
1	Ankle extremely rigid and struggling to flex
2	Large pillow or two required as prop between the bottom and heels
3	Small pillow/towel required as prop between the bottom and heels
4	Top of foot to floor, but some sign of discomfort/no sign of discomfort but a small gap between top of foot and floor
5	Top of the foot to the floor no sign of discomfort – no asymmetries present (both sides are balanced)

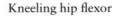

Kneeling hip flexor

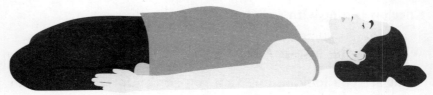

5 Kneeling hip flexor

From a toes-pointed kneeling position, how close can you get your shoulders to the floor when leaning back? See the illustration, and go very gently and carefully, as detailed below.

What does this assess? Hip extension

What are you looking for? Go gently and carefully with this one – it requires a fair amount of flexibility, so take it easy until you find your natural limit. You can put your hands behind you and use them for support, working your way down on to your elbows, if you can get that far. If this sounds a little complicated, look at the scoring chart and the illustration now, and you'll see what's wanted. The ultimate goal is to be lying on the floor, face up, with your legs tucked under you at the knees, and your arms resting comfortably by your sides. You can use props for your hands, but don't use anything to help your knees. If you can't kneel without pain or significant limitation, then your score is a 0 and the advice would be to not attempt this particular position for now.

Your everyday benefit Did you know that the hips hold emotion and stress? For most of us our hip flexors are chronically tight due to a modern lifestyle that asks us to sit at 90 degrees for large amounts of the day. Working on your hip extension will help with posture, efficient gait mechanics and, perhaps most notable of all as we age, it will help to relieve lower back pain. And that's huge for a lot of people. Imagine if you could alleviate it by starting work on your hips right now.

Coaching points:

1 Look for complete comfort with your head and shoulders resting on the floor, but more importantly, your hip line should be as close to straight as possible with no large curve in your back.

2 If necessary, straighten one leg to assess one side at a time and check for asymmetries.

3 Focus more on spine angle and alignment than the position of your hands and arms.

4 Keep your knees together. If you can't stop your knees splaying out to the side, then the last point at which they are still together is your score.

5 If there is shoulder restriction preventing your hands/ elbows from being placed behind you for support, you'll need props to discover your score. (See the score table for details.)

6 At every level, ensure that your knees are not rising off the floor. When they start to come up, this indicates that you have reached your limit in your range of motion and your score is wherever you were before your knees lifted.

7 Remember not to use any props for your knees on this one.

Scores for kneeling hip flexor

0	Pain
1	Barely able to lean back at all/go back past upright
2	Hands on floor behind to help support
3	Hands on floor comfortable but not able to reach elbows yet
4	Elbows resting on floor
5	Head and shoulders resting on floor, but more importantly, hip line as close to straight, no large curve – no asymmetries present (both sides are balanced)

Crossed-legs test

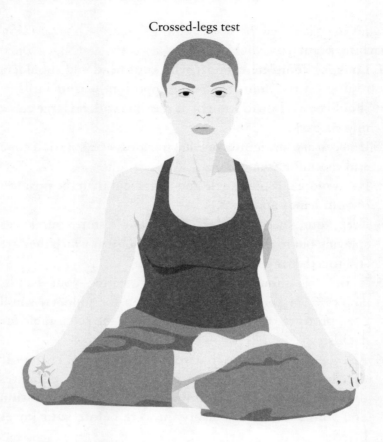

6 Crossed-legs test

Can you sit on the floor with your legs crossed? Now see below
to obtain the position in the illustration.

What does this assess? Hip rotation

What are you looking for? How close are your knees to the floor
in a cross-legged seating position? You'll see the final pose is
often referred to as a 'quarter lotus'. This is where you cross
your legs and then bring one foot onto the opposite thigh, while
the other rests comfortably under the opposite leg.

Your everyday benefit Sitting on the floor in a cross-legged
position (or any other position) should be part of your

everyday activity. (See the box at the end of this chapter to find out why.) When you sit cross-legged, you're helping to keep your hips mobile, which will guard against hip and lower back pain.

Coaching points:
1 Test both sides by changing which leg is on top.
2 Ensure your back is straight and not rounded.

Scores for crossed-legs test

0	Pain
1	Barely able to sit in position. Having to hold on to legs to keep up
2	Knees up high, no sign of comfort in position
3	Fist can be placed in the gap between floor and knee, some degree of ability to sit there for a short while
4	Both knees close to floor either straight away or within a few minutes of sitting
5	Quarter lotus pose – no asymmetries present (both sides are balanced)

Reverse table top (parts I and II)

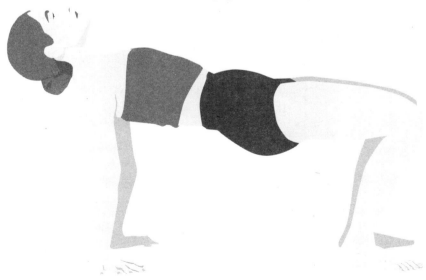

7 Reverse table top (part I)

Can you raise yourself into a table-top position as in the illustration?

What does this assess? Wrist flexion

What are you looking for? In a reverse table-top position, how close to 90 degrees is the bend in your wrists; that is, the angle between your flat hand, fingers pointing towards your toes, and your straight arm? (See the illustration for guidance.)

Your everyday benefit Modern life doesn't ask us to bear much weight through our hands, so we can start to suffer with sore wrists as we age. Wrist flexion comes into play in many daily activities: brushing your teeth, eating, driving, writing, playing sports, and even typing this chapter. Wrist flexion is also important for things that involve bearing weight, for example getting up from the floor or a chair and carrying heavy shopping.

Coaching points:
1 Look for your wrist to reach 90 degrees with no discomfort.
2 Be careful not to over-stretch or shift your weight too far forward. If it hurts, or there is any discomfort in the wrist, make sure that you have not gone past 90 degrees and shift back if need be.

Scores for reverse table top (part I)

0	Pain
1	Wrist barely able to bend
2	0–45 degrees
3	45 degrees onwards
4	Wrist just short of 90 degrees
5	Wrist comfortably at 90 degrees and able to hold body weight in this position – no asymmetries present (both sides are balanced)

8 Reverse table top (part II)

Take the reverse table-top position as part I above and see below for details of how to retract your shoulder blades.

What does this assess? Shoulder extension

What are you looking for? In a reverse table-top position (have a look at the illustration for guidance), can you fully and comfortably retract your shoulder blades to hold this pose? (That means squeezing both blades together and pulling them in towards your spine. By the way, each blade is known as a scapula, together they are scapulae.) Your ultimate aim is to have an angle of 90 degrees in your armpit area; that is, between your straight arm and your flat back with raised hips and a straight line from your knees to the crown of your head.

Your everyday benefit Shoulder extension will be used specifically in daily movements that involve reaching your arm down and behind you. But your shoulder also has multiple planes of motion, so to function fully in everyday life (reaching, lifting, carrying and stretching) it also needs to have a full range.

Coaching points:
1 Check and address your wrist flexion first (using test 7) to ensure that any issues with your wrists do not detract from testing your shoulders.
2 Look for complete comfort with your hips up, and holding a straight line along your body from your knee to the crown of your head.
3 Have your hands with your fingers facing your feet.

Scores for reverse table top (part II)

0	Pain
1	Hips from just off the floor to ankle height. Able to hold for just a few seconds

2	Hips from just off the floor to ankle height. Able to comfortably hold
3	Hips mid-shin height. Able to hold comfortably
4	Hips in line with shoulders (fully extended), 90 degrees in shoulder. Able to hold comfortably, but not yet able to retract scapula (some asymmetries may be present)
5	Scapula retracted, 90 degrees in shoulder, hips fully in line with shoulders – no asymmetries present (both sides are balanced)

Overhead range

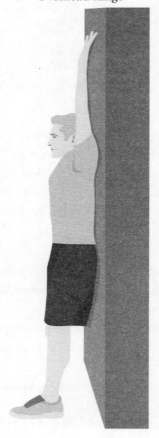

9 Overhead range

Stand a foot's length away from a wall, then raise your arms as described below and in the illustration.

What does this assess? Overhead range, lats (*Latissimus dorsi*, the large fan-shaped muscles in your mid and lower back – your wings) and scapula function.

What are you looking for? How far can you raise your arms so that your hands are touching, or nearly touching, the wall above your head?

Your everyday benefit Life has become more convenient, requiring much less reaching and stretching (especially overhead), which means a lot of us are losing our overhead range. A loss of overhead range will affect movements such as taking something from an upper shelf, putting on/taking off a jumper, and even some sports (your tennis serve, for example).

Coaching points:
1. To set up, place the heel of your left foot against the wall. Then line the heel of your right foot up with the toes of your left. Now bring the left foot forward so that they match. Lean back against the wall.
2. Keep your elbows straight.
3. Raise your arms directly in front of you, not out to the side.
4. Be conscious of your back position. As soon as your back starts to curve, you have reached your limit. The last point before curvature appears is your true score.

Scores for overhead range

0	Pain
1	Arms at 45 degrees
2	Arms between 45 degrees and temple
3	Arms to ear
4	Knuckles to wall
5	Hands to wall with external rotation (i.e. back of hands to wall)

Use it or lose it, Hannah explains

You've heard the adage 'use it or lose it': a scenario that is increasingly true in our lives today. As the modern world eliminates the need for certain movements, our bodies adapt, losing patterns that are no longer needed for daily life. Take the resting squat position for example (that low, heels-down easy squat you associate particularly with people in Asia and Africa). Since the development of chairs, toilets, car seats, sofas and anything else that stops our hips and knees at 90 degrees, the majority of Westerners have lost the ability to achieve this comfortable, deep squat. Our ankles, knees and hips have become tighter and more limited in range, and our lower backs ache, simply because life no longer asks us to go beyond 90 degrees and use the full intended range of our joints.

Each of the positions above have been chosen because they cover the ranges of motion we use going about the ordinary business of living. The extent to which you can access these ranges will be the extent of the freedom you have to navigate life and the challenges it throws at you. The ranges must be used as often as possible, so that we don't lose them, along with our physical capacity for meeting challenges as we age.

These positions are particularly important when we are looking to embark on a journey of new physical challenge through exercise. Some bodies are simply not ready to take on the rigours of mainstream fitness training, which means that jumping in at the deep end has as much potential to be detrimental as it does to be helpful.

In other words, consider these movements as the start line and not a final target. Going through them regularly as part of your morning routine or as a warm-up to an exercise session will allow you to see where your body is on any given day, or at any given time, highlighting where your attention should lie.

Think of it like this: if you want to improve the speed and performance of your car, what would you do first, add a turbo or just take the handbrake off? If you struggle with these positions, you're effectively going around with your handbrake on. Although you can still move, your brakes and wheels won't last long, and your freedom will be limited.

What your scores indicate

Use the table below as a guide to the meaning of your scores. Keep in mind that human beings are vastly different, so this table is very much a guideline. Some people may never score all 5s because of injuries or disabilities, and that is OK.

The meaning of your scores

Your score	A brief summary of where next
0 and 1	If your scores are at this level, you need to focus on the position and pattern in question. When our scores are here, the dysfunction will be having a negative effect on our lives, whether we realise it or not. Strip your movement back to the basics and take a minute to ask yourself about your everyday habits. As a priority, start to understand why your scores are like this. Is there an injury that you know about or an underlying dysfunction that has not been highlighted until now? Either way, focus your attention on the position and pattern at fault and spend more time there to help improve. (Here we would not be looking to load these positions or patterns with external weight.)
2, 3 and 4	Working on the individual positions and patterns is still needed with these scores, particularly if you are scoring at the lower end. At this stage, however, your body should be more open and able to take on bigger challenges through increased complexity of movement, range or load. Be aware that your body may end up compensating in ways that you don't want. If this happens, don't be afraid to return to the 0–1 basics.
Consistent 5s across the board	Your body is ready for greater challenges. Be mindful, however, that scoring all 5s only shows that you can achieve these ranges of movement. Before progressing, you need to ensure that you have the ability to tackle a greater challenge – and to do it without restraint or dysfunction.

Are you sitting comfortably? Now stand up

More from Hannah on the exercises:

Reading through the positions in this chapter have you noticed that seven out of the nine involve sitting on the ground either throughout or, in the case of the table top, at the beginning? A coincidence, you might think – well, not quite.

You see, your ability to sit on the floor, the amount of time you spend there and your ability to get back up again, are all directly related to your longevity. Societies that eat, socialise and rest on the floor (such as in Japan) tend to live longer than those who don't (in the UK and the USA, for example).

Sitting on the floor reverses the effects of all the chair sitting that we do. It stretches and mobilises our bodies and stimulates our brains, keeping them alert with varying patterns of movement. Perhaps the most important benefit is how we make ourselves stronger *simply by standing up*. This develops new neural pathways (think of it as a mini puzzle for your brain) and builds confidence in the knowledge that if we fall over at any point, we can get up safely and efficiently.

This will one day prove invaluable, since the damage done by a fall in old age is often not about the tumble itself but the fact that you get stuck down there.

Beneficial as it would be to sell all our furniture and adopt a floor-based lifestyle, it's not a realistic solution if you live in Europe or America where the majority of life is spent sitting at 90 degrees. What you can do, however, is incorporate floor sitting into your day by making the movement patterns above a part of your normal routine. Try sitting cross-legged or kneeling to rest, eat or socialise. Perhaps even to work.

Go ahead and channel your inner child! Get on the floor more, move around and switch it up. Move wild to live free, and longer.

Aaron Parsley's dynamic duo

. . . or why your grip gives your health a leg up.

Did you know that you can tell a lot about someone's likely healthspan and longevity by their grip? Aaron Parsley (the brilliant trainer at Hooke) does, and he even has a gizmo to take precise measurements.

Along with leg strength, grip is a huge predictor of how well we will be in older age. I asked Aaron to share the science here because, crucially, both of those things are trainable: you can improve them, or at least reduce their rate of decline over time.

Aaron Parsley talks about muscular strength

Aaron: A 2018 paper analysing data from approximately two million men and women found that muscular strength is a predictor of all-cause mortality in an apparently healthy population.[1] Given that strength is both easily measured and trainable, could this Herculean quality, so revered by the ancient Greeks, be an elixir for a longer life?

As it turns out, the answer is not that simple. Strength itself does not cause a longer life, but frailty and sarcopenia (age-related muscle loss) are linked to higher rates of cardiovascular disease, along with other major determinants of all-cause mortality, such as diabetes, Alzheimer's disease, and cancer.[2]

Within the scientific community, two particular measures – leg strength and grip strength – have revealed some especially compelling findings. A meta-analysis published in the *Archives of Physical Medicine and Rehabilitation* found that greater knee extension strength reduced the risk of mortality by 14 per cent, with further studies highlighting the equal importance of hamstring and gluteal strength.[3]

What explains these findings, and how does it work?

The quadriceps, hamstrings and gluteal muscles are all essential for mobility. The more muscle mass we maintain as we age, the more mobile we remain, the brisker our walking pace, the better we can climb stairs, the more efficiently we burn fat, and the stronger our heart and lungs become. Losing these abilities leads to the deterioration of our cardiovascular system and overall health.

The same principles apply to grip strength. Grip is a simple yet effective measure of overall strength and has been shown to be another useful predictor of mortality.[4] Studies have found that weaker grip strength is associated with functional decline and an increased risk of all-cause mortality, whereas those with higher grip strength in midlife are significantly less likely to experience disabilities in old age.

Again, this is correlation, not causation – it's not as though you could sit at a desk all day with a hand gripper and expect to live past 100. The key point is that those with stronger grip strength tend to have more muscle mass, greater functional independence, and a more physically active lifestyle. This leads to better nervous-system function, improved metabolism, and enhanced cardiovascular health, while also lowering the risk of insulin resistance and type-2 diabetes.

In for the long run

As Hannah has explained to us, this chapter is about building a foundation for later life, ensuring that you can access fundamental patterns and everyday moves with ease and safety as we head for OUR golden years. This means having joints that can flex and turning them into a set of legs that lunge, jump, balance, bound and sprint at will; a pair of shoulders that can climb, swing, lift and carry; wrists that do what you need; and, yes, a back that doesn't hurt. It's about independence and freedom.

If this is not for you at present, but you're keen to try something else, please know that it's never too late, and perhaps check out Pilates classes near you for the over-sixties, or search online 'Pilates video for beginners' for a 45-minute session from the NHS.

Happy hacks

- **I have now installed a pull-up bar** across our son's bedroom doorway for the whole family to hang off to help with back stretching and to improve our grip strength. We have competitions to see who can hang on for the longest. So far, one of the ten-year-old twins is the runaway winner. I can manage one minute thirty-five seconds. Why don't you try to find somewhere you can safely do the same thing?
- **Never miss the chance to strengthen your legs** Climb stairs two at a time, power walk up a hill, do squats and lunges or a wall sit (slide down a wall into a seated position and stay there until your thighs are on fire).
- **Remember to squat**, crouch and sit on the floor – anything to get your legs past 90 degrees – as often possible.

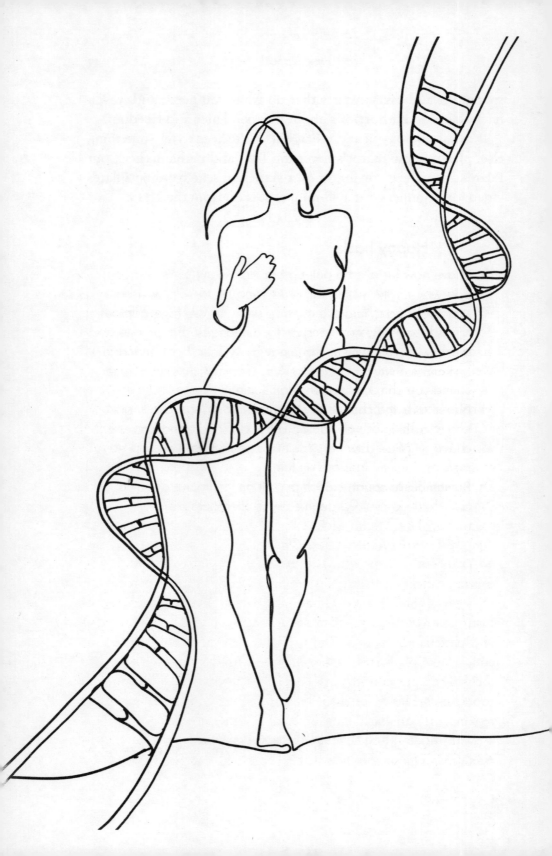

Chapter 15

Breast Cancer, Drugs and DNA

What if I told you that there was a way to find out which medications work for you, how stress might impact your physical and mental health, or even if you're likely to have fertility issues? Well, there is a way.

When I was diagnosed with breast cancer in 2021, I wanted to learn as much as possible, not just about cancer but also about health overall. Suddenly, healthspan became important to me, which led to *Hack Yourself Healthy*. I started diving into books and asking lots of questions. My curiosity steered me towards Dr Nasha Winters (and many other of the experts who have shared their knowledge with me in this book). She is the co-author *The Metabolic Approach to Cancer*, and *Mistletoe and the Future of Integrative Oncology*.

A cancer thriver herself (after being sent home to die with stage-4 ovarian cancer aged 19), Nasha has made integrative oncology her life's work. She is one of the founders of the Metabolic Terrain Institute of Health (a non-profit organisation focusing on research and patient access to integrative care) and Metabolic Regen (an educational platform), whose mission is to transform cancer care, focusing on prevention, personalised treatments and addressing the root causes. Her vision is to create a global whole-person approach to cancer treatment that becomes a standard of care.

Many doctors and health professionals have trained as Integrative Metabolic Oncology specialists – I've worked with one over Zoom based in South Africa, Dr Jen Levin. Now I'm working with Jo Gamble who you will read more about in this chapter.

I've got to know Nasha over four years; her opinions are controversial to some, and what follows are some of the topics we've covered while we've been discussing my case. **Please note, however, that what follows is not medical advice and it relates to my case only. I have included details so that you can get a first-person insight into what is involved and what the tests can show. If you are considering any tests yourself, please first consult with your doctor who is aware of your medical history and your current situation.**

Before we dive in, you need a little understanding of something called SNPs (single nucleotide polymorphisms). Think of them as the building blocks of our DNA. (See a full explanation in the Appendix, page 310, where you will find the Lifecode Gx DNA test I have taken too.) Personally, I think that getting your DNA tested is one of the best tests we can all do, because our DNA doesn't change – it is therefore a lifetime test. These fragments of DNA – SNPs – can subtly influence how your body works. Nasha started educating herself about SNPs in 2003 and began teaching others about them in 2009.

Even though I am talking about breast cancer specifically here, this conversation is about so much more than that. It demonstrates how a whole-person approach, taking into account personal history, testing and exploring the link between conditions can create a personalised effective treatment plan for many health problems. It gets technical, and you may want to skip parts, but I think there is a lot of valuable information tucked into these pages.

SNPs, breast cancer treatment and endometriosis – my conversation with Dr Nasha Winters

Julia: During one of our meetings you said to me, 'For you tamoxifen would do one of two things: not do very much at all, or actually cause problems in addition to the known side effects.'

Why wouldn't tamoxifen have worked for me?

Nasha: Firstly, they wouldn't have offered you tamoxifen, because you were post-menopausal; secondly, your (Lifecode Gx) DNA test revealed that you are what is known as a poor metaboliser (explained below); and thirdly, you've had endometriosis.

Tamoxifen (a medication used to treat certain types of breast cancer that works by blocking oestrogen) would have added insult to injury to a uterus that has already been overgrowing for years because of your history of endometriosis. You already have a vulnerability to hyperproliferative patterns in this part of your body. One of the things we have learned is that women should be screened for endometrial thickening before they are put on tamoxifen. We are told as patients that there is a 'slight' risk increase of endometrial hyperplasia – but it's not slight in my experience, and this can lead to endometrial cancer.

Endometriosis – still no fix?

Julia: Let's talk more about the treatment of endometriosis. Globally, an estimated 10 per cent of women of reproductive age (around 190 million women), are affected by it, and it still takes about eight years to diagnose.

Nasha: The inflammation caused by endometriosis can lead to an imbalance in the immune system, and women with endometriosis have a higher risk of developing an autoimmune disease. It is now recognised as more than just a hormonal or gynaecological condition. Instead, we need to understand its metabolic and immune-system involvement. Chronic inflammation, gut dysbiosis (an imbalance in the gut micro-organisms), and environmental toxin exposure play significant roles in its development and progression.

Rather than defaulting to symptom suppression with hormonal therapies or surgery alone, women should take a wider approach. You know that I'm going to talk about testing: comprehensive testing can help to identify immune dysfunction, any inflammatory markers, and metabolic imbalances that could be contributing to the endometriosis. Taking care of the gut and optimising microbiome health is key. Gut issues drive systemic inflammation, which can exacerbate symptoms. Stool-testing, microbiome support and personalised nutrition can be game-changers.

I'm a little slow . . .

(Relevant SNP: CYP2D6)

Julia: My DNA test showed that I'm a 'slow metaboliser' of tamoxifen – what does that mean and why should I care?

Nasha: Doctors can now assess how your body is likely to process tamoxifen. If you're a slow metaboliser like you, they might adjust your treatment plan and choose a different medication to ensure the best possible outcome. This is a perfect example of personalised medicine in action: tailoring treatment to your unique genetic terrain.

Tamoxifen works by blocking oestrogen's effect on cancer cells, but here's the catch: it's not fully active at the point when you take it; your body needs to convert tamoxifen into its more powerful form, called endoxifen, to make it work effectively. This conversion is done by an enzyme in your liver, which is produced by the CYP2D6 gene.

If there's a SNP (a small variation) in your CYP2D6 gene, it can change how well your body produces or uses this enzyme. People can fall into different groups:

- **Normal metabolisers,** who convert tamoxifen into endoxifen efficiently, so the treatment works as expected.
- **Poor metabolisers,** who have a less-active version of CYP2D6, so they produce much less endoxifen. This might reduce the effectiveness of tamoxifen.
- **Ultra-rapid metabolisers,** who convert tamoxifen very quickly, which might cause side effects or other unexpected responses.

For you, Julia, tamoxifen (if you weren't already post-menopausal) would do one of two things: not do very much at all or actually cause problems in addition to the known side effects. And another interesting discussion is that drugs such as SSRIs (selective serotonin reuptake inhibitors – a class of antidepressant) can also impact the response to drugs such as tamoxifen because they share the same drug detox pathway.

In the US, if you have particular SNPs, they give you endoxifen instead of tamoxifen, which doesn't use that same pathway – that's a rational choice, and woman should have that choice.

What's really cool is that there is even a new study about baby tamoxifen: a lower dose, taken from the standard dose of 20 to 25mg (milligrams) a day to 5mg a day. In fact, you could take 5mg every other day and get just as good a benefit. That's what I've been telling my patients to do for 20 years. Today, we have the evidence to support it.

Sad effects

Julia: Lots of women are put on SSRIs/antidepressants along with tamoxifen to help them to manage the emotional impact of a cancer diagnosis, so are you saying that they might be working against each other?

Nasha: Certain SSRIs block CYP2D6 activity. If you're already a poor metaboliser and then you take one of these SSRIs, the problem will get worse and your body might not activate tamoxifen effectively, thereby reducing its ability to prevent cancer recurrence.

Some SSRIs, such as citalopram (Celexa) or venlafaxine (Efexor), don't significantly inhibit CYP2D6. Choosing these alternatives ensures that the SSRI won't interfere with tamoxifen activation.

One more thing on cancer

(Relevant SNPs: ESR1 ESR2)

Julia: Before we move on, can similar testing be done if aromatase inhibitors are suggested?

Nasha: Aromatase inhibitors (AIs, for example: anastrozole, letrozole, exemestane) work by blocking the enzyme aromatase, which converts androgens (the hormones that trigger male characteristics) into oestrogen. This reduces oestrogen levels in the body, depriving oestrogen receptor-positive (ER+) breast cancer cells of the fuel that they need to grow. This would be your option as a post-menopausal woman with an oestrogen-positive cancer. (Folks with clotting history/disorders should not use these drugs, however, because there is a much higher risk of blood clots.)

We can check SNPs to test the suitability. We look at the ESR (oestrogen receptor) SNPs. It's called pharmacogenomics – the study of how a person's DNA affects their response to drugs.

Some SNPs are associated with higher oestrogen-receptor activity, potentially making AIs less effective (because even small amounts of oestrogen can continue to drive cancer growth). Other SNPs might reduce receptor sensitivity, which could enhance AI effectiveness.

SNPs in ESR1/ESR2 may also affect how women tolerate AIs, influencing risks such as bone loss, joint pain or cardiovascular changes. For example:

- ESR1 variations linked to bone density might worsen AI-induced osteoporosis.
- ESR2 SNPs affecting vascular function could exacerbate cardiovascular side effects.

ESR SNPs, for the most part, quite simply make AIs ineffective. Patients with ESR1 mutations often experience poorer outcomes and shorter progression-free survival (PFS) when treated with AIs. Therefore, detecting these mutations (you don't have any, by the way) can help guide treatment decisions and lead to the consideration of alternative therapies. These include selective oestrogen receptor degraders (SERDs) like fulvestrant or newer oral SERDs, or a combination of therapies involving endocrine agents and targeted therapies, such as CDK4/6 inhibitors.

Infertility and IVF

(Relevant SNP: CYB1B1)

Julia: I had four rounds of IVF, which gave me beautiful twin girls. Could that have been a driver of my breast cancer in your opinion?

Nasha: It certainly increased your risk. Your CYB1B1 SNP combined with a ton of others means that you were not the person designed to take exogenous hormones (hormones taken through medication, for example) because you weren't even processing your internal ones well.

Most women I work with have their beautiful children, but now they're afraid that they're not going to live to see their children grow up. You're good. You're clear of cancer, but do you know how many aren't? I want people to know that this data is life-changing and life-saving.

The effects of IVF

Julia: What else, with hindsight, could I have done to counteract the effects of IVF?

Nasha: We would have really adjusted your metabolomics (see below). We would have tested your liver, we would have worked on those things so that your body could process this and head things off at the pass.

Meta-whats?

Nasha: Metabolomics is like a snapshot of how your body is functioning at a microscopic level. It's the study of metabolites, which are tiny molecules produced when your body processes food, hormones and chemicals during normal metabolism. It's another route to help us understand how well your body is producing energy, balancing hormones, detoxifying harmful substances, managing inflammation, and responding to stress. You can use things like the DUTCH test to assess this (see Appendix).

Diet and lifestyle: the conductors of your metabolic symphony

The beauty of metabolomics is that it shows us how diet and lifestyle choices directly impact your metabolic and hormonal health. Here's how you can fine-tune the symphony:

1 **Eat nutrient-dense foods** A diet rich in whole foods such as vegetables, fruits, healthy fats and lean proteins provides the raw materials your body needs to create energy and to balance hormones. It's possible to manage aromatase levels and the reabsorption of harmful 4-OH oestrogens on your own by incorporating plenty of foods rich in phytoestrogens, such as cruciferous vegetables, broccoli, cabbage, brussels sprouts and berries. These compounds have been shown to inhibit aromatase activity and lower oestrogen production in the body.

2 **Support detoxification**
   - Include cruciferous vegetables (such as broccoli and kale) to help detoxify harmful hormone metabolites. Eating plenty of fibre can also enhance oestrogen detoxification. This shift promotes a healthier oestrogen balance and reduces the risk of DNA damage, oxidative stress and cancer progression.
   - Drink plenty of water to flush out waste products.

3 **Balance blood sugar** Focus on low-glycemic foods such as berries, greens and nuts to keep insulin (a key hormone) steady and to reduce inflammation.

4 **Prioritise gut health**
   - A healthy gut microbiome helps metabolise hormones and eliminates excess oestrogen through the digestive system.
   - Add probiotics, prebiotics and fibre to your diet.

5 **Get quality sleep** Sleep restores hormonal balance and allows your body to repair metabolic pathways.

6 **Manage stress** Chronic stress disrupts hormonal and metabolic harmony. Incorporate mindfulness, yoga, or other relaxation techniques, to calm the system.

7 **Move your body** Exercise improves insulin sensitivity, supports hormone balance and reduces toxic metabolites.

In short, metabolomics helps us to understand how our body is performing, and simple, intentional changes in your diet and lifestyle can fine-tune your metabolic and hormonal health, creating a symphony of energy, balance and vitality.

Nasha enlarges on IVF – injected with hope

Julia: How can women protect themselves during IVF?

Nasha: It's important to make sure that the organs of elimination (the kidneys, lungs, liver, skin and large intestine) are functioning efficiently. Ensure the liver is performing well by doing the hormone metabolite test (DUTCH test, see Appendix) to show how your hormones are being metabolised, so that you're not pushing a pedal in the wrong direction.

If a woman has a strong family history of cancer or a personal history of cancer, I would strongly encourage against IVF and would suggest choosing a different route.

This is a heavy and intense conversation, but also an ethical one; people need to be aware of it. Julia, you have a good story and these two beautiful girls, plus you have your health. But, as I said earlier, most of the people I have this conversation with don't enjoy the same positive outcome. And that is really hard.

Do IVF and HRT cause cancer?

(Relevant SNPs: COMT, GSTP1/GSTM1, VDR, CYP1B1, CYP1A1)

Nasha: When you have the SNPs above, which you do, Julia, it can impair your body's ability to process and eliminate hormones safely, potentially increasing the risk of carcinogenesis through the accumulation of toxic hormone metabolites or oxidative stress.

Rather than jumping into hormone therapies (including HRT and IVF) without understanding your genetic terrain, focus on modulating and supporting your hormonal health through diet and lifestyle. Strategies such as optimising liver detoxification, supporting methylation pathways (see box

below for an explanation of methylation), reducing
inflammation, balancing blood sugar, and managing stress
can naturally enhance hormone metabolism and reduce
risks. By testing your SNPs, you can have a proactive way to
tailor your approach to hormonal health, avoiding potential
harm and fostering a more balanced, resilient system.

Methylation

Methylation is a biochemical process that takes place more than a
billion times a second in every cell of the body. It's a bit like putting
a stamp on a letter: a tiny chemical group – a methyl group – is
added to your DNA, proteins or other molecules. This simple act
changes how your body reads instructions. It's not rewriting your
genes; it's changing how loudly (or quietly) they are read.

Methylation is at the heart of so many vital things. It helps your
body to process nutrients and vitamins, especially B vitamins
such as B12, B6 and folate (you might have heard of meythl B
vitamins, perhaps). These nutrients are methyl donors: they hand
over those little methyl stamps so that your body can keep running
smoothly.

Every time your body wants to build brain chemicals, detox
harmful substances, or even create energy, it needs methylation.
It's involved in: detoxing your liver, balancing your mood and
brain function, healthy growth during pregnancy, switching
genes on and off (without changing the DNA itself), creating
new cells and repairing damage.

If methylation isn't working properly – perhaps you're low in
folate or B12, for example – you might feel tired, foggy or low
in mood. Over time, poor methylation has even been linked to
conditions such as heart disease or cognitive decline.

You're not saying that HRT or IVF causes cancer?

Nasha: No. To be clear – our endogenous hormones do not *cause* cancer. It is when they are *out of balance* that the terrain becomes vulnerable. Exogenous supplementation (such as HRT and IVF hormones), however, can be playing with fire, especially if there is already an internal imbalance at play. Today, we are swimming in a pool of endocrine disruptors (plastics, pesticides, cleaning products, birth-control medication) and that is adding complicated and confusing messages to our hormone receptors, making us more out of balance and more vulnerable than ever.

We didn't know this in the 1970s. We didn't know this when we started using IVF, and we didn't know that when we started pumping women with HRT how it would impact them individually, but now we do, and the data is compelling.

Why do you think that I needed IVF?

(Relevant SNPs: MTHFR)

Nasha: Well, in addition to everything above, you have the MTHFR mutation (which stands for methylenetetrahydro-folate reductase. It's known as the Mother F***er gene!) This gene is responsible for the production of the MTHFR enzyme, and a mutation causes a reduction in the production of the MTHFR enzyme. In your case, Julia, you have a 70 per cent reduction in the production of the enzyme because you're homozygous (there are two mutations).

It's complicated, but with a poorly functioning MTHFR enzyme, the body cannot efficiently convert folate into its active form (5-MTHF). Active folate is crucial for DNA production and repair, which are necessary for egg and sperm health, proper embryo development, and its implantation in the uterus. Poor MTHFR function can lead to elevated homocysteine levels (homocysteine is a building block of protein, but elevated levels lead to ill-health), which can impair blood flow to reproductive organs, negatively affecting egg quality, ovulation and health of the uterine lining. There's an increased risk of miscarriage due to poor implantation or inadequate blood supply to the placenta and this creates oxidative stress and inflammation, damaging reproductive cells.

Julia: It sounds hopeless.

Nasha: Infertility is a symptom of a root pattern; it is an *expression* of the problem; *not* the problem itself. In my 17 years of private practice, if I get a woman's insulin under control, with cortisol modulated, oxytocin levels up and optimised D3, she will get pregnant or rid herself of her PMS and peri/post-menopause issues. We have focused on their terrain; we never needed exogenous hormone input. I have a best friend who has MTHFR mutations and also had fertility issues – we worked on her, and within three months she conceived after six years of previously trying. She now has two children.

How to address MTHFR-related infertility

(As stated previously, this is Nasha's recommendation to me and does not represent advice to others. If you wish to look into this subject for your own health, please consult your own doctor.)

1 Supplementation
  - Use active folate forms such as 5-MTHF (instead of synthetic folic acid) to bypass the MTHFR enzyme and ensure sufficient folate levels.
  - Include methylated forms of vitamin B12 (methylcobalamin) and B6 to support methylation and homocysteine metabolism.

2 **Dietary support**
- Eat folate-rich foods such as leafy greens, avocados and lentils.
- Avoid fortified foods with synthetic folic acid, which can build up and block active folate in people with MTHFR mutations.

3 **Lower homocysteine** Ensure adequate intake of nutrients such as magnesium, zinc and choline, which support homocysteine metabolism.

4 **Improve detoxification** Support liver health with antioxidants (such as glutathione, NAC) and avoid environmental toxins – for example, BPA, pesticides).

5 **Stress and lifestyle management** Chronic stress and poor lifestyle habits exacerbate methylation issues. Practices such as mindfulness, adequate sleep and regular exercise help to optimise overall reproductive health.

The bottom line

Poor MTHFR function affects fertility by disrupting folate metabolism, increasing homocysteine levels and impairing DNA repair, hormonal balance and detoxification. By identifying MTHFR mutations and addressing these pathways through diet, lifestyle and supplementation, couples can significantly improve their chances of conceiving and sustaining a healthy pregnancy.

Natural-born stressor

(Relevant SNPs: ADRB2 SNP, COMT)

Julia: I'm obviously a big advocate for nature as a healing source, I write about the science behind it, I live and breathe it, but the SNP science agrees doesn't it?

Nasha: You, Julia, are literally wired for stress! It can be your drive, but people with this SNP never turn off the stress, and they end up having heart attacks. You take stress right to the heart, so checking your stress response, managing your sleep cycle and circadian rhythm alongside light exposure are really important for you.

That's why walking in nature is so good: that's your antidepressant, alongside your breathwork and meditation.

You also have a slow COMT SNP, which means that your body is slower at clearing stress-related hormones, making you more reactive and sensitive to stress. This can enhance creativity, focus and drive, but it also makes stress-management essential. By balancing your lifestyle, diet and environment (which you're working hard on), you can help your body to process stress more effectively and build resilience.

Support this with magnesium and vitamin C. Magnesium is critical because you have an increased need to assist oestrogen detoxification. You're also not going to be good at processing caffeine, quercetin, green tea or wine, so it's a good job that you no longer drink alcohol! Don't have beta blockers any time soon, either, and work on calming that overzealous brain. You're a researcher and an over-thinker – always revving that sympathetic overdrive – and you might have some mood issues. Does this sound like you?!

Note: please remember that this advice is tailored for me and it won't be relevant for others. I have included these descriptions so that you can see how each individual differs in their needs for supplementation, for example, although the general advice about exercise, diet and finding ways to relax are essential for everyone to maintain good health, plus you can see that a tailored supplement regime can have huge benefits for the individual.

The menopause: how to benefit from the metabolic-approach way

Nasha lists below her tips for bone, heart and brain health:

As we transition through peri-menopause, the menopause and then post-menopause, supporting our bones, heart and brain isn't about replacing hormones but optimising our metabolic health and terrain. Rather than relying on bioidentical or conventional hormone-replacement therapy (bHRT/HRT), I focus on restoring cellular resilience through lifestyle, nutrition and targeted therapies.

- **Bone health** Strength training and eating adequate protein and essential nutrients (such as vitamins D3, K2, magnesium and boron) supports bone remodelling. Pairing this with metabolic strategies, such as therapeutic ketosis and fasting, enhances mitochondrial efficiency, reducing oxidative stress on the bone cells. (There are many books available that explain the benefits of therapeutic ketosis and fasting – I suggest you buy Nasha's, see page 251, if you would like to dig deeper.)
- **Heart health** Blood sugar regulation is the key to heart health. Avoiding insulin resistance through cyclical fasting (as mentioned above), low-glycemic nutrition and omega-3-rich fats (see Chapter 1) helps to maintain arterial flexibility and lowers inflammation. Stress management and circadian alignment also regulate blood pressure and cardiovascular function.
- **Brain health** The brain thrives on ketones (used for energy by the body). Implementing metabolic flexibility, prioritising sleep, and engaging in neuroprotective strategies such as cold therapy, sauna and mindfulness, all enhance cognitive function and neuroplasticity, reducing the risk of dementia.

Dr Mindy Pelz's approach (*The Menopause Reset* and *Fast Like a Girl*) deeply resonates with me, and aligns beautifully with my work on metabolic health and terrain-based healing. My podcast, Metabolic Matters, and my books, offer a deep dive into optimising health beyond just menopause – addressing longevity, cancer prevention, and whole-body resilience.

Eyes and sleep

(Relevant SNP: SNP [CTH])

Julia: Why do I need reading specs and my phone torch to read labels at night now?!

Nasha: This SNP is your glutathione pathway and it plays a crucial role in eye health. The CTH enzyme contributes to the production of glutathione, which is your body's master antioxidant. Glutathione is especially important in the lens, retina and cornea to protect these tissues from oxidative damage caused by light exposure, ageing and environmental toxins. Keep on taking the vitamin E.

Sleep it off

(Relevant SNP: MTNR1B)

Julia: Sleep is such a big topic for so many people. I've been working hard on paying more attention to sleep and trying to improve the quality and duration of my sleep.

Nasha: (You have only just realised this – after almost 30 years of not giving it much attention at all!) The MTNR1B gene encodes for the melatonin receptor 1B. Your circadian rhythm, Julia, really needs to be dialled in. Time-restricted eating (no late-night snacking), light exposure, reducing exposure to EMFs (electromagnetic fields emitted from various sources, from power lines and Wi-Fi routers to microwaves and mobile phones), all these things should be prioritised by you. This gene is linked to longevity, or a lack thereof.

Melatonin's dual role as a natural SERM (selective oestrogen receptor modulator, such as tamoxifen and raloxifene, which are both used to treat breast cancer in different ways) and AI (aromatase inhibitors, as explained on page 256) makes it a valuable tool in preventing and managing hormone-driven cancers. Its ability to block oestrogen receptors, reduce oestrogen production, and provide antioxidant and anti-inflammatory effects, positions melatonin as a holistic and integrative cancer therapy.

You might consider daily dosing of 20+mg melatonin at bedtime. I personally take between 60mg and 180mg for its therapeutic effects, depending on my schedule/travel/stress levels.

Look up Dr Shallenberger and Dr Russel Reiter and Doris Loh, who are big on melatonin. Your personal anti-cancer strategy, Julia, would be to take 150–180mg of melatonin every night.

Melatonin, of course, isn't available easily in the UK, so you are going to stir up a hornet's nest.

Nasha: This is precisely the time to push back around the melatonin issue; it is such utter hogwash that this supplement is difficult to get, given that it is the most studied, second only to mistletoe, in oncology. To date, in PubMed there are over 3,700 studies on melatonin and cancer alone – and mostly are all favourable! Dr Russel Reiter is a world-renowned melatonin researcher (who's also on the staff at NASA). His research on melatonin protecting against radiation poisoning is vast. I would use this as an opportunity to question the rationale of keeping this from the UK public. It is used commonly around the globe. And there is no alternative.

There are studies showing melatonin as an alternative SERM dating back to 2008. Also, since 2006 it has had a role as an aromatase inhibitor as well as supporting AI side effects – especially the musculoskeletal side effects of these drugs. It should be available in the UK. (See also Sleepy Foods, that contain melatonin, in Chapter 6.)

Iron (wo)man

Nasha: Your genetics show you have the gene for familial hemochromatosis, which means your body is naturally inclined to absorb more iron from your diet than most people's. Normally, this can lead to iron overload and might require you to have iron removed through phlebotomy (like a blood donation) to keep levels safe.

However, in your case, you also carry an SNP (single nucleotide polymorphism) in the TFR2 gene, which is linked to an increased risk of iron-deficiency anaemia. This means that even though your body has the *potential* to absorb too much iron, your iron transport and regulation system is also genetically wired in a way that could make it harder to actually hold on to enough iron for healthy function.

In other words, it's as if your body has its foot on the gas *and* the brake at the same time when it comes to iron levels – one gene tells your body to absorb more, while another may interfere with how that iron is managed and stored. You have to keep a close eye on your iron levels, as too much or too little iron can be problematic.

Julia: My Hooke report showed that I have low transferrin saturation levels at 18 (normal range is 20–55). This means there is not enough iron available in the blood to bind to the transferrin protein, which is responsible for transporting iron throughout the body, and could add to fatigue or sleep issues. They are suggesting a daily iron spray, but you're not convinced this is right for me?

Nasha: Your body has a complex relationship with iron. Direct iron supplementation can push your system toward iron overload (like stepping on the gas pedal), and it doesn't address how well your body regulates and uses that iron.

Instead, I would suggest that lactoferrin or IP6 (inositol hexaphosphate) are more aligned with your needs. Lactoferrin (found in bovine colostrum), for example, helps mobilise *and* regulate iron in the body, rather than simply adding more fuel to the fire. IP6 acts as a natural iron chelator, helping to liberate stored iron from tissues and making it available for the body to use appropriately. In essence, these help your body balance iron.

Finally, while it is important to recognise that iron is crucial for healthy red blood cell production and oxygen transport, it can also act as a double-edged sword in the context of cancer. Cancer cells often have an increased demand for iron because they rely on it to fuel their rapid growth and proliferation.

Several studies have shown that excess iron in the body – whether from high dietary intake or supplementation – can contribute to tumour growth and metastasis by:

- Generating **reactive oxygen species** (**ROS**) through the Fenton reaction, which can cause DNA damage and support cancer progression.
- Upregulating **transferrin receptors** on cancer cells, increasing iron uptake and promoting proliferation.
- Altering the **tumour microenvironment**, fostering angiogenesis and inflammation that aid tumour survival and spread.

Because of this, I generally recommend avoiding routine iron supplementation in people with active cancer unless there is a clear, confirmed iron-deficiency anaemia – and even then, we approach it carefully, ideally by supporting the body's own iron regulation, as outlined above (e.g., with lactoferrin or IP6).

How to choose the most beneficial foods

Not all foods contain the same quantities of pesticide residues. An organisation called the Environmental Working Group in the US compiles a list that is updated each year of foods considered 'clean' or 'dirty' with regard to pesticide residues. (Note that this list relates to foods grown in the US, although it's relevant to the UK as well.)

The Clean 15 (produce with lower pesticide residues):
Avocado, sweetcorn, pineapple, onion, papaya, frozen peas, asparagus, honeydew melon, kiwi, cabbage, carrot, mushroom, watermelon, sweet potato and mango.

The Dirty Dozen (produce with higher pesticide residues):
Strawberry, spinach, kale, spring greens, peach, pear, nectarine, apple, grape, pepper, chilli, cherry, blueberry and green beans.

Should I go organic?

(Relevant SNP: PON1)

Julia: I try to follow the Dirty Dozen and the Clean 15 lists when I do my grocery shop, and buy organic where possible.

Nasha: You have a susceptibility to organophosphates, because of your particular mutation of this SNP, which protects against oxidative stress. That means you should try to avoid pesticides, because you have a reduced ability to detoxify certain toxins, particularly pesticides and other chemical residues found in non-organic foods.

Julia: Eating organic is expensive and not possible when I travel for work. I do, however, soak my veggies in vinegar for 20 minutes or use bicarbonate of soda to try to reduce the pesticide residues.

Nasha: You can also use what are known as 'binders' with fulvic or humic acid, or something with a little charcoal, or you can take oral vitamin C to flush out the system. If you tolerate glutathione, you could also take that. Other than that: sweat it out, move it out, flush it out, sauna. And be careful with the hair dye – the dark colours are the worst!

Julia: I use a water-based organic dye that doesn't have PPD in it and has ingredients that are gentle enough for people to use during chemo. (PPD – paraphenylenediamine – is an oxidiser used in dark hair dyes and dark clothing dyes. A build-up in the body caused by frequent hair dyeing with dark colours – and always wearing black – can be dangerous, causing a range of serious allergic reactions.) My hairdresser also uses this great detox powder, which contains asorbic acid, after each session to close off the hair follicles and stop the colouring after the application. I use it on my girls when they've been swimming in chlorine too.

Nasha: Foods such as watercress, broccoli sprouts, and supplementing with sodium selenite would be really good ongoing tools to help you detoxify, because of your SNPs. If you have the double SNP (which you do) your children will have at least one variant; therefore it might be beneficial for everyone in your family to take sodium selenite: once a week for the children; three times a week for you.

The end but not the end

Nasha: Your case highlights a critical and often overlooked truth: genetics are not our destiny: our *terrain* determines our trajectory. In your case, Julia, despite having many SNPs that could have made you more vulnerable to severe COVID-19 complications, inflammation and hormonal disruption, your commitment to a metabolically supportive lifestyle appears to have overridden many of these risks. This is a powerful testament to the ability of epigenetics (which we discussed in Chapter 3) – through diet, lifestyle and environmental choices – to shape our health outcomes.

You're very lucky for lots of reasons. Your lifestyle and the changes you've made really speaks to the overriding of your SNP expression. I want to highlight that. It's not set in stone. This is testament to how clean living on all your levels can override these expressions.[1]

What the func?! – a dip into functional medicine

Hippocrates was on to something when he said 'all disease begins in the gut'. Functional medicine focuses a lot on the gut, which you've read plenty about in this book. It's also known as 'root cause medicine' – and, perhaps surprisingly, how we digest and absorb our food, how our enzymes are activated, and even how we poo, lie at the root of many seemingly disconnected health issues.

Rather than just treating symptoms, functional medicine aims to understand a person's individual health history and lifestyle. It's more personalised, and you often start by filling in a lengthy document to trace your health throughout your lifetime. My timeline shows: a near fatal stint in hospital aged 13 with salmonella food poisoning, continuous episodic tonsillitis, painful periods, endometriosis, multiple amalgam fillings, a miscarriage . . . the list goes on. Suddenly, more serious health issues later in life don't seem so surprising when you see everything laid out like this.

A functional-medicine doctor will often try to find alternatives to pharmaceuticals, and will instead use personalised supplements and lifestyle modifications to address issues.

The road to health discovery

Jo Gamble is a metabolic practitioner, functional medicine practitioner and fellow in integrative oncology. She started working with autistic children at the age of 17. When her 19-month-old daughter became ill with multiple autoimmune diseases, which required a four-year chemotherapy regime, she wanted to support her but was told there was nothing she could do. That wouldn't do for Jo, so she studied nutritional therapy and took a fellowship in integrative oncology with The American Academy of Anti-Aging Medicine (a4m). Eventually, Jo became the first UK certified functional-medicine practitioner. She managed to support her daughter to full health, by the way, who is now 22 and has just graduated with a biochemistry first-class honours degree. As with so many in this world, Jo's research started with MeSearch.

What I'm learning as we work together is that, just like the landscapes we walk through, our bodies need balance, nourishment and care – and it begins in the stomach region. When we look after our inner ecosystem, we're laying the path for lifelong health vitality and resilience.

Jo talks about Julia

Julia and I first met at the first IPM (Integrated and Personalised Medicine) conference in 2023, when she was hosting and I was lecturing. The next year we were talking in the exhibition hall when I felt I should mention to her the coating that I had noticed on her tongue. The microbiome is not just limited to the gut, but the mouth and oral microbiome is massively influential on our wellness, especially for those who have had cancer.

Julia was by now aware of metabolic health, but she hadn't gone deep enough into all areas of imbalance in her body, so I took on the baton and told her that we were going on a deep dive. I knew Julia was seeing Dr Victoria Sampson to explore her oral microbiome (see Chapter 5 and Appendix), but I wanted to get to her gut. She took the Invivo Clinical GI Ecologix test, which is a comprehensive stool test that analyses the gastrointestinal microbiome. The gut can impact inflammation, immune function, digestion and gut-barrier health. We looked at the bad bacteria, but just as importantly, the balance of the good bacteria.

Gut instinct

Here are a few highlights pertaining to Julia, but they are also relevant to most of us.

Julia had very low levels of *Bifidobacterium* (a healthy bacteria found in the intestine which helps to digest fibre, prevent infection and produce important compounds). A depleted gut microbiome, including low *Bifidobacterium* levels, can lead to increased inflammation, which can contribute to tumour growth and the reduced effectiveness of treatments. It also plays a role in oestrogen metabolism, which is particularly relevant for hormone-sensitive breast cancers.

Energy for gut cells

Julia also had a below-detectable level of *Akkermansia*. (Dr William Li speaks about the importance of this in Chapter 3.) This bacterium helps to reduce inflammation and strengthen the immune responses. It's important for all of us: it helps to strengthen gut-barrier function and promote the production of short-chain fatty acids (SCFAs). SCFAs are crucial for gut health, providing energy for the gut cells – and they have known cancer-protective properties too.

Let it grow (but not too much)

Julia also had overgrowth of some opportunistic bacteria (*Citrobacter freundii*, *Enterobacter cloacae*, and *Klebsiella oxytoca* to name a few). When these bad-guy bacteria become overgrown, they can produce endotoxins. This can trigger a continual pro-inflammatory state, which can contribute to DNA damage and create a microenvironment that supports cancer (due to tumour-cell survival and proliferation).

Naughty bacteria

Testing also showed evidence of *Helicobacter pylori*. When *H. pylori* goes rogue, it is predominantly known for its role in gastric diseases, including stomach cancer. It can interfere with iron absorption (causing anaemia), disrupt the balance of the gut and cause chronic inflammation and therefore a number of diseases. Hormonal imbalances might contribute to an environment that could increase breast cancer risk, so it was important to address this.

The standard treatment for *H. pylori* infection is a triple therapy, which consists of two antibiotics and the use of a proton pump inhibitor (PPI).

We wanted to avoid antibiotics, because they kill gut bacteria indiscriminately, meaning that they wipe out not only the harmful bacteria causing infection but also the beneficial microbes that help with digestion, immunity and mood regulation. Julia did not use a PPI, as we didn't feel comfortable using a pharmaceutical acid-lowering medication when she was showing no symptoms. PPIs can reduce stomach-acid production, which can impair the absorption of nutrients, particularly B vitamins (which are essential for methylation, the clearance of oestrogen and the breakdown of homocysteine), amino acids (which are incredibly important for muscle-building and muscle-repair – especially in post-menopausal women), and calcium and magnesium (which are needed for optimal bone density).

We used supplements from a trusted specialist dispensary called Amrita Nutrition UK, who we work with regularly. Firstly, we began an antimicrobial protocol over a two-week period using the following supplements:

- **Serrapetase** – a proteolytic enzyme to break down the biofilm (the protective shell around the bacteria).
- **Renew Gut** to support fortifying the gut lining and tight junctions (the junctions in the gut that act as a barrier) to promote a healthy intestinal mucosal barrier.
- **Astragalus** Used for thousands of years in traditional Chinese medicine, astralagus is known as a 'superior herb' to optimise white blood cells and to support the immune system.
- **Bio.Revive Mucin +** has been formulated specifically for the mucosal layer of the gastrointestinal tract and contains arionia berry, which has been shown to increase the healthy bacterium *Akkermansia*.
- **Pylori-X** contains mastic, bismuth, zinc-carnosine and berberine sulfate, which jointly kill off *H. Pylori*.

After the gut cleanse, we wanted to repopulate and rebuild Julia's gut microbiome to create a more balanced environment where the good bacteria outweigh the bad. To do that we used:

- **Astragalus** We continued using this for the cleanse. *Astragalus membranaceus* (or Huang Qi) has been used for thousands of years in traditional Chinese medicine for its impressive abilities as an adaptogen (a substance that helps the body adapt to and manage stress) and an immune-system restorer.

- **Bio.Me Barrier** is a multi-strain live bacteria combination for the gut–brain microbiome and for intestinal barrier health.
- **Pylopass (*L. reuteri* DSM 17648)** Each capsule delivers 5 billion CFU (colony-forming units) of the *Limosilactobacillus reuteri* strain (proven to survive through stomach acidity) to support the repopulation of good bacteria post-*H. Pylori*.
- **Polyphenol Booster**, by Pendulum, supports the diversity of the gut microbiome. Polyphenols are considered prebiotics (non-digestible dietary fibres to feed the good bacteria) and can benefit the good bacteria such as *Akkermansia*.
- **Tributyrin 350** to support diversity of the colon microorganisms because of its advanced colon bioavailability.

Moods, microbes and mayhem

In summary, you can see that gut health plays a pivotal and multifaceted role in our health. For Julia, certain bacteria can affect her protection against a breast cancer recurrence. There's a collection of gut bacteria called the 'estrobolome', which affect oestrogen metabolism and ensures that oestrogen is properly processed and eliminated. This is important for all women, and a specific issue for Julia (see the DUTCH test and DNA Test Lifecode Gx in Appendix).[2]

The breast-cancer link

This is key for reducing the stimulation of hormone-sensitive breast cancers. An imbalanced microbiome, or dysbiosis, can disrupt this delicate hormonal balance, and even alter the breast tissue microenvironment through changes in immune cell behaviour, which might facilitate metastasis. Additionally, a healthy gut enhances the efficacy of cancer therapies – particularly immunotherapies – by ensuring a robust immune response. Julia and I are continuing our work on repairing her gut, addressing vitamin absorption issues and dealing with her emotional health.

Functional practitioners currently don't work within the NHS in the UK (although more and more health coaches are being enlisted to help in similar ways); they can be found through the Institute for Functional Medicine (https://www.ifm.org).

Conclusion: From north to south

'Good mooooorning everyone, welcome to Marguerite Bay. Our coordinates are: 68 17' 36"S, 67 09' 21"W and right now we are the most southern passenger ship on the planet.' Expedition leader Brad Siviour's mellow Australian voice came over the ship's tannoy system, and a ripple of applause and some whoops rang out in the dining area.

In March 2024, I fulfilled a lifetime ambition to visit Antarctica, journeying there in my role as patron of Whale Dolphin Conservation, a charity dedicated to the protection of endangered whales, dolphins and marine areas around the world. It had already been a thrilling trip on the *Ocean Endeavour*. After crossing the Antarctic Circle on the first of the month, through the infamous Drake Passage with a storm licking at our heels (yes, I was sick), we set foot on Antarctic land at a promontory called Red Rock Ridge, which is home to a penguin colony.

We landed on the rocky shore in our Zodiac (a type of rigid, inflatable boat) under full instruction: stay five metres away from the penguins; no kneeling down for photographs; no eating; no placing anything down on the ground – not even a tripod or a backpack. Our boots had been disinfected in a walk-through dip on the ship, and the day before we had hoovered out our kit to reduce the risk of any contamination.

I'll never forget taking those first steps, walking up to the crunchy ice and finding myself seconds later face to bill with some fluffy (they were moulting) juvenile Adelie penguins, which are only found in Antarctica. Almost everything here is named after an explorer or has a connection with one; Jules Dumont d'Urville discovered these sea birds in 1840 and named them after his beloved wife, Adele. They are so endearing that it is easy to get lost in their antics, and I almost forgot to look up.

When I did, I gazed out to the surrounding frozen mountains and took a deep breath in through my nose and then exhaled a long '*Wow!*'. I smiled to myself, my eyes scanning slowly from left to right taking in the dark, glassy water covered in tiles of floating white ice, the reflections of huge peaks, and icebergs shimmering across the surface. White, blue and even green, icebergs are mesmeric: how they float, move and crack, each one unique.

This ancient frozen landscape has been sculpted by wind and time, the great glaciers and rivers of ice are centuries in the making. This is one of the most extraordinary places on the planet. 'I've seen Antarctica,' I said to myself, and in that moment, despite being thousands of miles from home in an utterly alien place, I had never felt a closer sense of oneness with the earth.

Over the 14 days at sea and on other landings, we saw scores of humpback whales, showing off their tail flukes as they dived deep into the icy waters below, startling us with their trumpeting blowholes, sometimes close enough to touch.

We witnessed an extraordinary crabeater seal feeding frenzy of krill (they don't eat crab!), when hundreds of them churned up the waters, popping up with enormous curious eyes around us. We even had a rare sighting of two emperor penguins that had strayed into the bay.

It seems as if Antarctica is teeming with life, but you have to ask for how long, since every year the sea ice arrives later and melts away sooner. The British Antarctic Survey (BAS) reported that the sea ice has now shrunk to record lows, startling even to the most seasoned scientists.

The impact of reduced sea ice over 20 years would be profound; influencing local and global weather patterns and the unique ocean ecosystem here (including, of course, the whales and penguins, and much more). It's estimated that around 230 million people living in coastal communities would be displaced.

On a social-media post just after my trip, I shared a sad story about more human damage inflicted on Mother Earth. Studies have revealed that microplastics have been found in penguin poo. This indicates the widespread presence of microplastics throughout the Antarctic marine ecosystem. We're only just beginning to understand how harmful these chemicals are (phthalates, bisphenols and PFAS (polyfluoroalkyl substances) to name but a few), so this is not good news.

I came home from Antarctica with a renewed determination to expose calamities such as this and highlight the link between planetary health and human health. You know me as a green (and blue) evangelist, not a violent activist, but I promise you, unless we make the Earth well again, our own health has little chance of survival in a way that we recognise today.

This book, I hope, highlights the very real connection between the two. From my nature experiments in Cornwall to my time at Ananda in the Himalayas, and even listening to birdsong at Wormwood Scrubs, the impact on our health is undeniable.

Briefly, here is another marvellous story. Stanford professor Dr David Furman has reversed his biological age by ten years through a radical lifestyle change. He traded in urban life for a forest cabin with his family, where they embraced nature, candlelight, organic food and screen-free living. After just three years, his biological age had dropped from 42 to 32. (His actual chronological age was 39.) Yet another testament to the power of Vitamin N.

So, the conclusion we must draw is that the natural environment is a powerful anti-ageing tool, and one we can all reach for in our quest for healthspan. It's free and it is all around us, albeit diminishing rapidly (as re-emphasised by my findings with the penguins). It might seem that there is no connection between having your own veg patch, herb pot or flower bed and the white wastes of the icecap, but I promise they are all interlinked parts of one bigger whole – just like our bodies.

So, take care of all the green and blue spaces in your life and your community, as well as yourselves. I hope there has been plenty in these pages to help you.

I have undergone multiple tests and scans which I know are not accessible and affordable to all but, as I have said throughout, many of these pioneering procedures will become more normal and affordable in the not-too-distant future. A case in point is the emergence of a brand-new AI full-body scan backed by Daniel Ek, the entrepreneur who brought us Spotify.

Remember how novel it felt to be able to play your own music from a near-infinite back catalogue anywhere you wanted? That's what's going to happen to healthcare, and it's why I have written this book. (The scan is called Neko, which is Japanese for 'cat' (as in nine lives). It takes an hour and costs around £300.) Already there's a waiting list of tens of thousands of curious humans. In addition, the UK government recently announced that it will test the DNA of every newborn baby in England in a drive towards predicting and preventing illness, investing £650 million in DNA research by 2030.

If you remember, back in the Introduction, I had a full-body MRI scan that discovered a cyst bang in the middle of my brain. Luckily, it's benign, but something to watch and I'm glad I know it's there. As Joseph Malins suggested in his 1895 poem 'A Fence or an Ambulance', it is better to spend your efforts building 'a fence round the edge of the cliff' rather than having 'an ambulance down in the valley'.

Build your fence.

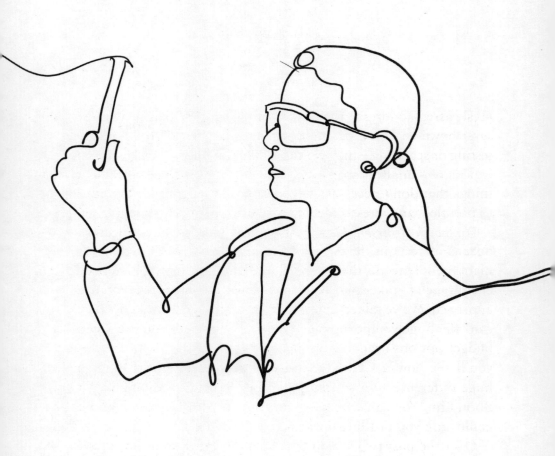

Appendix

Testing, Testing 1, 2, 3 – The Science of Self

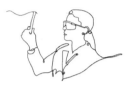

'Test, assess, address', that's what my friend Dr Nasha Winters says; however, some people don't like the idea of preventative testing or scanning – they would 'rather not know'. And it can be expensive – unaffordable, even. One also runs the risk of finding things that don't necessarily need discovering, and this can lead to pointless and stress-inducing exploration and treatment.

For *Hack Yourself Healthy* I've gone to extremes and taken dozens of tests in the name of research, but I wouldn't expect many people to do the same. I hope, though, that you've been encouraged to take some baby steps towards a more preventative approach. We've talked about tests from the NHS, and how they can offer hugely important insights into our health and suggested budget options available online. In this appendix, for example, you'll see how a CGM (continuous glucose monitor) made a huge difference to a seemingly fit and healthy cardiologist, Dr Boon Lim. You can wire up to one of those for fifty quid, and it could stop you heading towards type-2 diabetes.

Over the past two years of being a crash-test mummy, I have discovered:

- A cyst in my brain, luckily benign, after a full-body MRI scan, but it could have been life-changing.
- I now know that I'm genetically predisposed to insulin resistance, which could lead to type-2 diabetes and even cognitive

disorders such as Alzheimer's or dementia. I made the lifestyle changes of cutting out alcohol and sugar and eating a lower carbohydrate diet several years ago. The DNA results have galvanised me; I won't fall off the wagon and go back to my days of endless doughnuts, bags of sweeties and Friday-night cocktails any time soon.

- I can't turn back the clock, but I've discovered that the way my oestrogen pathways are plumbed suggests that IVF might have played a role in my breast cancer in 2021, and it also explains my endometriosis. These are compelling reasons to stay off the alcohol and eat plenty of fibre to help regulate my hormones.
- My gut (and my mouth) were overrun with bad bacteria, but good gut and oral health are crucial for overall vitality and immunity.
- Luckily for me (as you will read) my APOE gene is normal, which means that my risk of Alzheimer's or dementia is low.
- I'm also in possession of a fairly rare GG variant of the FOXO3 longevity gene, which apparently marks my longevity score as 'superhuman'. I'm assuming I inherited this from my Greek grandmother, Maria, who lived to be 103, but even this isn't a bullet-proof predictor when you take other variables into consideration.

I wouldn't have known any of this if I hadn't written this book, taken all the testing, or had breast cancer. I feel empowered and grateful. I'm fascinated by what's available in the preventative space today, and I'm curious about how this new approach is going to revolutionise healthcare and treatments in the not-so-distant future.

Alongside everything else I've explored in *Hack Yourself Healthy*, in this appendix I have run through some of the other tests that I have taken, and how the results have informed my decisions going forward. I hope you find them useful.

Over the years, I have become a believer. I believe in a personalised, rounded, holistic approach to health. One that integrates nutrition, exercise and genetics. Proactive medicine acknowledges the complex interdependent systems of the body, targeting root symptoms, not just the isolated symptoms. Although there are some universal truths (alcohol and refined sugar are bad for us; carrying excess weight increases the risk of other diseases; flossing our teeth and sleeping well are more important than we think), knowing what to focus on for the individual has huge value. The stories and information in this book emphasise that a rounded approach is the most effective. What is optimum for me may not be optimum for you, but I think we can all agree that the best day to start taking care of our health is yesterday. It's not about avoiding death, it's about optimising life.

What's your real age? – the telomere test

What is it?: Fagron Genomics TeloTest
Conducted via: Dr Ash Kapoor, Levitas Clinic (London, Guildford and Esher)
Telomeres are protective caps at the tips of DNA; they protect the chromosomes from damage. The presence of, and length of, these telomeres reduce as we age. Measuring their length can help to determine on a cellular level your biological age.

Studies have shown that brisk walking, or even just faster walking, is linked to longer telomeres. This suggests that brisk walking could help to slow down the process of telomere shortening and potentially delay the onset of ageing-related health issues. Some studies suggest that the relationship between walking speed and telomere length might be causal, meaning that brisk walking might directly influence telomere length.

Why test?

A telomere test can help us to understand how our cells are ageing internally. This is known as your biological age and can be different from your chronological age.

My results

The telomere test shows that my biological age is exactly the same as my actual age: 54 years. This means that my cells are ageing at a healthy and expected pace. I am doing well in terms of how my body is holding up at a cellular level, which is valuable after a cancer diagnosis. Nevertheless, it is possible, and typically desirable, to reverse our biological age to support longevity, health and wellness.

How to reverse biological ageing

Dr Ash Kapoor is a longevity and regenerative medicine doctor. He explains about my tests. Although detailed and specific to me, I think his commentary gives an outline of the kinds of things that can be helped through supplementation and detoxification, for example:

Longevity protocol The principles of this plan are to ensure that the body is well equipped to feed the cells and protect itself. This is based on the foundations of longevity medicine: if the pathway between DNA and the cell is controlled, the tissues and organs will look after themselves, and biological age should improve. To restore the body, we would focus on the body's infrastructure and cell-communication pathways.

Key micronutrients and hormones to restore include vitamin B12 and D (if the level is below 175).

Mitochondrial energy will be restored with NMN (nicotinamide mononucleotide, a compound naturally derived from vitamin B3, and known as an anti-ageing supplement to increase energy and improve sleep quality). This is expected to stabilise the immune system, hormones and adrenal gland.

A detoxification phase involves detox of the small intestine, liver and neuroendocrine pathway through autophagy (the cell's recycling system, which helps to remove damaged or unnecessary parts and re-utilise the materials). For the small-intestine detox, we will use a fibre supplement and glutathione to help to detoxify the liver.

I also recommend a turmeric/curcumin supplement.

After six weeks, we will carry out a controlled medically supervised autophagy fast. This is broken down into a two-day water and mineral fast, and five days of one meal a day (consisting of plant food). There will be micronutrient support during this.

To repair your body after the fasting phase, we would recommend supplements such as ashwagandha, KSM, melatonin, seriphos and magnesium.

Gut health will be also be addressed with probiotics and collagen peptides.

Finally, the renewal phase involves bioregulator peptides (short-chain amino acids) to feed the epigenetic space around the DNA, including pineal peptides (for longevity), thymus peptides (for the immune system), adrenal peptides and gut peptides – cycled over three months.

I would recommend repeat testing in six months to one year after implementing the plan.

With consistency and commitment, it is often possible to reduce one's biological age significantly – in some cases by several years. The true goal, however, is not just to measure time differently, but also to feel stronger, more resilient, and better equipped to thrive.

A detailed health check for the whole body

What is it?: MRI scan, including chest, abdomen, pelvis, spine and brain
Conducted via: The Scan.com, Full Body MRI Scan
A full-body MRI scan is a safe, detailed health check that looks inside your body from head to pelvis. It checks the major organs and blood vessels – such as your brain, liver, kidneys and more – to spot any signs of disease or problems early. You lie in an MRI machine for 60–90 minutes while it takes detailed images using magnets – not radiation. Before and after the scan, you speak with a doctor who explains the process and walks you through your results.

Why do this scan?

An MRI can detect early signs of things such as tumours, cysts or aneurysms – often before you have any symptoms. Catching these early gives you more options for treatment and peace of mind. Following something like a breast-cancer diagnosis, as in my case, this type of surveillance scan can check for other changes.

Julia's Results

Doctor Abhinav Singh, who performed the MRI, said the following:

Chest, abdomen and pelvis Julia previously had a left-sided mastectomy (breast removal surgery) and now has a breast implant on that side, which appears as expected. There are no signs of swollen lymph nodes in the central chest, armpits or lungs. A few small spots were seen in the liver that look like harmless fluid-filled sacs (cysts), which are common and not usually cause for concern.

Brain Julia's brain scan was clear. There were no signs of blocked or damaged blood vessels, brain swelling or bleeding. All the main arteries and veins looked open and healthy. The scan also showed no signs of brain degeneration (such as Alzheimer's or Parkinson's), inflammation or infection.

A small 13mm cyst was found near the pineal gland (a tiny area deep in the brain). It's thin-walled, looks benign (non-cancerous), and is not affecting nearby brain tissue.

Spine The scan of Julia's spine showed mild wear-and-tear changes, which are common with age and usually not serious:

- Minimal disc osteophytes were seen – these are small bone spurs that can form along the edges of the spine. They're usually harmless unless they press on nerves.
- There were mild disc bulges (slight outward movement of the soft discs between the bones of the spine) in the neck and upper back. These weren't severe.
- Some mild joint inflammation and early signs of wear were seen in the lower back (specifically between the L2 and L5 bones).
- One of the lower back bones (L3) was slightly out of place, but not in a way that would typically cause major issues.
- There were small tears in some of the discs in the lower spine (L3 to S1), but no signs of any unusual masses, growths, or fluid build-up in those areas.

Summary

Despite the unexpected discovery of a benign 13mm pineal cyst on the brain, overall, my brain scan showed no other negative issues. Most pineal cysts do not cause any harm. In rare cases, larger cysts can lead to symptoms due to pressure on surrounding structures. Dr Singh recommends a follow-up brain MRI in six to twelve months' time to ensure that it is not growing.

Regarding the whole spine, Dr Singh said, 'a few mild degenerative changes in the lumbar spine were found, and are early
signs of wear and tear in the lower back often associated with
ageing. It's a common finding, especially in people over 30, and
nothing unusual for someone of Julia's age.'

(See also Introduction for my consultation with consultant
neurosurgeon Kevin O'Neill about my brain.)

Breast health

What is it?: Thermocheck – a breast-screening method
Conducted via: Dr Nyjon Eccles at The Natural Doctor (London)
Thermocheck is a revolutionary approach to breast health
created by Dr Nyjon Eccles. It is a non-invasive breast-screening
method that complements traditional techniques such as
mammograms. It is suitable for women of all ages, including
those with dense breast tissue, twin implants or a family history
of breast cancer. (It cannot, however, be used on women like me
who have had a mastectomy and a single breast implant because
the breasts are compared to each other, and mine don't match,
so I sent my friend Sarah.)

Whereas mammograms use X-rays to detect structural
changes (such as lumps), Thermocheck uses digital infrared
thermal imaging to detect subtle temperature changes in breast
tissue. Increased heat can indicate inflammation, increased
blood flow or abnormal cell activity – all potential early signs of
concern.

It's not recognised as an alternative to a mammogram, because
it is approved as an adjunct, for use in conjunction with other
technologies; however, since heat changes are visible six to ten
years before a mammogram would detect a lump, this kind of
scan can lead to earlier interventions. Dr Eccles's personalised
breast-health plans turn an abnormal Thermocheck rating into a
normal rating in approximately 80 per cent of cases. Patients use

nutraceuticals (supplements from food sources that are understood to help fight disease in ways beyond nutrition) and are encouraged to make lifestyle changes to reduce their cancer risk.

Key differences include:

- No radiation exposure, therefore safe for frequent monitoring.
- No physical compression, therefore more comfortable for sensitive breasts.
- Empowering: a normal Thermogram indicates that you have physiologically healthy breasts, unlike a mammogram, which shows only the absence of a lesion. It helps you take charge of your breast health.

Sarah's results

Sarah writes:

This is a no-contact examination. It's conducted in the comfort of a chair, undressed to the waist and with your arms above your head, your torso turning to give the infrared camera front and side views. There's an initial scan, then a ten-minute wait in a cooled room (it's 18°C in there, and Michelle, the highly experienced scanner, wears a bodywarmer) followed by a second scan. The whole process takes about 20 minutes.

Afterwards, I receive a report of my Thermocheck findings. On a rating of TH1–5 where 1–2 is normal, 3 is equivocal/low risk, 4 is abnormal/moderate risk, and 5 is suspicious/high risk, my left breast scores a TH2 and my right is a TH3. Dr Eccles recommends a regime of specific nutraceuticals and that I should get my vitamin D levels checked, since low vitamin D is a known risk factor for breast cancer. He will see me again in six months when he hopes that my right breast score will also be within the 1–2 category.

Understand your blood glucose level

What is it?: continuous glucose monitor testing – tests the level
of your blood glucose for a period of time
Conducted via: Dr Boon Lim, One Wellbeck Heart Health
(London)
Dr Boon Lim MB BCHIR PhD FRCP IBHRE is the consultant
cardiologist at Hammersmith Hospital and One Wellbeck Heart
Health. He is slim, energetic and at the top of his game. He had
a COVID scare, which wiped him out – at one stage he didn't
think that he would fully regain his health. Now, he takes exercise and nutrition seriously, he meditates and has tried to even
out his work–life balance.

Dr Boon says, 'I have been experimenting on myself as I approach
my mid-life, to understand how to keep myself in optimal shape.
I'm 49 now, and I have worn a CGM (continuous glucose monitor)
three times. I was completely shocked to see my high glucose levels.
I'm slim, I consider myself fit and healthy (walking 10,000–15,000
steps a day) and I had always been very strict with my diet: low-
carb and mainly low-GI foods; I've also followed some intermittent fasting for the best part of three to four years.'

What shocked Boon was that his CGM profile showed that he
was close to what is sometimes called a 'pre-diabetic state': 'I
was not quite in the pre-diabetic range, but a few points away.
And I nearly fell off my chair, because I see a lot of my patients
who are much larger than me, less healthy, but with much better,
normal range HbA1c levels and I thought: *What the hell is going
on?*'

HbA1c is the measure of your average blood glucose levels.
The normal range is from 20 to 39 mmol/MOL (millimoles per
mole) (or 4–5.6 per cent). Bear in mind that normal isn't necessarily optimal, and many health experts and medics advise keeping it closer to the 20 range (roughly equivalent to 4 per cent).
Someone with an HbA1c level of 48mmol/mol (6.5 per cent) is
considered diabetic.

Boon says, 'I thought to myself: *I've got good diet, I generally rest well, I meditate, I breathe . . . But the thing I did not do, or I hadn't fully done, for a long time, is zone-2 exercise.*'

Zone 2 exercise, also known as LISS (low-intensity steady state) cardio or base training, involves maintaining a heart rate between 60 and 70 per cent of your maximum heart rate. Think steady, low-intensity exercise that you can comfortably sustain for extended periods, such as a brisk walk or a light jog. You should be able to hold a conversation in an out-of-breath way.

Boon recognised that this was missing from his routine and started to do some zone-2 aerobic activity three times a week. And it worked. 'That really brought it down,' he says 'and the second thing I realised is that doing zone-2 also brought my HRV (heart rate variability) *up*. So, above and beyond the science of wellness and the science of eating and nutrition, there is an element that can be personalised, which I found for me worked very well. I did three days a week of running or zone-2 aerobic training for 30–35 minutes, and that's all it took to tip the scales! You have the CGM, you follow your glucose trends for two weeks and you do the experiments. Had I not done this experiment on myself I would never have known.'

Oral microbiome

What is it?: the Ammp8 point-of-care saliva test by Dentognostics
Conducted via: a dental practice
Ammp8 testing is a saliva test that takes five minutes to perform. Ammp8 stands for 'activated matrix metalloproteinase 8', which is an enzyme that breaks down a certain type of collagen found in the gums. (We have lots of different types of collagen in our body – hair, skin, nails – but our gums are a different type.) Gum disease is essentially the breakdown of this collagen. The problem with gum disease is that by the time it's detected the destruction has already occurred and can't be reversed, only managed.

It can start up to six months before clinical signs show in the mouth.

Dr Victoria Sampson, BDS (Lond) MFDS RCS Ed Pg Dip, is a functional dentist. She says, 'If you already have gum disease, this test is still super-useful as it puts a "number" on your gum disease, telling us how rapid and aggressive it is.'

My results

In the collagen breakdown, my result was 25.8 mmol. This suggests moderately elevated collagen breakdown and early signs of gum disease. Thankfully, despite high levels of ammp8 there were no clinical signs of gum disease. Victoria recommended a retest within three to four months after two guided biofilm therapy sessions (explained in Chapter 5), and I have followed a new oral hygiene protocol including a hydroxyapatite toothpaste, probiotics (a combination of *Streptococcus salivarius* M18, *Lactobacillus reuteri* and *Lactobacillus paracasei*) and propolis drops.

Track your oral bacteria and genetic mutations

What is it?: ORALIS 1 – an oral microbiome test
Conducted via: TSH Labs https://thslabs.co.uk/
This is an innovative test to look at over 500 different bacteria, 10 genetic mutations, and inflammation in your mouth. The idea behind the test is that it is not just bacteria that causes disease, but also how your body responds to it and how bacteria is acting in your body (which will be different from your partner, for example). This includes the mouth in whole-body health.

My results

The results revealed that I had generalised gum inflammation, high levels of bacteria associated with gum inflammation and elevated levels of collagen breakdown. High levels of *Fusobacterium periodonticum* were detected: a bacterium associated with gum inflammation and general inflammation. I have no genetic mutations associated with increased risk of inflammation or gum disease although I have two genetic mutations associated with decay: GALK2 and DEFB1 gene mutations mean a higher risk of decay and sugar cravings.

After following a bespoke protocol for three months, my results showed an improvement in the levels of good bacteria and a more balanced oral microbiome. I was also able to reduce the collagen breakdown to zero in my mouth and reduce the levels of bad bacteria – all amounting to a more balanced microbiome.[1]

Lab rats

Today, there are labs and places sprouting up all over the world to test everything from our blood to our DNA. Some work only directly with practitioners, whereas others operate a direct-to-consumer service. A professional can unravel results and explain tests fully, which can get technical, and I've found that invaluable when writing this book. For *Hack Yourself Healthy*, I've been working with multiple practitioners and Regenerus Labs in the UK. If you'd like to do any of the following tests you need to be working with a practitioner. Here's a link – http://q-r.to/FindAPractitioner – to help you choose a qualified medical practitioner that can help you. Most will offer a discovery call.

Julia's tests

Jo Majithia, BA (Hons), DipION, BANT registered nutritionist and head of clinical education at Regenerus Labs explains below about the tests:

Understanding the comprehensive adrenal stress test with CAR

This test provides valuable insight into how your body responds to stress by measuring key hormones and immune markers.

Your adrenal glands help your body to respond to stress by producing hormones such as cortisol and DHEA (see the box below for these terms). If these hormones are out of balance, it can lead to symptoms such as fatigue, trouble sleeping, anxiety or a weakened immune system.

Key terms for the adrenal stress test

- **Cortisol**, released daily by the adrenal glands in a circadian rhythm, helps to regulate blood sugar, mood, metabolism, inflammation and memory. It increases in response to stress.
- **DHEA** (dehydroepiandrosterone), a pro-hormone mostly converted into androgens and oestrogens, supports muscle, bone, sexual health, brain function, immunity and cardiovascular health.

What does the CAR test measure?

- **Cortisol awakening response (CAR)** measures how your body reacts to stress first thing in the morning. A strong CAR suggests a healthy stress response, whereas a weak or exaggerated CAR might indicate issues such as burnout or chronic stress.
- **Salivary secretory IgA (sIgA)** is a marker of immune function in the saliva. Low levels may indicate that stress is suppressing your immune system.

- **Cortisol and DHEA levels** The test tracks your cortisol at six points throughout the day, along with DHEA, to assess overall adrenal function and stress levels.

Why is this important?

This test helps to identify whether stress is affecting your overall well-being and if your body needs extra support.

My results

I have been working with Michael Ash (see Chapter 9) to navigate these tests and results. They show how my body responds to stress over time by measuring cortisol at specific time points across the day, DHEA and secretory IgA (sIgA) (an antibody that plays a key role in immune defence, protecting mucosal surfaces from pathogens).

My key findings, as listed by Jo Majithia, were:

- **Morning cortisol response (CAR)** Your free cortisol levels (the active form of cortisol able to enter tissues and have an effect) are below optimal on waking and 30 minutes after waking. This might explain why you sometimes feel sluggish or grumpy after waking up. They rise to an optimal level after 60 minutes, which is encouraging; however, your cortisol awakening response (CAR) is exaggerated at 71.88 per cent (optimal is 35–60 per cent), and even after reaching your peak your levels continue to rise rather than returning to baseline. This pattern suggests that your stress response may be overactive in the morning, possibly due to disrupted sleep, anticipatory stress or a sensitised nervous system.
- **Afternoon cortisol levels** Your cortisol drops below the normal range in the afternoon, which may contribute to fatigue and low energy.
- **Diurnal cortisol pattern** Your results refer to 'Phase 2 HPA axis dysfunction', meaning that chronic stress might be affecting your body's ability to regulate cortisol. This can lead to

blood sugar imbalances, weight gain (in some), immune suppression and increased susceptibility to infections.

- **DHEA levels** Your DHEA levels are normal, which is beneficial for muscle, bone, brain, immune and cardiovascular health. DHEA naturally declines with age, but reducing stress and eating a balanced diet can help to maintain healthy levels.
- **Secretory IgA (sIgA)** Your sIgA levels are normal, which is good news, as this antibody is essential for immune defence on mucosal surfaces.

How you can support your health

- **Manage stress** An exaggerated CAR can be linked to job-related or anticipatory stress. A calming morning routine is important for you. Try CBT, meditation, breathwork or journaling to help regulate your response.
- **Improve sleep quality** Address sleep disturbances to support a healthier cortisol rhythm.
- **Balance blood sugar** Ensure stable blood sugar levels by eating protein, fibre and healthy fats (such as those found in extra-virgin olive oil, oily fish, avocados, flaxseeds, chia seeds and nuts), and avoiding excessive sugar and processed foods.
- **Exercise wisely** Moderate exercise such as brisk walking or cycling can help to regulate afternoon cortisol levels and improve overall well-being.
- **Consider nutritional support** Vitamins B5, B6, C and E, along with adaptogenic herbs (such as ashwagandha or rhodiola), might help to support adrenal function.

Understanding the Mercury Tri-Test

Mercury is a toxic heavy metal that can build up in the body over time, potentially affecting brain function, the nervous system and overall health. Today, we are exposed to mercury through sources such as certain seafood (for example, tuna and other large predatory fish), dental fillings, pollution and some cosmetics. Too much mercury in the body can lead to fatigue, memory problems, mood changes and other health issues.

What does the Tri-Test measure?

The Mercury Tri-Test is a unique way to assess mercury levels in the body by analysing three different sample types:

- **Blood** Helps to identify the source of mercury exposure by distinguishing between inorganic mercury (mainly from dental fillings and industrial sources) and methylmercury (mainly from seafood).
- **Hair** Shows long-term methylmercury exposure and how well your body is eliminating it.
- **Urine** Helps to assess how efficiently your kidneys are removing inorganic mercury from the body.

Unlike older challenge-testing methods, which use chemical agents to force mercury excretion, this test directly measures both inorganic mercury and methylmercury. It gives a clearer picture of mercury exposure, how much is stored in the body, and how effectively it is being eliminated.

Why is this important?

Chronic mercury exposure can contribute to neurological issues, fatigue, immune dysfunction and more. Identifying your mercury levels can help to guide you to the appropriate detox strategies. A healthcare professional might recommend dietary adjustments, targeted supplements or lifestyle changes to help reduce mercury exposure and support natural detoxification.

My results

- **Total mercury in my blood** is moderately elevated – higher than the Centers for Disease Control and Prevention (CDC) recommended levels in the US, and Quicksilver Scientific averages.

- **Methylmercury levels** (primarily from seafood and fish consumption) are also moderately elevated.
- **Inorganic mercury levels** (mainly from dental amalgams) are in the low-normal range, which is good news.

How our body processes mercury

My key findings, as listed by Jo, are:

The body eliminates inorganic mercury primarily via the kidneys and through urine. Your test results suggest that your kidneys are effectively excreting the low-normal level of inorganic mercury you are exposed to. This means that the low mercury exposure from sources such as dental fillings is not accumulating in your body.

Methylmercury is primarily excreted via the liver into the bile and out through your bowels. We can examine the levels in hair and compare this to the level in your blood to provide a proxy for your elimination via the liver. Your hair-to-blood mercury ratio suggests that your body may not be efficiently clearing methylmercury. This can lead to a build-up over time.

How you can support your health

- **Reduce high-mercury fish** Limit larger fish such as tuna, marlin and swordfish, as they contain higher levels of methylmercury. Opt for smaller oily fish such as anchovies and sardines, mackerel, or sustainably fished white fish instead.
- **Consider dietary history** If Julia ate more fish than usual before the test, it might have temporarily lowered her hair-to-blood ratio.
- **Support detoxification** Eating a nutrient-rich diet and maintaining good liver and kidney health can aid mercury elimination.
- **Monitor exposure** If you are concerned, continue tracking mercury levels over time and adjust your seafood intake accordingly.

Understanding the DUTCH Complete test

Hormones play a vital role in energy, mood, metabolism and overall well-being. When hormone levels are imbalanced, they can contribute to symptoms such as fatigue, weight changes, sleep issues, mood swings and more.

What does the DUTCH test measure?
The DUTCH Complete test provides a comprehensive look at 35 key hormones, including:

- **Sex hormones** Oestrogen, progesterone, testosterone and their metabolites, which influence reproductive health, mood and metabolism.
- **Adrenal hormones** DHEA and cortisol, which help to regulate stress, energy levels and inflammation, including daily cortisol and cortisone patterns, which reveal how well your body manages stress throughout the day.
- **Melatonin** A key hormone that regulates sleep–wake cycles.
- **8-OHdG** A marker for oxidative stress and DNA damage, which can indicate poor cellular health.
- **Organic acids** These assess nutrient status, neurotransmitter activity and metabolic function. Key markers include vitamins B12, B6, biotin and glutathione, which are important for energy, detoxification and overall health.
- **Dopamine, norepinephrine and epinephrine**, which are neuro-transmitters that affect mood, focus and stress response.
- **Neuroinflammation**, which indicates potential inflammation in the nervous system.
- **Gut dysbiosis marker** Reflects imbalances in the gut bacteria, which can contribute to gut-health issues and impact your hormone clearance.

Why is this important?

This test offers valuable insights into hormonal and metabolic health, helping to identify imbalances that could be affecting mood, energy, weight, sleep and digestion. It can be used to help address hormone-related conditions, stress management, nutrient deficiencies and gut-health concerns.

How to access the test

If you're interested in testing, please note that these tests should be ordered through a qualified healthcare practitioner (as noted previously) who can help interpret the results and recommend the appropriate next steps for you. By working with a practitioner, you will gain a clearer understanding of what your results mean and you will receive personalised guidance on how to address any imbalances.

To find out more or connect with a practitioner, please visit Omnos Find A Practitioner.

My results

Below are my initial test results dated July 2023 (at age 52) as explained by Jo.

Adrenal health and cortisol DHEA was lower than expected for Julia's age but still within range. Low DHEA can impact energy, mood and resilience to stress.

Cortisol (stress hormone) Total metabolised cortisol was lower than expected, indicating lower overall adrenal output. Free cortisol (the active form) was within range, but the afternoon cortisol drop was below normal, which can contribute to fatigue and low energy. Your body showed a preference for storing cortisol as cortisone, which can happen under long-term stress or during recovery from illness. This suggests that stress management and adrenal support are key areas to focus on.

Oestrogen levels and detoxification Oestrogen levels were very low, even for a menopausal range. Although low oestrogen is expected post-menopause, very low levels can contribute to:

- Hot flushes, night sweats, insomnia.
- Joint pain, dry skin, brain fog.
- Vaginal dryness, low libido.
- Increased cardiovascular and bone-health risks.
- Low oestrogen levels would be beneficial with regarding oestrogen-driven cancer, however.

Oestrogen detoxification pathways Oestrogen is detoxified in two phases in the liver:

- Phase-1 detoxification (conversion of oestrogen into metabolites): your results show less than optimal activity down the CYP1A1 pathway; this is the preferred phase-1 route, as it produces a safer metabolite (2-OH-E1).

    CYP1B1 pathway was more active, which increases production of 4-OH-E1 – considered a 'naughty' metabolite due to its association with DNA damage and increased breast cancer risk.
    Typical activity for the CYP3A4 pathway produces 16-OH-E1, which can promote tissue growth and may increase risk for fibroids and breast-tissue proliferation.

- Phase-2 detoxification (methylation – see box on page 261): this step processes oestrogen for elimination. Your methylation activity looked good, meaning that your body was effectively clearing phase-1 oestrogen metabolites.
- Supportive strategies: to shift oestrogen metabolism toward the safer CYP1A1 pathway, a diet rich in cruciferous vegetables (broccoli, Brussels sprouts, kale), flaxseeds, fish oil and antioxidants (sulforaphane – broccoli seeds are a particularly

rich source – resveratrol) may be beneficial. Reducing sugar and alcohol also helps.

Progesterone and androgen levels Progesterone, which is mostly made by the adrenal glands after menopause, was low. Low progesterone can contribute to fatigue, irritability, anxiety, insomnia and low bone density. Supporting adrenal health with adaptogens (for example, ashwagandha or rhodiola) and stress management could help.

Androgens (testosterone and metabolites) were within range, supporting mood, motivation and muscle maintenance.

Nutrient, neurotransmitter and oxidative stress markers, vitamins B12 and B6 levels: there was a potential need for B12, which is essential for energy, brain function and red blood cell production as well as to support methylation activity. Good sources include lean meats, fish and eggs.

Both your neurotransmitter metabolites are at the lower end of the normal range, suggesting a potential for lower production, which might contribute to feeling tired. Eating sufficient protein-rich foods and a nutrient-rich diet can support production.

Oxidative stress marker (8-OHdg) This marker, which reflects DNA damage risk, was on the higher end of normal. Given your history of oestrogen-receptor-positive breast cancer, reducing oxidative stress with antioxidant-rich foods (berries, greens) and appropriate supplements might be helpful.

My results (retest)
Below are my retest results, in summary, dated October 2024, (at age 54) as listed by Jo:

Key improvements Oestrogen levels have improved, although still below typical menopausal levels. This balance is important:

whereas too much oestrogen can increase breast-cancer risk, very low oestrogen can worsen menopause symptoms and affect bone, brain and cardiovascular health.

Most encouragingly, the 'naughty' oestrogen phase-1 detox pathway (CYP1B1) has normalised, reducing the production of potentially DNA-damaging 4-OH-E1. This significantly lowers the risk of oestrogen-related cancers.

The preferred detox pathway (CYP1A1) is now dominant, meaning this first part of oestrogen clearance is being processed in a safer way.

The second step, the methylation activity, is still looking good.

Adrenal and cortisol function DHEA and androgen levels: a slight improvement, which is encouraging, as levels typically decline with age.

Progesterone metabolites are now in a normal postmenopausal range, suggesting that adrenal support and stress management have been beneficial.

Total cortisol production has improved, and the body's balance between cortisol and cortisone is more regulated.

Afternoon cortisol levels remain slightly low, but overall adrenal function has strengthened. Continued stress management, moderate exercise and a nutrient-dense diet will help.

Nutrient and oxidative stress markers B12 levels still need monitoring, but neurotransmitter markers have normalised, indicating improvements in dopamine and norepinephrine balance. This suggests better energy, mood and focus.

Oxidative stress (8-OHdg) has decreased to a normal level, which is a great sign for DNA protection and long-term health.

Next steps and recommendations

- Continue stress management and adrenal support (adaptogens, good sleep, mindfulness).

- Maintain a nutrient-rich diet to support hormone detoxification (cruciferous vegetables, antioxidants, flaxseeds, omega-3s).
- Monitor B12 levels and ensure sufficient intake for brain and energy support.
- Keep an eye on cortisol levels in the afternoon – avoiding excessive caffeine and sugar while including a balanced protein intake might help.

Celebrate the progress – these improvements are a fantastic result!

Test for body fluids to detect and monitor cancer

What is it?: TruBlood Test +, a liquid biopsy: The Datar Cancer Genetics Blood Biopsy and ESR genetic test
Conducted via: Dr Vineet Datta at Cancer Track Monitoring, https://uk.datarpgx.com/contact-us
The TruBlood Test + is a liquid biopsy. A liquid biopsy is a minimally invasive test that analyses body fluids, such as blood, to detect and monitor cancer. The blood harbours various types of cancer fragments, including circulating tumour cells (CTCs), DNA or other biomarkers that are shed by tumours. The real-time monitoring of tumour dynamics and detection of genetic mutations, makes it a valuable tool in personalised cancer management.

Genetic research has rapidly transformed the utility of testing over the past decade with the benefits of the science getting more established. There now exists a phenomenal ability to isolate fragments of cancer and cancer cells that can be picked up from a simple blood draw.

Dr Vineet Datta, MD, FRCP(Glasg), FRCP(Edin), MRCP(UK) MCEM FIMSA, undertook the testing and says: 'Julia underwent a novel blood-based test that analyses cancer cells, which aids in the diagnosis of cancer, in the absence of a physical biopsy. This new approach is revolutionary, as it doesn't just detect the presence of cancer fragments in a blood draw, but it also finds where the cancer is coming from. A common challenge for doctors is to determine if the cancer is spreading from the original site or if it's a new cancer.' Dr Vineet explains further:

Julia's results

Julia's tests revealed no evidence of any cancer cells or fragments in her blood, indicating that no cancer mutations were found. This would suggest, thankfully for her, the absence of cancer or, rarely, a very low tumour burden, below the levels that can be detected by the technology. Cancer cells and/or fragments may have many alterations in their make up that a specific targeted therapy is designed to attack. Her liquid biopsy fortunately did not detect these errors. The liquid biopsy would have showed, in the presence of active disease, if she was a good candidate for certain types of targeted therapy treatment or not. Targeted therapy is a type of cancer treatment designed to destroy specific types of cancer cells.

What are ESR SNPs?

SNPs are differences in your genetic code that are inherited and that you are born with. We also tested Julia for both ESR1 and ESR2 SNPs (single nucleotide polymorphisms, as explained in the Lifecode Gx test below). An ESR mutation is a change in the oestrogen receptor gene that can cause breast cancer to become resistant to hormone therapy. These mutations are a common cause of resistance to endocrine therapy, which is the primary treatment for hormone receptor-positive breast cancer. These alterations can be detected with a liquid biopsy, and ESR1 mutations are associated with a more aggressive disease and a shorter progression-free survival. There are specific targeted therapies to treat ESR1-mutated breast cancer. While an ESR1 mutation is generally considered more clinically significant in cancer treatment, ESR2 mutations are less frequently studied and may have a subtler impact on cancer progression. Julia tested negative.

Test your saliva to analyse genetic markers

What is it?: The Lifecode Gx Nutrigenomics DNA test
Conducted via: Emma Beswick, Lifecode Gx Nutrigenomics (available through https://www.lifecodegx.com/public, direct to the consumer, or https://listing.lifecodegx.com/, via a practitioner)
These tests analyse cheek cells via saliva to examine how genes interact with nutrition and lifestyle, offering personalised health insights. A simple cheek swab collects DNA in order to analyse over 200 genetic markers. This provides insights into areas such as metabolism, detoxification and hormone balance. The goal is to optimise your health and well-being by aligning your lifestyle choices with your genetic predispositions.

Emma Beswick CEO and co-founder of Lifecode Gx, MBA, and registered nutritional therapist, mBANT, explains:

Nutrigenetics is a subset of genetics which examines how diet and other lifestyle factors (sleep, stress, emotion, exercise) interact with our genes to impact health. Understanding our genetic needs enables us to tailor our environment to optimise health in a personalised way rather than damaging it. Some aspects of nutrigenetics are straightforward: one genetic variant can confer a need for more or less of a vitamin or nutrient, but the real power is in examining clusters of genes in contexts. What is 'good' in one context, or for one person, may be 'bad' for someone else.

What are SNPs?

Every one of us has a genetic blueprint, like a personalised instruction manual, written in a language of four letters: A, C, G and T. These letters are the building blocks of our DNA, strung together in precise sequences to guide how our bodies grow, function and repair.

Sometimes, though, a single letter in this sequence can vary between people. Think of it as a typo in a book. If this typo (called a 'single nucleotide polymorphism', or SNP) shows up in more than 1 per cent of the population, it's considered a natural variation rather than an error. These SNPs can subtly, or not so subtly, influence how your body processes nutrients, detoxifies chemicals, responds to inflammation, or even manages energy; for example, some SNPs may affect how well you metabolise vitamins or handle certain medications. Others might influence your likelihood of developing conditions such as heart disease or cancer – but they don't cause the condition on their own. Instead, they act as clues, showing where your terrain might need extra support.

Two terms that you might encounter when discussing SNPs are heterozygous and homozygous. They describe whether you inherited the same or different versions of a SNP or 'letters' from your parents:

- **Heterozygous** means that you inherited one version from one parent and a different version from the other. It's like having a mix of two recipes.
- **Homozygous** means that both parents passed down the same version, so you're working from one consistent recipe.

Emma explains further:

My results

There is so much to discuss, I have kept it to some of the key genes that play a role in Julia's breast-cancer diagnosis. Her CYP17A1 and CYP19A1 (also known as aromatase) genes confer a default to making more oestrogens, and her COMT gene confers slower removal of them (to do with a process called methylation [explained on page 261]) – a combination which can result in higher oestrogen levels. Chronic, long-term high oestrogen can be a factor in breast and gynaecological cancers. Once the risk is identified, it can be reduced, very effectively, through diet and lifestyle. Reducing alcohol has a direct, lowering effect on oestrogen synthesis. Oestrogen deactivation (the COMT methylation step) can be supported with B vitamins and zinc, and the inclusion of sulphur foods, such as broccoli, garlic and leeks, can be a game changer in a positive way. The benefits post a breast-cancer diagnosis are to reduce the risk of excess oestrogens.

Tamoxifen is a medication used to treat certain types of breast cancer. It works by blocking oestrogen's effect on cancer cells, but it's not fully active when you take it. Your body needs to convert tamoxifen into its more powerful form, called endoxifen [as explained on page 254], to make it work effectively. The CYP2D6 SNP is the gene that converts tamoxifen into its active forms, and it impacts how your liver converts tamoxifen to endoxifen. This conversion is done by an enzyme in your liver, which is produced by the same gene.

CYP2D6 is quite complicated; there are a number of different SNPs that should be looked at in combination to determine if someone is a fast or slow metaboliser. About 25 per cent of people of white European heritage and 50 per cent of Asian people are slow metabolisers (the official terms are 'intermediate' or 'poor'. Julia fits into the poor category (see below), whereas about 30 per cent of East Africans are fast metabolisers (the official term is 'ultra-rapid' metaboliser).

Julia is a poor metaboliser, and it's actually quite rare to have this particular SNP (only 2.5 per cent frequency).

By testing for CYP2D6 SNPs, doctors can assess how your body is likely to process tamoxifen. If you're a poor metaboliser, like Julia, they might adjust the treatment plan. The implication is that you would not receive enough of the active form in a dose, so a different medication (such as an aromatase inhibitor) might be offered, to ensure the best possible outcome. This is a perfect example of personalised medicine in action: tailoring treatment to your unique genetic terrain.

- **Normal metabolisers** convert tamoxifen into endoxifen efficiently, so the treatment works as expected.
- **Intermediate or poor metabolisers** have a less-active version of CYP2D6, so they produce much less endoxifen. This may reduce the effectiveness of tamoxifen, meaning that it might not work as well to prevent cancer recurrence.
- **Ultra-rapid metabolisers** convert tamoxifen very quickly, which might cause side effects or other unexpected responses.

The CYP1B1 SNP promotes 4-OH (4 hydroxy-oestrogen), which has more potential to increase semi-quinones (harmful free-radical molecules), which in turn can cause DNA damage, and therefore a potential for cancer. Julia's result indicates a predisposition for higher activity.

Sulforaphane, famously found in broccoli sprouts, can help with this, but all cruciferous vegetables, as well as mustard, cabbage and horseradish help to reverse this via the NQO1 gene.

Julia's vitamin-D genetics looked as if they could be a problem both in terms of transporting vitamin D (the GC gene) and sensitivity to it (the vitamin D receptor, VDR, gene), but a blood test showed robust vitamin D levels. Vitamin D is hugely important for immunity and can help to see off cancer before it starts or takes hold anywhere. We concluded that Julia's lifestyle – of being active in sunlight – was already compensating for her vitamin D genetic vulnerability. She was 'walking herself happy' physically as well as literally; however, it could also be that her vitamin D levels were high when she tested them because of exercise and activity, which raises them. This is why regular testing is important.

With the less-sensitive receptors that Julia has, we recommend supplementing 150nm/l (nanomoles per litre) or more, although NHS guidelines say that 50–75nm/l is adequate.

It is possible to overdo vitamin D supplementation and it can be toxic, so be careful to avoid excessive supplementation, which can only be confirmed by functional or blood testing as each person is different. The best food sources of vitamin D are oily fish, such as mackerel, salmon, tuna and sardines. Smaller amounts can be found in beef, pork, chicken, cheese, egg yolks and mushrooms. It is also very important to consider taking vitamin K alongside vitamin D to avoid excess calcium deposits in the arteries, and Julia's VKORC1 gene indicates a significantly increased need for vitamin K anyway.

Julia's 'metabolic' genetic results (particularly her TCF7L2 gene, which is responsible for insulin release) showed inefficiencies in processing sugar so that it is more likely to stay in her blood (circulation) for longer, rather than being transported efficiently into muscle cells. Being 'thin on the outside' does not equate to being metabolically healthy. Julia has cut out alcohol and sugar, which will be beneficial.

Gut feeling

Julia's UGT1A1 SNP is related to the gut. It means that her liver makes less UGT1A1 (a UDP-glucuronosyltransferase) and is less efficient at attaching the glucuronic acid to oestrogen (in this case) for it to be removed. Glucuronic acid is derived from glucose and found in fermentation products such as kombucha.

Apples, alfalfa and broccoli are good sources of glucuronides. *But* if you have too much of a certain bacteria (beta-glucuronidase) in your gut, this unpicks the oestrogen from the glucuronides, frees them up and they can then be reabsorbed and recirculated – adding to the oestrogen excess and the wrong kind of, or 'dirty', oestrogens.

Julia's FUT2 SNP suggests a genetic predisposition for a less diverse microbiome, so the potential is there for less of the good bacteria to outplay the beta-glucuronidase. We can support microbiome diversity by eating a varied diet including prebiotics – dietary fibre found in many vegetables, fruits and whole grains (making it food for the good bacteria) – and probiotics, such as yoghurt, kimchi, fermented pickles such as sauerkraut, which contain good bacteria to help outnumber the bad.

Summary

Nutrigenetics testing helps to identify a personalised need for specific nutrients and types of foods that will benefit you individually. Often several genetic SNPs will highlight the need for the same nutrient and lifestyle factors, such as in Julia's case less sugar and more fermented foods, enabling you to focus on incorporating a smaller, manageable amount of change that you know is right for you. It is never too early or too late to test, and as your genes don't change, you will have the benefit of self-knowledge throughout your life.

I want to include Emma's story for you below, because it demonstrates so clearly how this kind of test can improve everyday life, not just in relation to cancer.

Emma Beswick – a case study: run Emma run

In 2003, I had run the London Marathon. It was a big dream, but I ended up hating it, and I hit the wall at about the halfway point, and finished in just over five hours. In 2014, I faced it again, but this time I loved every minute, and finished in 3:49:24 – 11 years later (aged 45). My training was personalised this time around, and it was informed by my genetics and the testing I did. Instead of guessing, I confidently fuelled with fats over starchy, sugary carbs, against the 'popular' advice of 'carb loading'. With the knowledge that I'm ultra-sensitive to caffeine, I ditched it completely, but the 'big' one was iron. My genetics predispose me to iron-deficient anaemia, which hugely impacts delivery of oxygen to muscles and the ability to make ATP (energy). I followed up with a blood test to assess iron, so that I could safely increase my levels.

In addition to improving my running, these changes had knock-on effects on my overall health. Cutting out caffeine reduced my stress levels and jitteriness. Optimising my iron status supported my dopamine levels – helping me to focus – and my less 'addictive'-type behaviours (typical of a low-dopamine type), and probably it also protected me from a whole range of other health issues.

DNA test and longevity report

What is it?: saliva test for health reports to increase healthspan
Conducted via: The DNA Company (Canada), https://thedna-company.com/products/dna-360-report-with-longevity-report
Founded by entrepreneur Kashif Khan (when he was trying to get to the root cause of his own health issues), the DNA 360 test scans your saliva and uses 4.7 million data points to create a series of comprehensive health reports unique to you. Everything from the type of exercise suitable to you, supplement suggestions and nutritional advice are included in the reports.

Why test?

There are multiple DNA tests available globally, but the focus here is very much on health and lifestyle adaptations that can be made to increase healthspan. The millions of data points offer comprehensive insights.

My results

The APOE gene plays an important role in the health of your brain. Mine carries the 3/3 version of the APOE gene. This is considered 'normal'. Variations influence the risk for the deposit of amyloids, which are mutated proteins, in your brain. The increased presence of amyloids in your brain can increase your risk of cognitive disorders such as Alzheimer's disease, dementia and mild cognitive impairment (MCI).

Engaging in brain-boosting activities such as learning and speaking in a foreign language or playing chess, sudoku, and other logic-based activities can keep the mind sharp throughout our life.

Note: famously, the actor Chris Hemsworth discovered that he has two copies of the APOE4 gene when he was filming the health series *Limitless*. This genetic variant is linked to an increased risk of Alzheimer's. He has since made lifestyle changes and now campaigns to increase awareness.

My key findings, as listed by Kashif Khan, were:

- **Julia carries the GT version** of the TCF7L2 gene. This suggests an increased predisposition towards insulin resistance, which could lead to both type-2 diabetes and cognitive disorders such as Alzheimer's or dementia. (If you also carry the 3/4 or 4/4 version of the APOE gene, which Julia doesn't, you need to be extra careful with your sugar, carbohydrate and fat intake in your daily diet.)
- **Diet, going forward** Julia needs to watch carbohydrates, being mindful of starch (pasta, rice, bread) and sugar consumption by seeking out low-carb or no-carb alternatives to starchy carbohydrates and sticking to more complex carbohydrates such as sweet potatoes or nuts. She should aim to eat her carbohydrates during the morning and afternoon, but skip them for dinner.
- **Longevity** The FOXO3 gene is popularly known as the 'longevity gene'. FOXO3 helps to initiate DNA repair, kill off mutated or dying cells, respond quickly to inflammation, maintain healthy stem-cell production, and attack infectious organisms. Carrying at least one G allele in your FOXO3 result greatly increases your potential for longevity by reducing your body's oxidative load; Julia carries two (GG). This marks her longevity level as 'superhuman'! (While the GG variant is linked to certain health outcomes, however, it's not a definitive predictor of longevity or disease.)
- **Julia's superhuman longevity gene** obviously isn't a gold pass or a guarantee. She needs to take care of all areas of her health, because what you don't want is to be very old hanging on in poor health.

Acknowledgements

Writing each book is such an intense, all-encompassing experience, and everyone in your life has no choice but to live through it with you. Thank you to my family (ZXZ) for putting up with me tapping away on the laptop at the kitchen counter, on the beach and in the car over the past two years. Holidays, weekends and late evenings have been consumed by writing *Hack Yourself Healthy*: adding last-minute details, doing research and verifying facts. Thanks to my partner, G, for holding the fort while I've been away on field trips and filming, and thanks to other G in my life for being everywhere I could possibly need her.

Sarah Oliver, my co-writer, is a friend, colleague and someone who I admire greatly. Her emotional stability, steadfast nature and eye for detail are invaluable. There are very few humans on this planet with whom I have shared so many intimate moments. Many are in this book.

A huge, grateful hug to Anna Dixon at YMU Literary for sharing her extensive knowledge of the book world and being a reliable sounding board, always there with great advice. Thanks to my wonderful agent, Vanessa Fogerty, and the Curtis Brown team for taking care of me and helping me to manage that all-important 'work-life balance' thing!

Thank you to my publisher, Jillian Young, for all of her support, guidance and patience. Pinning me down for dates is always a trial! Rebecca Sheppard (managing editor), Louise Harvey (audio editor), Jan Cutler (copy-editor) and Charlotte

Ridings (proofreader) have pored over this book, correcting, tweaking and probing – painful and necessary tasks.

I'm grateful to Charlotte Stroomer, the cover designer, for working tolerantly through our ideas, and to David Venni for the beautiful photography and lighting. All of the images you see associated with this book are by him, with hair and make-up done by Alice Theobold, styled by Gayle Rinkoff. Thanks to Terry and the Hair Organics team and Daniel Field for the water-based safe hair colouring that I discovered four years ago. And thanks to my team at Hunter & Gather for keeping me fuelled.

If you're reading this, it is because Laura Vile, Clara Diaz and Narjas Zatat did a great job with the publicity.

A huge thanks to all of my contributors, labs, clinics, spas and wellness hubs that let me explore so many protocols and tests: Ananda, Broughton Sanctuary, Hooke London, HUM2N Lab, Oxygen Advantage, Levitas Clinic, Embracing Nutrition, Sixth Senses Douro Valley, Conscious Breathing, Regenerus Labs, ArminLabs, Invivo Healthcare, ORALIS 1, Lifecode Gx, Datar Cancer Genetics, PhlebPro, Amrita Nutrition, Thermocheck, Scan.com, The Health Society, Colab Services, The European Centre for Environment & Human Health at the University of Exeter, Clinical Education and the University of Vienna.

Finally, once again, I want to thank my parents, Chrissi and Michael Bradbury. They're both in their late eighties and they don't biohack, but they have both survived cancer. Throughout my own health trials, they have been a constant source of inspiration. The importance of love and social connections is highlighted in this book, and to be loved the way I am makes me feel very lucky indeed.

References

Chapter 2

1 Bourne, A., 'Why walking backwards can be good for your health and brain', *BBC Future*, 11 November 2023, https://www.bbc.com/future/article/20231110-why-walking-backwards-can-be-good-for-your-health-and-brain

Chapter 3

1 'Why are bowel cancer rates rising in younger adults?', The Royal Marsden, 25 March 2024, https://www.royalmarsden.nhs.uk/private-care/news-and-blogs/why-are-bowel-cancer-rates-rising-younger-adults
2 Routy, B., et al., 'Gut microbiome influences efficacy of PD-1-based immunotherapy against epithelial tumors', *Science*, 2 Nov 2017; 359, 6371: 91–7
3 Li, L., and McAllister, F., 'Too much water drowned the miller: *Akkermansia* determines immunotherapy responses', *Cell Reports Medicine*, 17 May 2002; 3(5):100642
4 Derosa, L., et al., 'Intestinal *Akkermansia muciniphila* predicts clinical response to PD-1 blockade in patients with advanced non-small-cell lung cancer', *Nat Med.*, Feb 2022; 28(2):315–24
5 Grajeda-Iglesias, C., et al., 'Oral administration of *Akkermansia muciniphila* elevates systemic antiaging and anticancer metabolites', *Aging*, 2 March 2021; 13(5):6375–405
6 'Fructose intake enhances lipoteichoic acid-mediated immune response in monocytes of healthy humans', *Science Direct*, 11 June 2025; 85:103729

Chapter 5

1 X.S., He and W.Y., Shi., 'Oral microbiology: Past, present and future', *Int J Oral Sci*, June 2009; 1(2):47–58

2 'Periodontal disease and cardiovascular risk', American Heart Association, 2012, Circulation

3 Barutta, F., et al., 'Novel insight into the mechanisms of the bidirectional relationship between diabetes and periodontitis', *Biomedicines*, 16 Jan 2022; 10(1):178

4 Beydoun, M., et al., 'Clinical and bacterial markers of periodontitis and their association with incident all-cause and Alzheimer's disease dementia in a large national survey', *Journal of Alzheimer's Disease*, 2020: 57–172

5 Eaton, K., et al., 'The WHO Global Oral Health Action Plan 2023–2030', *Community Dental Health*, 2023

Chapter 6

1 Ghosh, Pallab, 'Why do we sleep?', BBC News, 15 May 2015

Chapter 8

1 Stern, C., 'Is walking BAREFOOT the secret to a better life?', *Daily Mail*, 6 April 2017, https://www.dailymail.co.uk/femail/article-4387742/Gwyneth-Paltrow-swears-earthing-therapy.html

2 https://www.instagram.com/naomieharris/p/BWt8TclDYzC/

3 Chevalier, G., et al., 'Earthing: Health implications of reconnecting the human body to the earth's surface electrons', *National Library of Medicine*, 12 Jan 2012; 291541

Chapter 9

1 Exposure to mild heat-stress (heat shock) can significantly increase the life expectancy of the nematode *Caenorhabditis elegans*. Wu, D., et al., 'Multiple mild heat-shocks decrease the gompertz component of mortality in C. elegans', *Experimental Gerontology*, September 2009; 44(9): 607–12

2 Mołoń, M., et al., 'Effects of temperature on lifespan of *Drosophila Melanogaster* from different genetic backgrounds: Links between metabolic rate and longevity', *Insects*, 25 July 2020; 11(8):470, https://pmc.ncbi.nlm.nih.gov/articles/PMC7469197/

3 Heim, S., and Keil, A., 'Too much information, too little time: How the brain separates important from unimportant things in our fast-paced media world', *Frontiers for Young Minds*, 1 June 2017, https://kids.frontiersin.org/articles/10.3389/frym.2017.00023#ref1

4 Bohn, Roger E., and Short, J., 'Measuring consumer information', *ResearchGate*, January 2012; 6(1):980–1000

5 Bohn and Short, 'Measuring consumer information'
6 Laukkanen, T., et al.,'Association between sauna bathing and fatal cardiovascular and all-cause mortality events', *JAMA Intern Med*, 2015; 175(4):542–8
7 Laukkanen J.A., and Laukkanen, T., 'Sauna bathing and systemic inflammation', *Eur J Epidemiol*, March 2018; 33(3):351–3
8 Bearne, S., ' "There are so many benefits": why more and more Britons are building a home sauna', *Guardian*, 4 May 2024, https://www.theguardian.com/money/article/2024/may/04/there-are-so-many-benefits-why-more-and-more-britons-are-building-a-home-sauna
9 Palc, C., 'Heat therapy may lead to better outcomes in treating depression than cold exposure', *Medical News Today*, 9 February 2024, https://www.medicalnewstoday.com/articles/heat-therapy-sauna-better-outcomes-treating-depression-cold-exposure
10 Garolla, A., et al., 'Seminal and molecular evidence that sauna exposure affects human spermatogenesis', *Hum Reprod*, April 2013; 28(4):877–85; Rettner, R., 'Sauna visits may lower sperm count', *LiveScience*, 25 March 2013, https://www.livescience.com/28157-sauna-sperm-count.html
11 'A sauna session is just as exhausting as moderate exercise, study finds', *Science Daily*, 12 June 2019, https://www.sciencedaily.com/releases/2019/06/190612093900.htm

Chapter 10

1 'Brain Drain: The mere presence of one's own smartphone reduces available cognitive capacity', *Journal of the Association for Consumer Research*, 2017; 2(2)
2 Kaplan, R., and Kaplan, S., *The Experience of Nature: A Psychological Perspective*, Cambridge University Press, 1989
3 de Keijzer, C., et al., 'Residential surrounding greenness and cognitive decline: A 10-year follow-up of the Whitehall II Cohort', *Environmental Health Perspectives*, 2018; 126(7), 077003
4 Steininger, M.O., et. al., 'Nature exposure induces analgesic effects by acting on nociception-related neural processing', *Nature Communications*, 2025; 16, 2037

Chapter 11

1 Boccia, M., et al., 'The meditative mind: A comprehensive meta-analysis of MRI studies', *Biomed Res Int.*, 2015:419808

Chapter 12

1 'PTSD linked to increased risk of ovarian cancer', Harvard School of Public Health, 5 September 2019, https://www.hsph.harvard.edu/news/press-releases/ptsd-linked-to-increased-risk-of-ovarian-cancer/

2 'Stress and heart health', available on the American Heart Association website, this article outlines how stress and poor mental health contribute to cardiovascular disease risk

3 Whooley, M.A., and Wong, J.M., 'Depression and cardiovascular disorders: The American Heart Association Statistics', *JAMA Psychiatry*, 2013. Research links depression to higher rates of cardiovascular events, particularly in those with long-standing depression

4 Cohen, S., et al., 'Chronic stress, immune changes, and susceptibility to upper respiratory infections', *Psychosomatic Medicine*, 2012; 74(2): 227–32

5 American College of Gastroenterology, 'The impact of stress on gastrointestinal disorders', Findings discussed at their Annual Scientific Meeting. American College of Gastroenterology, (n.d.). 'Stress and Digestive Health'

6 Mezuk, B., et al., 'Depression and Type 2 diabetes: A meta-analysis of the association', *Diabetes Care*, 2008; 31(12): 2383–90

7 'Leisure activities and the risk of dementia in the elderly', *New England Journal of Medicine*, 2003; 348:2508–16

8 Melinda Maxfield Research on rhythmic beat of the drum and inducing the theta state

9 Van der Kolk, B.A., *The Body Keeps the Score: Brain, Mind, and Body in the Healing of Trauma*, Penguin: London, 2014

10 'Effect of exercise for depression: Systematic review and network meta-analysis of randomised controlled trials', *BMJ*, 2024; 384:e075847

11 Porges, S.W., *The Polyvagal Theory: Neurophysiological Foundations of Emotions, Attachment, Communication, and Self-Regulation*, W. W. Norton & Company: London, 2011

12 Move Dance Feel: https://www.movedancefeel.com/the-evidence

13 Delaney, B., 'Why I swapped my wellness obsession for Stoic philosophy', *The Times*, 12 February 2024, https://www.thetimes.com/life-style/health-fitness/article/why-i-swapped-my-wellness-obsession-for-stoic-philosophy-jww8fhsnk

14 Brod, S., et al., 'As above, so below: Examining the interplay between emotion and the immune system', *Immunology*, Nov 2014; 143(3):311–18

Chapter 13

1 The Queen's Reading Room: https://thequeensreadingroom.co.uk/the-queens-reading-room-study/

Chapter 14

1 García-Hermoso, A., et al., 'Muscular strength as a predictor of all-cause mortality in an apparently healthy population: A systematic review and meta-analysis of data from approximately 2 million men and women', *Arch Phys Med Rehabil.*, October 2018; 99(10):2100–113.e5

2 Lopez-Jaramillo, P., et al., 'Muscular strength in risk factors for cardiovascular disease and mortality: A narrative review', *Anatol J Cardiol.*, August 2022; 26(8):598–607

3 García-Hermoso, A., et al., 'Muscular strength as a predictor of all-cause mortality in an apparently healthy population: A systematic review and meta-analysis of data from approximately 2 million men and women', *Arch Phys Med Rehabil.*, October 2018; 99(10):2100–113.e5; Lopez-Jaramillo, P., et al., 'Muscular strength in risk factors for cardiovascular disease and mortality: A narrative review', *Anatol J Cardiol.*, August 2022; 26(8):598–607

4 Rantanen, T., et. al., 'Midlife hand grip strength as a predictor of old age disability', *JAMA*, 1999; 281(6):558–60

Chapter 15

1 Systematic Review and Meta-Analysis (2019): This comprehensive analysis examined the relationship between endometriosis and autoimmune diseases such as systemic lupus erythematosus (SLE), Sjögren's syndrome, rheumatoid arthritis and multiple sclerosis. The findings indicated a significant association between endometriosis and these autoimmune conditions, suggesting shared immunological mechanisms. Exploration of Autoimmune Characteristics in Endometriosis: This study investigated the presence of autoantibodies and immune system abnormalities in individuals with endometriosis. The results revealed that endometriosis shares traits with autoimmune diseases, including abnormal immune responses and inflammation, supporting the hypothesis of an autoimmune component in its pathogenesis. Association Between Endometriosis and Autoimmune Diseases: This research explored the coexistence of endometriosis with autoimmune conditions like inflammatory bowel disease (IBD). The study found an increased prevalence of autoimmune systemic diseases and various autoantibodies in individuals with endometriosis, suggesting that endometriosis could be considered an authentic autoimmune or inflammatory disease. Garber, J.E., et al., 'Factor V Leiden mutation and thromboembolism risk in women receiving adjuvant tamoxifen for breast cancer', *Journal of the National Cancer Institute*, 7 July 2010; 102(13):942–9; Dean, L., et al., 'Tamoxifen therapy and CYP2D6 genotype', Medical Genetics Summaries 7 Oct 2014 [Updated 1 May 2019]; Lazzeroni, M., et al., ' "Baby-TAM" dose may be effective, but not for everyone', *Journal of Clinical Oncology,* Epub 14 March 2023; Cos, S., et al., 'Melatonin as a selective estrogen enzyme modulator', *Current Cancer Drug Targets*, Dec 2008; 8(8):691–702

2 Fan, S., et al., 'Akkermansia muciniphila: A potential booster to improve the effectiveness of cancer immunotherapy', *Journal of Cancer Research and Clinical Oncology*, Nov 2023; 149(14):13477–94; 'Akkermansia muciniphila can be a biomarker of response to cancer therapy, study suggests', Microbiome Post, 4 March 2022; Derosa, L., et al., 'Intestinal *Akkermansia muciniphila* predicts clinical response to PD-1 blockade in patients with advanced non-small-cell lung cancer', *Nature Medicine*, 2022; 28: 315–24; 'Gut microbiome may influence pancreatic cancer survival', Helio, 10 May 2023; Pei, B., et al., 'Bifidobacterium modulation of tumor immunotherapy and its mechanism', *Cancer Immunology Immunotherapy*, 2 Apr 2024; 73(5):94; Longhi, G., et al., 'Microbiota and cancer: The emerging beneficial role of Bifidobacteria in cancer immunotherapy', *Frontiers in Microbiology*, 2020; 11:575072

Appendix

1 Sanz, M., et al., 'Periodontitis and cardiovascular diseases: Consensus report', *Journal of Clinical Periodontology*, Mar 2020; 47(3):268–88; Preshaw, P.M., et al., 'Periodontitis and diabetes: A two-way relationship', *Diabetologia*, Jan 2012; 55(1):21–31; Wu, C. Z., et al., 'Epidemiologic relationship between periodontitis and type 2 diabetes mellitus, *BMC Oral Health*, 2020; 20, 204; Beydoun, M., et al., 'Clinical and bacterial markers of periodontitis and their association with incident all-cause and Alzheimer's disease dementia in a large national survey', *Journal of Alzheimer's Disease*, 2020; 75(1):157–72; Zhou, X., et al., 'Updated evidence of association between periodontal disease and incident erectile dysfunction', *Journal of Sexual Medicine*, Jan 2019; 16(1):61–9; Sanz, M., et al., working group 3 of the joint EFP/AAP workshop, 'Periodontitis and adverse pregnancy outcomes: Consensus report of the Joint EFP/AAP Workshop on Periodontitis and Systemic Diseases', *Journal of Periodontology*, Apr 2013; 84(4 Suppl):S164–9; Zepeda-Rivera, M., et al., 'A distinct *Fusobacterium nucleatum* clade dominates the colorectal cancer niche', *Nature*, 2024; 628: 424–32

THE NAVIGATOR

THE
NAVIGATOR

Robert Wales

HEADLINE

British Library Cataloguing in Publication Data

Wales, Robert
The navigator
I. Title
823'.914 [F]

ISBN 0-7472-0165-X

Typeset in 11/11½ pt English Times
by Colset Private Limited, Singapore

Printed and bound in Great Britain by
Richard Clay Ltd, Bungay, Suffolk

HEADLINE BOOK PUBLISHING PLC
Headline House,
79 Great Titchfield Street
London W1P 7FN

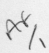

To John and Sybil

Prologue

On a morning in the world of snow and ice that was the New England February of 1832, twenty-one-year-old Jim McBain walked with rolling gait under the line of bowsprits that protruded over Boston's Long Wharf, his bag slung over his shoulder. Having just returned from France as mate on a Havre packet he was on his way to find cheap lodging in Purchase Street, but he was not too worried. His captain had promised him that he would sign him on again for the next sailing if the harbour did not ice up in the meantime and it was simply a matter of filling in time at the least possible expense. That was the loneliest time for him. He had long since discovered it was hardly worthwhile trying to make new friends ashore. You just started to get to know somebody and you were off again. At sea it was easier. Although crews changed all the time too, everyone fitted into their place to do their jobs, bound together by the way of life and communicating with the common jargon of seamen.

'Mr McBain!' the voice called and he turned his head. Outside the counting house of Kimball and Jay he saw their wharfinger beckoning him. He did not know the man to speak to but knew well enough who he was and the wharfinger clearly knew him. He went over to him.

'Yes, sir?' he said.

'Mr Kimball and Mr Jay would like to have a word with you. They asked me to keep an eye open for you.'

'Me?' Jim queried. 'What for?'

'You'll have to ask them that,' the wharfinger said, 'I'll tell them you're here,' and leaving Jim standing there he went inside and up the stairs. Jim had no idea what it might be about. Kimball and Jay were small, independent operators running a packet carrying passengers and freight between Boston and Liverpool in England. The wharfinger was not long in returning.

'They'll see you now,' he said and directed him to go up the stairs. Jim dumped his bag, went up, knocked on the door and was invited to enter.

1

The two men were seated at opposite sides of the same desk.

'I'm Mr Kimball,' said the larger of them.

'And I'm Mr Jay,' said the much smaller one.

Although Jim had seen them in the past getting into their separate carriages he had never seen them together. He judged them to be in their late thirties, or maybe forty.

'How do you do, sirs,' Jim said and was invited to sit on a chair at one end of the desk. It was clear to both Mr Kimball and Mr Jay that Mr McBain lacked polish but that was something which could be acquired with a bit of practice.

'How long have you been at sea now, Mr McBain?' Mr Kimball asked him.

'Since I started as a cabin boy at ten, sir,' Jim replied.

'A long time,' Mr Kimball noted.

'A very long time,' Mr Jay added.

In fact Mr Kimball and Mr Jay had already made it their business to find out all about McBain and had had their eye on him for some time. They already knew he was self-taught, could navigate, could speak French and Spanish which was a necessary qualification, that he was a moderate drinker and was solid and reliable.

'You have any family, Mr McBain?' Mr Kimball enquired and Jim hesitated.

'Relatives,' Mr Jay encouraged.

'None to speak of, sirs,' Jim replied, curious as to what it was all about.

'Why is that?' Mr Kimball said.

'My father was killed in an accident in the granite quarry at Quincy when I was eight, sirs,' Jim explained, 'and I suppose because there were ten of us to feed my mother married again soon after. But we started to split up after that and my mother and stepfather moved away. Being away at sea so long I lost touch with them and don't know where any of them are now.'

After several more questions which were simply to help them make a personal assessment of the mate Mr Kimball said, 'Do you mind waiting downstairs for a moment, Mr McBain?'

Jim rose, well aware that he had been closely scrutinised.

'Do you mind telling me, sir, what . . .?' he began, only to be interrupted.

'In a little while,' Kimball said.

Jim made his way back down and confronted the wharfinger.

'What in the hell do they want?' he wanted to know. 'If they're looking for a mate why don't they just say so? I've never had to be interviewed by ship owners before. That's a captain's duty.'

2

'But their captain isn't here, Mr McBain, is he?' was all the wharfinger said.

Across their desk Mr Kimball and Mr Jay looked at each other.

'What do you think?' Mr Kimball said.

'What do you?' Mr Jay returned.

'He's very young, only twenty-one,' Mr Kimball opined.

'But older than his years,' Mr Jay pointed out.

'A little rough.'

'There is that,' Mr Jay agreed.

'We could be taking a risk with him.'

'There is that, too.'

But although it worried them a little that McBain was unfashionably clean-shaven they thought they could tolerate that and each knew the other had already made up his mind. So, after a short while, Jim McBain was called back and found himself seated again, more curious than ever.

'You know our ship the *Nantasket*, Mr McBain?' Mr Kimball questioned.

'I've seen her several times, sir,' Jim replied, 'but I've never been aboard her.'

'A fine vessel,' Kimball assured him.

'A very fine vessel,' Mr Jay added.

'Did you know her master, Captain Tyler, is retiring?' Mr Kimball said.

'No, I did not, sir,' Jim told him, and even then it did not strike him.

'Well, he is,' Mr Jay confirmed, 'when he gets back. In about a month to six weeks' time.'

'And we wish to offer you command of our ship as his replacement, Mr McBain,' Mr Kimball said.

It took a few moments to sink in and Jim looked from one to the other, stunned. In all his years at sea he had regarded ship's masters as gods, even if some of them were mortal and had bits of clay sticking to their feet. At sixteen he had been an able-bodied seaman aloft, serving before the mast, at seventeen a foremast hand, at eighteen a second mate for little extra in wages, at twenty a first mate on a packet for not much more. Since the age of twelve he had spent every penny he could save on books, studied hard through fair weather and foul in stinking, ill-lit, unruly fo'c'sles amongst hard men on his off-watch, aiming towards what often seemed like the unachievable goal. And he knew exactly what competition he was up against, the college-educated men and the sons and nephews of owners who, after only a year aboard as trainee deck officers, were given command for a year or so more before joining fathers and uncles in the counting houses. He had thought that if he worked hard enough, in a few more years he just might be able to attain the unattainable. Not in his wildest imaginings did he dream that without any warning whatsoever the opportunity would be presented to him at the age of twenty-one. It was almost unbelievable.

'Master of the *Nantasket*, Mr McBain,' he heard Mr Jay say further. It was not often Jim McBain was at a loss for words but he certainly was now.

'I don't know what to say, sirs,' he finally managed. 'I don't know how I can thank you enough.'

'You can do that by making sure our vessel is well run, makes respectable passage times, does not sink and returns a decent profit, Mr McBain,' Mr Kimball informed him.

'I'll do all that and more,' Jim got in eagerly.

'Your primage will, of course, be the normal five per cent and the money for carrying the mail will be your own as is the practice.'

'You have any questions?' Mr Jay enquired.

'No, sir, none.'

'Then keep closely in touch with our wharfinger and be ready to take over the *Nantasket* on her return, Mr McBain,' Mr Kimball said finally and he and Mr Jay rose to their feet, bringing Jim quickly to his. They held out their hands in turn and Jim shook them firmly. 'I'll do my utter best for you, sirs,' he said and, knowing he was dismissed, made his way out in a haze. Kimball and Jay sat down again at their desk, facing each other.

'I think he was most appreciative, don't you?' Mr Kimball said.

'Very,' Mr Jay replied.

Jim McBain was more than appreciative. He was ecstatic and had he been a man of lesser control he might have danced. As it was, his feet were at least six inches off the ground. It was the very peak of his career and there was not another thing in life he wanted. Nothing. He was a god, looking down on the less fortunate mortals who would never know what it was like to stand on a quarterdeck in supreme command. After a few words with the wharfinger during which he could hardly contain his excitement, he picked up his bag and walked out on to the freezing wharf, no longer to head for Purchase Street but for lodging in Summer Street that would befit his status. His life was totally and utterly complete. The small boy who had once not even had a pair of boots to his feet had reached the very top. Soon he would buy a new suit and a fine tall hat for his shore clothes. He would be a gentleman or he would be nothing.

In Summer Street he did find lodging in the house of the ageing

4

widow of a retired captain. Then, feeling desperate to find some-body with whom to share his news, he took the coach to Cambridge to tell a bosun's mate with whom he had once sailed for two years, a man who had given up the sea and borrowed money to start a small turkey farm. There he spent a most pleasant evening with the turkey farmer who could not have been more delighted for him. It was dark when he left although his old acquaintance had pressed him to stay the night. With half a moon rising into the broken sky, he decided he would walk all the way back to Boston and save money. He was going to need every bit of that to see him through. He made his way across the deep white of a field, enjoying every moment of the fresh crunching sound the virgin snow made under his feet with childlike pleasure. The world was his. But then, as he almost reached the Boston Road, it happened.

Chapter One

Amelia Hall felt herself being tumbled over in the darkness. She remembered cries of fright, the sound of cracking wood, the images of shadows on the moonlit snow coming towards her and the bare, outstretched limbs of trees. And that was all.

When she woke she did not know how long she had lain there but became aware she was not on the ground, rather on a couch with a blanket over her in a lamplit room with a fire burning in the grate. Then she saw the two figures standing back a little way, observing her. One was a grey-haired, grey-whiskered man in a suit, with pince-nez halfway down his long nose. The other was a young man in a heavy broadcloth jacket with a hint of steam rising from the lower end of his trousers which were wet and drying in the warmth. What was unusual about him was not so much that he wore no whiskers about his face but his colouring. Although he had dark hair his eyes were of a strong blue. Even although her head was hurting she could not help but think him handsome. Then Pince-nez came forward to her, bent over her and gently prised her eyelids further open to examine her. Her large, deep brown eyes appeared clear and undilated.

'Good,' he said, letting her go. 'Now just rest for a time and when you feel like it you can tell us all about yourself.'

'I'm Amelia Hall,' she said without waiting, 'I was in an accident. The coach turned over.'

'Yes, we know,' said Pince-nez. 'This gentleman reached it only a minute after and when he found there was no family with you quickly fetched a man with a cart and got you back here to Cambridge.'

'Oh,' she uttered, at least knowing where she was, but not understanding why she began to feel embarrassed.

'You've had a little bit of a shock,' Pince-nez said, 'I'll mix you a draught that will ease it,' and he had gone from the room before she could gather her wits enough either to answer, ask him who he was or thank him.

'Don't worry, you'll be all right now,' the man in the broadcloth

7

offered with a reassuring smile. 'I'm sure the doctor knows what he's doing.' To Amelia, even his voice bore strength and confidence.

'It's not like me to be knocked out, sir,' she said. 'Not like me at all.'

'Isn't it?' the man said, and she could tell he was amused by that. 'Well, it does happen now and then. I've been knocked out myself before now.'

'Have you?'

'Oh, yes, several times.'

For a moment she looked at him directly but found herself having to glance away. Her eye caught the bag with which she had been travelling and that was reassuring too.

'What about the others with me?' she asked with concern.

'No need to trouble yourself about them either, Miss Hall. No one else was badly hurt and even the horses were quick back on their feet as soon as they were cut free. They were all taken on in a wagon and are probably in Boston by now.'

'I must thank you kindly, sir.'

'No need, it was my duty and my pleasure. I'm Jim McBain by the way. Captain Jim McBain.'

Intended to impress the very pretty girl to whom he was already taking more than a liking it did just that. And although only sixteen Amelia was not so ignorant she could not tell the difference between a soldier and a sailor.

'A sea captain,' she said unnecessarily.

'Of a Liverpool packet.'

'A Liverpool packet. How wonderful for you, sir.'

Again their eyes met, Amelia finding she swiftly had to avert her gaze.

'At least I should be soon,' Jim corrected, it somehow seeming important to tell this girl the truth. 'In another month to six weeks I'll be a captain.'

'A captain tomorrow, a captain today, it's surely all the same, sir,' she found herself saying in a moment of sheer inspiration and was aware out of the corner of her eye he was amused again. But a further exchange had to wait as Pince-nez returned with his mild draught of laudanum.

'No need to sit right up,' the doctor told her as she made the move.

'But I want to, sir, I'm perfectly all right,' she insisted, swinging her feet to the floor and sitting upright before sipping her medicine with the sophistication and dignity of a lady.

'How old are you, young lady?' old Pince-nez asked.

'Seventeen, sir.' She found herself lying by a year without hesitation.

'And where did you come from and where are you going to?' the nosey doctor questioned further over the top of his spectacles.

'I was on my way from my father's farm,' Amelia explained. 'That's four miles this side of Worcester and I'm going to stay with my aunt, Miss Dorothea Jackson, for a few days. She has a cottage in Boston in West Street.'

'Ah, *that* Hall,' Pince-nez said with recognition. 'Your father is a fine upstanding gentleman by all accounts although I don't think I've met him. I've heard of your aunt, too. A very charitable lady, I believe.'

'Yes, she is,' Amelia confirmed. 'She does a lot of good things for people.'

Jim was beginning to feel unreasonably resentful of the doctor having Miss Amelia Hall all to himself but could find no excuse for intervening.

'Isn't your father the one at present planning to move away?' asked Pince-nez with a questioning lift of his grey eyebrows.

'Yes, we're going to take up new land near Erie as soon as the thaw comes.'

Why, on the most successful day in all his life, Jim felt somewhat dismayed at that he could not have explained.

'Well, it's too late for you to go on to Boston tonight, young lady,' Pince-nez said, 'and in any case you may not be fully recovered. You'll stay here for the night and I'll arrange for you to go on in the morning.'

'I can look after that,' Jim heard himself say quickly before Amelia had time to reply. 'I'm staying in Cambridge for the night and *I* can escort Miss Hall safely to her aunt's tomorrow.'

'You're very kind, sir,' Amelia said in acceptance and felt excited at the prospect although she could not show it and cast her large eyes shyly down.

'Then I think,' Pince-nez said to the sailor, 'it might be better if you took your leave now and allowed the young lady a good night's rest.'

'But I'm not in the least tired, sir,' Amelia meekly tried to protest.

'I would thank you, young woman,' Pince-nez said with some severity, 'if while you're here you do as I tell you.' And with that he began to show the sailor out.

'I'll return sharply at eight with transport for you, Miss Hall,' Jim informed her over his departing shoulder.

'Thank you, Captain, I'll be ready,' Amelia returned.

9

At the outside door, Jim dipped into his jacket for money. 'She seems a bright young lady and will no doubt ask about settlement. Just tell her that under the circumstances the expenses are being waived. You understand, sir?'

Old Pince-nez accepted the money with graciousness and bid him goodnight.

But in the morning eight o'clock came and went. And only fifteen minutes later Amelia Hall was plunging from the heights of expectancy into doubt and despair. Over and over she went to the front window and looked out, only to see nothing but the white-clad roofs of a few other houses, the bare elms, a smoking chimney and the snow.

'Perhaps your escort's been held up, Miss Hall,' Pince-nez's wife offered in comfort, but as Amelia had once heard someone say that nothing delayed a good sea captain unless he'd been dismasted, it was no comfort at all. But she was quite wrong about that since there were other things that could hold a sailor up and only a little while later there was Jim McBain with it, approaching the house, leading on foot what was a shaggy horse pulling an old buggy with a much-patched hood. And Amelia threw open the door and hurried out to meet him, full of smiles. He looked sheepish and more than a little upset.

'I'm very sorry, Miss Hall,' he greeted her apologetically, 'but this beast I borrowed from my friend is either a damned yardarm furler or its tops'ls are missing and I don't know which. Either it wants to do nothing or take me into a tree at a gallop. There's no in-between with it. Without an anchor or a gale behind I had no choice but to walk. If you can please be a bit more patient with me, I'll take it back and make other arrangements.'

'I'm sorry you've had so much trouble over me, Captain,' Amelia said and went up to the horse to rub it on the forehead.

'It doesn't deserve that, it should be dog meat for keeping you waiting,' Jim hastened to tell her. 'If you can give me another hour.'

Amelia, judging the horse to have a kind enough eye, said, 'Let *me* try it.'

'No, no, don't, Miss Hall,' the sailor warned but before he could stop her, Amelia hopped nimbly up on to the buggy and slapped the reins across its rump. The scraggy horse walked obediently away and she drove it around in a circle, Jim watching anxiously, ready to spring to her rescue, but there was no need. Amelia made it trot, stop, back up, walk forward again and do as she liked with it. In other circumstances, Jim might have been annoyed by the showing up of his inadequacy. Instead he felt most appreciative of the cleverness of this very pretty girl.

'No damned malingering or losing its rudder with you, Miss Hall,' he said when she pulled up alongside him and Amelia, eager to relieve him of any embarrassment he might have felt, replied, 'You must have taught it a good lesson on the way, Captain, and knocked all its contrariness out of it.'

The Pince-nezs stood looking on from their doorway, both concerned.

'*There's* trouble brewing if I ever saw it,' Pince-nez commented to his wife. 'The man is making a fool of himself and so is she.'

They saw the girl smile, her large brown eyes shining like stars, and like a child asking for a special favour, say, 'Would you let me drive it, Captain? Please? I love to drive,' and heard him reply, 'I'm in your hands, Miss Hall.'

Shortly after, their thanks and brief farewells said to the Pince-nezs, Amelia, reins in hand, frayed blanket over her lap and the sailor squeezed into the restricted space beside her, drove on to the track to head for the wooden bridge and the road to Boston. At first they went in silence, simply enjoying each other's presence and the wonderful shared secrecy of being alone. It was not until they reached the river that Amelia was suddenly struck with worry. She had always been inclined to act impetuously and it had got her into trouble before, but it did not stop her now.

'I lied to you last night,' she blurted out without warning and in surprise Jim looked at the profile of her adorable, anxious face, her eyes fixed straight over the horse's ears.

'I'm sure you had a perfectly good reason,' he replied forgivingly, but he had to wait a few moments to find out in what way she had deceived him, and he too worried.

'I'm not actually seventeen until much later in the year,' came rushing out and Amelia felt she might throw herself from the buggy and over the rail of the bridge to drown in the icy water below if the captain saw her differently because of her age. She heard the laugh that was from relief as much as anything and she turned her head to him.

'Goddamnit, Mis Hall,' he said, 'seventeen tomorrow, seventeen today, it's surely all the same, isn't it?'

And not having to drown all life returned to her and they laughed together in pleasure, the very first tiny pain of their relationship over.

As there was no cause for hurry, particularly on the rough, icy surface, they took their time, the sailor, on her questioning, telling her where he had been on his travels. Many times in New Orleans and down in Rio, several times down around Cape Horn and all the way up the Pacific to the Columbia River for cargoes of furs. Hawaii, Australia, England, France, Italy.

'My goodness, you've seen all of the world, Captain!' Miss Hall exclaimed in wonderment.

'Not all of it by any means,' Jim admitted modestly, 'and I wish you'd call me Jim instead of Captain.'

'I could never call you that,' Amelia told him firmly, disappointing him.

'Why not? It is my name.'

'Because I don't think it's dignified for a man of your position, that's why.'

'But it's what I've been called all my life, Miss Hall.'

'Maybe so, but I shall call you James.'

'James?' Jim repeated, amused.

'It's either James or Captain and nothing else,' she insisted, 'it's for you to decide.'

'Is it, now?' James answered, even more amused.

'Yes,' she stated, 'you're the captain.'

So charmed was Jim McBain by Miss Amelia Hall, it is entirely possible he might seriously have considered changing his name to Ebenezer the Tenth to please her. 'Then James it is, Miss Hall,' he consented.

'Thank you,' she smiled. 'And you shall call me Amy. I've always hated Amelia.'

It was a voyage of discovery, that slow road to Boston, during which James was not only enthralled by the girl's eloquence but by the extent of her general knowledge which was highly unusual for any woman and he questioned where she had got it all from.

'It wasn't really intended for me,' she explained. 'Although my father's a very religious man he has little faith in churches and instead of sending my six brothers to church school in Worcester he got them a tutor to teach them at home, a Mr Hayne, and I was allowed to join the lessons when I was old enough, although my five sisters never bothered. But I can do mathematics.'

'You can what?' James queried almost in disbelief, and in case the captain thought she meant only arithmetic, Amy added, 'And a bit of geometry and trigonometry as well.' For a few moments, James was speechless. For years in heaving fo'c'sles he had struggled and suffered until his brain was about to burst trying to get a grasp of these things and here was this lovely-looking girl talking as if it had come as naturally to her as breathing.

12

Amy worried again. She knew full well the risk she had been taking with her admission since there were many men who bitterly resented a woman having knowledge. If there were many local boys who had eyed her with lust and longing, they shied clear of her because of it. 'That girl's touched by the Devil and can be nothing but trouble,' frightened fathers had warned them. 'A woman who has anything else in her head but knowing a woman's duties and proper place in the home is headed for Hell and taking all with her. If she ever snares some poor fool then may the good God help him. He'll be the one after a hard day's toil in the field who'll find his weary bones stirring the pot to feed her and be carrying her half-starved children up the stairs in the dark while she sits with the lamp and her nose stuck in a book. A man would be better off dead than suffer the likes of it.'

In truth, the sailor had never given a thought as to what damage it might do for a woman to know so many things. When the subject of women arose on the decks of ships at sea, education was certainly not amongst the attributes or failings they considered.

'You've been very lucky, then, Amy Hall,' he said at last to Amy's great relief since she could tell he was sincerely impressed and not in the slightest resentful.

'There now,' she said, happily restored, 'I've confessed all my sins and have no more to tell.'

It was not until the semaphore signal tower of Telegraph Hill came into view that the cold reality of the immediate future loomed like an insurmountable obstacle, but there seemed to be no way around it. A parting there had to be and they were thrown back on their own dependencies, already separated without any kind of resolution. And the closer they got to West Street, the worse Amy Hall felt since her Captain James McBain made no suggestion and offered no comforting remedy. She had always been a self-sufficient girl but it was not helping her now. Not that James was without thoughts. Indeed there were far too many of them and he struggled to clarify the essence of their meaning. Only the day before he had been the happiest man in all America, now because of Amy Hall he was becoming the most disturbed. The two events falling one on top of the other were simply not compatible. Amy Hall was shortly to be taken away by her family to Erie, an impossible distance away, while he would soon be taking over as Master of the *Nantasket*. Common sense alone should have been telling him which was the more important, yet common sense and reason did not seem enough. A storm at sea he could handle with confidence, but not this. Nothing would come to him.

'That's it there,' Amy said, trying to conceal the tremble in her voice as she pointed out the cottage.

'That one there,' James said, at a loss as to what to say and simply nodding his head towards it, feeling an idiot. He determined to make his feelings known to her, no matter what, but he did not get the chance. The moment Amy pulled the horse up outside, she leapt from the buggy and, stricken as if to die, was through the gate and hurrying up the path. At the same time, Miss Dorothea Jackson who had seen the approach of the buggy from her window opened her front door to step out in her black dress, welcoming arms wide, with a cry of 'Amelia!' But all was confusion as Amy, head lowered, did not stop at her, but rushed past to go inside and release her tears where neither James McBain nor anyone else could see them, leaving her aunt standing there in mystification. Not only at her niece's behaviour but at the man in the broadcloth jacket hastening towards her with Amelia's small travel bag, looking pained from his head to his boots and in the deepest apprehension.

'Whatever's the matter?' Miss Jackson demanded to know of him and since there was no possibility of him making any other kind of explanation, he started to say, 'Miss Hall was in an unfortunate accident last night when her coach overturned and . . .' It was as far as he got but if he thought that was all Miss Jackson understood he was wrong.

'Accident?' she cut in. 'The poor child!' And, grabbing Amelia's bag from him, turned to go inside to attend to her, James desperate to stop her.

'Wait a minute, wait a minute – please!' he pleaded, 'I'd like your permission to call on her while she's here.'

'Call on her, call on her?' Miss Jackson came back quickly almost as if anticipating his request. 'I'm not at liberty to give you any such permission, sir. Good day to you.' And with that, she closed the door on him. Shut out, he stood for a few moments in dismay but had no choice other than to make his way back down the path. With no one on whom to vent his anger against himself, he glared at the horse.

'God damn and curse you, you stupid, lop-eared ass,' he swore at it and led the indifferent shaggy animal away to find a stable where it could be fed and sheltered, not knowing if he would ever see Miss Amy Hall again.

Chapter Two

James McBain got no proper rest. The disembodied head and face of Amy Hall kept coming towards him in the dark and would not go away. Not that he wanted it to. There had been the odd occasion at sea at ten or eleven years of age when, with no one to turn to in troubled moments, he had buried himself in some ship's locker and secretly wept with loneliness, but that had been a long time ago and he had become used to it, learning to handle it every bit as well as sheets, braces, halyards and sail. As a man not much given to introspection he rarely gave it a thought any more. Yet after having spent only one day in the company of Amy Hall, a sense of loneliness was beginning to smoulder in him like a fire and he could not put it out.

It was still dark when his widowed landlady gave him breakfast.

'Do you know of a Miss Dorothea Jackson who lives in West Street?' he questioned her.

'I know *of* her,' the widow told him, 'and know her by sight. A very fine lady. Does much charitable work and is greatly concerned by the plight of our poor lunatics, I'm told.'

That sounded very encouraging to James. Any woman kind enough to be concerned about lunatics would surely not turn him away if he presented himself properly. His breakfast finished, he walked out into the frozen streets to walk all of Boston, impatiently waiting for what he thought the charitable lady, Miss Jackson, might consider to be a respectable and convenient hour. Although still dark, merchants were already arriving from their homes in their carriages to converge on the Post Office for their mail before heading for their counting houses. The wharves were already becoming busy with activity in the dim, winter light rising from the Atlantic. It was not yet eight when he knocked on the cottage door, prepared, determined, buoyed up in expectation.

'Good morning,' he said brightly, but the black-clad figure quickly put a finger up to her lips and seemed not at all surprised to see him. 'Sh,' she whispered, 'She's still asleep. I gave her a little something to help.'

15

'I'm sorry,' James apologised, keeping his voice down as low as he could, and felt her bony fingers grasp his hand as she raised a smile he did not expect.

'Mr McBain, Mr McBain,' she whispered, 'how can we ever thank you? And how can you ever forgive me for dismissing you like that yesterday? I didn't know what you'd done for her.'

James, more used to yelling his lungs out on deck against the wind, felt a little awkward having to engage in whispers on a doorstep.

'It was no more than my duty, Miss Jackson,' he voiced quietly, 'but if you'll understand my intentions are nothing but honourable, maybe you'll let me come back and see her when she wakes.'

Miss Jackson raised her mouth much closer to his ear as if in the greatest secrecy. 'Oh, Mr McBain,' she hushed with sympathy, 'would that I could so easily.'

'But I just want to talk to her, Miss Jackson.'

'Oh, Mr McBain, you must be a man of the world and will not be upset when I'm honest and say I think it's courting you have in mind?'

'I just want to see her,' he persisted.

'Oh dear, oh dear, I know, Mr McBain, but what would her father say when I'm meant to be acting responsibly and taking good care of her?'

'Miss Jackson . . .' he managed further and suddenly she was grasping his hand again like a willing conspirator.

'All right, listen, listen, I tell you what I'll do. You come back in three days when our minds are more settled and we can all have afternoon tea together,' and she leaned so close to his ear again she was almost touching him, adding, 'I'll bake you some very special tea rusks.'

If James McBain had been thinking more clearly, he might have asked Miss Jackson why, if Mr Hall was so protective of his daughter, he had let her travel alone from Worcester in a public coach. Neither did he notice from the damp around the hem of Miss Jackson's dress and on her black boots that she had already been out that morning. All he could see was that the lady appeared to be favouring him and was doing her very best for him.

'Thank you, Miss Jackson,' he said quietly in appreciation.

'Until Friday then, Mr McBain,' she smiled and turned to go back inside, giving him a little wave before softly closing the door.

For the next three days, James did all he could to keep himself busy. He arranged to have the horse and buggy returned to Cambridge with a letter of thanks, bought his new sea clothes and shore clothes and spent an interminably long day in the shops of instrument-makers looking for the cheapest sextants, chronometers and deck watches. He had hardly enough money left to cover them and was unable to make up his mind. There were many older captains who refused to go to such expense for their navigation, relying on dead-reckoning and experience alone, but James knew he was going to need all the help science could give him. Several times he presented himself at the small warehouse of Kimball & Jay on Long Wharf. And there, amid the lingering smell of cheeses, spices, freshly cut lumber, Madeira wine and other produce with clerks sitting writing out lists and accounts and apprentices laboriously making out copies in the same hand, he discussed with the wharfinger freight, stowage, and what passenger bookings there might be for the next sailing out of the *Nantasket*. But through it all, it was Miss Amy Hall who was uppermost in his mind and he could not wait to see her again. He had met other pretty girls in ports around the world and had even had the luck to have bedded two of them, but there had been little genuine sorrow in the partings. With Amy Hall it was all quite different and he ached to have her back by his side every bit as much as he longed to take over the *Nantasket* as her master.

It was in the highest of expectations that James, all dressed up in his black suit and fine tall hat, turned up on the Friday afternoon at the door of Miss Dorothea Jackson's cottage.

'My dear Mr McBain,' she greeted him, looking a little solemn, 'come in, come in,'

Hat in hand, James entered, controlling his excitement and keeping his reserve like a proper gentleman should. The aroma of fresh baking was seductively warm and sweet, the blazing wood fire crackled with hospitality and the table gleamed with fine china set on the whitest of linen.

'Sit down, sit down, Mr McBain,' Miss Jackson offered. 'The kettle's near to the boil and won't be a minute.' And he sat, missing the touch of gravity in her voice, eyes alert for any movement, ready to spring to his feet with a smile the instant Amy appeared.

'I hope Miss Hall is fully recovered,' he said.

'Oh, yes,' she replied, 'a bump and a bruise is nothing to the young.'

'Good,' said James.

'Oh, Mr McBain, Mr McBain,' she suddenly lamented, 'what could I do, Mr McBain, what could I do?'

'About what, Miss Jackson?' he asked anxiously, now sensing something was badly wrong.

'Miss Amelia isn't here. Two of her brothers arrived early this morning and whisked her away back home. She didn't want to go, of course, but neither she nor myself had any say in the matter. Oh, Mr McBain, I'm so sorry.'

Mr McBain, his sails in tatters, his holds awash, ready to go down, sat there and stared at her. The lid of the iron kettle rattled and spat water to steam on the hot surface of the stove.

'I'll make the tea, Mr McBain,' Miss Jackson said quietly as if not to desecrate the sadness, and took the teapot away.

What neither James McBain nor Amy Hall knew, or were ever to know, was that on the very morning three days before when the sailor had so impatiently walked the early streets, it was not a Boston merchant who had been first to the Post Office but Miss Dorothea Jackson, hurrying to have a letter sent to Mr Hall. In it she told a rather confused story of a captain who was not a captain and of the coach accident. Cleverly she said that the man seemed quite presentable to her but on making discreet enquiries there were those who thought him to be a most unsavoury gentleman. Needless to say, she knew exactly what Amelia's father's reaction would be and the timing of it. But no one, not even those who knew her best, would have believed the satisfaction she got from the outcome.

'You can come to the table now if you would, please, Mr McBain,' she said politely and with an unmistakable tone of sympathy. 'I do so much hope you like the tea rusks I made specially for you.' And James had no option but to impose some self-discipline and re-seat himself, even if he did feel like a man wallowing on the lee shore of distress. More than painful, it was excruciating for him, but it would have been the height of rudeness and ingratitude to the kind lady to have picked up his hat and left.

'I'm very, very sorry, Mr McBain,' she said, offering her plate of warm rusks, 'very sorry. Take as many as you like, go on.' He took one, and she went on, 'But we can't question the ways of the Lord. He giveth and He taketh away and there's no help for it. Sugar?'

It was only with the greatest difficulty that James managed to sip the tea that had gone mouldy on its long voyage, get through a rusk, and be polite. He wanted to nurse his loss on his own, get shot in the neck in a rum mill, anything.

'You see, I'm not really Miss Hall's proper aunt, being only first cousin to her father,' he heard her say, 'but I've been aunt to all of them all their lives. Used to take a cottage for two weeks in the summer out on Long Island and take some of them there with me. They used to love going out to see the light on the headland there.

18

You must know it very well, Mr McBain, sailing in and out of the harbour so many times.'

'Yes, Miss Jackson,' James managed.

'It's been a great joy to me to see those children grow, especially little Miss Amelia, my own and her father's favourite.'

The words had been carefully chosen but if Dorothea thought she was delivering her *coup de grâce* to the disabled mariner, she underestimated him. It was therefore perhaps just as well that, two unwanted rusks and two more cups of tea later, when he considered his duty to the kind and charitable lady done and began to take his leave, he did not mention his intentions. And considering his state of mind and the fact that Miss Jackson was well practised at courting confidences, he might well have done. As it was, she thought it was finished.

'It's a great pity you couldn't have seen Miss Hall again, Mr McBain, but there we are,' she said as she saw him to the door.

After thanking her, James put on his fine new hat and sailed out into the cold, leaden afternoon under jury rig. Dorothea stood there for a few moments watching the lonely figure go. At forty she looked somewhat older than her years, her hair already grey, and her small, round face seemed a little at odds with her thin but strangely wide frame. With seeming concern, she waited until her visitor was well down the road before she closed her door with pleasure. But as James walked on, determination rose in him with every step, and by the time he got back to his lodging in Summer Street he was ready to make a fight of it come hell or high water. He went straight out again and made his booking.

The following afternoon, all dressed up in his new suit and hat, he alighted from the coach a few miles before Worcester.

'That's it there,' the coach driver said as he pointed to the track leading to the Hall farm.

'Thank you,' James replied and the driver started his steaming horses up again to take his other passengers on.

The farmhouse was much bigger than he expected, more like some great mansion, but the terracotta-coloured paint on its clapboard was peeling everywhere and one of the supporting pillars to the once elegant porch had a slight lean to it. The impression it gave of a formerly wealthy family whose fortunes were now in decline was an accurate one. Three generations of bad management with a multitude of sons in each had scattered the original old money to the winds. Jim McBain knocked on the door but no one came at first and he knocked more loudly. Eventually, a poorly dressed black servant woman opened it and peered out. There was no way of telling whether she was a bonded slave or a freed one.

19

'I'm here to see Mr Hall,' he told her, 'I'm Captain McBain.'

For a moment the woman just continued to gaze at him.

'Yas, sah,' she finally said and closed the door on him. He waited a long time during which he could hear angry voices raised inside. Then the door opened to reveal a man standing there, his grey whiskers bristling with indignation. In keeping up the appearances of his ancestry he was dressed more like a rich Boston merchant than a farmer.

'Mr Hall?' James said, rightly taking it to be him. 'I'm Captain . . .'

'I know who you are,' Hall said, cutting him short, 'and if you don't get off my property it's buckshot you'll have in your trousers, sir.'

'Mr Hall, I'm just here to ask if . . .' James barely managed to get out before the door was slammed in his face. It was entirely unreasonable. James, flushed with humiliation, reacted in fury. 'And I mistakenly took you for a goddamned liberal, sir!' he shouted back in the hope that Hall might hear him. It was to be the one and only time he was ever to set eyes on Amy's father, or on any of the rest of her family. But if they thought they had heard the end of the supposedly unsavoury sailor they were wrong. Vowing to himself he would come back the following day, if it had to be with a battering ram, and force Mr Hall to listen, he turned away, now hoping to God the man had not heard his outburst. He did not know that Amy was watching him from an upstairs window and that he was the most wonderful vision she had seen in all her life. Knowing nothing about Aunt Dorothea's interference she had been in tears over the loss of her captain and never expected to see him again. Careful she was not being observed she hurried downstairs, slipped out the back then ran for all she was worth across a snow-covered field. Jim McBain had almost reached the road when he heard her call his name. Never had there been a sweeter sound. A few minutes later she was standing facing him over a broken fence, her bosom heaving as she panted bursts of steam into the air.

'You . . . came to see *me*, James?' she got out in order to remove any doubts.

'Yes, but your father didn't as much as let me get a word in.'

Amy dared not insult him by telling him that her father was determined to have her married only to a man of wealth and property since she had already guessed the captain's circumstances.

'I hate him,' she said for James's benefit although it was not quite the truth. Hate was not in her nature although she was old enough to see her father's social pretensions as his failing. As he looked at her, James was never more aware of how inadequate his life would be without her. And he knew without any doubt whatsoever that no other woman in the world could ever replace her.

'I have to talk to you,' he said, and Amy looked nervously back in the direction she had come.

'Can you meet me the day after tomorrow in Worcester, James?' she asked.

'I'll meet you any hour of the day or night wherever you want, Amy,' he replied, and even felt pleasure from speaking her name.

'Midday the day after tomorrow behind Erratt's store in Worcester,' she told him quickly, and with that suddenly turned and fled back across the field before she was discovered.

It was a much heartier captain-to-be in his black suit and fine tall hat who rolled the road into Worcester and he did not give a damn for Hall's threat or the problems that might still be facing him, nor gave any thought to the state of his finances. There he found a place to eat and a bunk for himself. And there he suffered in the doldrums, time dragging like molasses as he waited for the warm breeze to rise again.

Two days later, for half an hour before the clock struck twelve he hung around the back of the store where men were unloading supplies, then the warm breeze arrived in a dark cape over a green, silk dress. He did not believe that anyone could look so beautiful. Yet during the fifteen minutes of their meeting, not once did they as much as touch each other's hand, both fearing that any such move might break the spell and frighten the other away. And if they said nothing of any great consequence to each other they felt everything that was important.

It was with the greatest dismay that James learned it was to be another week before he could meet her again. But as there was no way around it he returned to Boston and presented himself once more at the warehouse of Kimball and Jay. There, news which only a week before would have brought him nothing but pride and joy only served to tell him that his time was running out with Miss Amy Hall.

'A ship just in said they sighted the *Nantasket* sailing into Liverpool Bay as they were coming out,' the wharfinger told him. 'Captain Tyler must have made a much faster passage than usual, so he could be back a lot sooner than we thought.'

It was not simply the pressing urgency of his situation James McBain felt during that week. Not even as a ten-year-old had he suffered such extremes of loneliness as a result of his enforced separation from Amy Hall. The captaincy that had been his life-long dream was now only part of it. Without Amy Hall he knew his life could never be fulfilled and that he would be the most isolated ship's master on the whole goddamned ocean. A day before the week was up he was on a coach again on his way back to Worcester, to stay the night there to make sure of being on time.

'Will you marry me?' were his very first words when Amy turned up at the back of the store.

'Yes,' she said without any hesitation, and still they did not touch each other. Serious of face they just stood looking at each other, committed, neither of them knowing what to say next.

'I mean before I sail,' James said after a little while.

'I realise that,' Amy replied.

'If your father finds out beforehand he'll probably lock you up.'

'I'll not tell him.'

'You're prepared for that?'

'Yes,' Amy replied firmly.

Their secret was well kept until the time came close and, after leaving a letter to her parents explaining her intention, Amy left home quietly in the dead of night with her only possessions: some highly fashionable clothes her father insisted she wear to attract the right man and a necklace she had inherited from her grandmother. An anxious James met her halfway up the track and hurried her to his hired carriage with its driver waiting on the road, and knowing just what risk he was taking, half expected his head to be blown from his shoulders. He felt like a thief but knew there was no other way. He was perfectly aware, too, that with all the expenses he had incurred his precious sextant had already been sunk to the bottom of the sea. It had crossed his mind that he might go to Mr Kimball or Mr Jay and ask for an advance on his primage, the percentage he would eventually expect from the freight and passenger fares from Liverpool and back, but it was not only his pride that stopped him. For all he knew, they might consider that to be penniless for love of a girl was a mark of reckless irresponsibility, change their minds about him and find another captain for their ship.

'We're going to be all right, Amy,' he assured her as they were driven through the night towards Boston.

'I'm not in the slightest worried, James,' she replied, seeming as happy as he had appeared confident, but there was deep apprehension in both of them.

It was in order to avoid a scandal and ensuing disgrace brought down on the heads of his family that Mr Hall, filled with impotent rage, saw no alternative but to give permission for his daughter to be married, pretending bare-faced to others that he had known the gentleman for some good time. Then, as his family packed up in preparation for their long trek to Erie, he ordered them never to speak her name again.

The wedding was probably the smallest ever to take place at King's Chapel in Boston and it grieved Amy that not one of her family came. Except Aunt Dorothea, a comforting presence Dorothea's ladies of charity who were in the know thought very charitable of her under the circumstances.

Aunt Dorothea stood smiling in her staid and practical costume and no one in the world knew of her strange and contradictory thoughts and feelings. She had always wanted to have Miss Amelia as her own and now with the Halls moving away and disowning their daughter, she realised she had been given the opportunity. But there was nothing so simple or straightforward about Miss Dorothea Jackson. At the same time as she raised her voice primly to the hymn with moistened eyes, no one could ever have guessed that she was consumed with a burning jealousy for her so-called niece. The truth was that Miss Jackson who had long ago learned to bide her time was far from finished with her Amelia. Or with her young captain-soon-to-be.

Chapter Three

Among the passengers staying on deck to watch Boston retreat under watery shafts of sunlight, those who knew about these things were rather surprised to see young Captain McBain at the wheel himself shouting orders directly to his crew. It was rare for a master to touch the wheel and he only spoke orders to his crew on the critical manoeuvre of taking a ship about through the eye of the wind. But it was not for their safety or to give them confidence in him that James was acting simultaneously as captain, mate and helmsman. It was simply to show off his skills to Amy and Amy could not have been more impressed as she stood close by.

'She's the best ship there ever was, Mrs McBain,' James smiled at her.

'I know, Captain,' Amy smiled back, flushed with joy, aware of how much he was at one with his environment.

All the way down Ship Channel with wind and tide, James hardly needed the red and black buoys that marked his way between rocks and shoals. And that was maybe just as well since he spent more time looking at his new wife than anything else. Not in all his life had he imagined he could have felt so complete.

'Oh, look!' Amy exclaimed as she pointed out the white-painted iron tower that supported Long Island Light, and soon they were swinging north-east towards Boston Light on the rocky 'Brewsters'. Then it seemed no time before they were making their way out into the Atlantic to head for the Gulf Stream.

That James saw the *Nantasket* as only a little less beautiful than his bride could have been excused by his having wildly distorted vision. The three-masted packet built years before at Charlestown upstream from Boston was a slow, heavy brute with broad, blunt bows that looked as if they had been designed to batter the sea into submission while, tapering back to pinched quarters and a narrow stern, she was very hard to steer in a following wind. In a stiff breeze, reduced sail and the sheer brute force of at least two men at the wheel were needed to stop the unruly bitch from going where she would. And downwind in a gale the only way of managing her was to strip her naked and let her lurch and slew before it under bare poles, like a mad drunk.

Amy, who was still to see that, had been fascinated by every detail of James's beautiful vessel.

'That,' he had told her, referring to the newly stocked 'barnyard' by the main hatch, 'is to make farmers' daughters feel at home,' and she had laughed. Partly roofed by the upturned jolly boat, the crammed pens contained a milking cow, pigs, chickens and sheep, some of which would barely find their sea legs before their necks were wrung or their throats cut. All the accommodation and facilities for crew and passengers were below under the main deck and, for the sake of trying to keep dry in heavy weather, were of necessity badly ventilated.

'It's wonderful!' Amy had said on first setting eyes on the captain's cabin and her new home which was all of eight feet by eight, including the bunk James had had extended to fit the two of them and a chart table. But if it was certainly much bigger than the passenger cabins of six feet by four, it was, nevertheless, a measure of her capacity for adaptability. She was hardly aware of the comparison with the very large house in which she had been born and raised. And she could not have complained of the tiny compartments that served as privies as there was no such thing as plumbing in Boston either and the only difference here, apart from the greater restriction, was that there were wooden handles to hang on to as the ship pitched and rolled. Saviour to it all was the comparatively large public saloon with its bronze-barred skylight, deeply varnished woodwork, gimballed oil lamps, shiny brass fittings, heavy dining table with chairs, and two hide-upholstered sofas. There, Amy had opened the door marked 'Library'. It was little more than a locker into which one could squeeze to select a book. Opposite, another door read 'Spirit Room', inside which it would have been very difficult to fall over, judged by many men in the past to be a most practical arrangement.

'Because you're my wife,' James had warned Amy, 'they'll expect you to be hostess, just as I'm expected to be host, but you don't have to if you don't want to. For me, it's very much part of a packet captain's duties and a lot of them do nothing else once they're at sea.'

'I'll be the best captain's wife a packet ever had,' Amy promised, all bright-eyed, and James had no idea that the new Mrs McBain had something entirely different in mind.

Only two worries kept intruding on James's total happiness. The first was whether Amy might get seasick. Several times he on

26

previous voyages had had to hold some elegantly dressed lady as she threw up the contents of her stomach into a bucket, pleading to be allowed to die and swearing to Almighty God that never again would she step on board a boat. If that happened he might stand the chance of losing her to the shore and the very thought of it was unbearable to him. The second was his own ability to make an accurate landfall across the other side of the ocean without a sextant. Worse. When he discovered that the first mate serving on the *Nantasket* did not navigate at all, he decided to ditch him and find one who could. But the retiring captain, on hearing of it, returned to Kimball and Jay's counting house to see him.

'I wouldn't do that,' he strongly advised. 'Mr Ludham might not be the brightest creature God ever created but he's much experienced on the Atlantic and knows every inch of the ship. He'll do everything you tell him without question and the crew will jump to his orders in the same way. If it's a well-run packet you want, sign him back on. He has no other ambition to do other than he does and he does it well.'

With that recommendation and plea for the whiskered, broad-faced Mr Ludham of the huge, raw hands who was ten years his senior, James felt obliged to take him back on and prayed that he might not regret his decision. Even a tiny fraction of a compass point off course could mean the difference between going north of Ireland or to the south of it, and, if he did not know which, he stood to make a laughing stock of himself on his very first command.

At least the retiring captain had been right about Mr Ludham's amenability. While James took the ship out from Boston, calling orders over the mate's head, Mr Ludham had stood patiently by like a large, obedient dog, questioning nothing of his master's strange behaviour.

'Take over, Mr Ludham,' James instructed him at last, thinking Amy might be getting too cold, and Ludham bellowed by name for a helmsman to come aft. James ordered the speed to be measured every hour around the clock, but if the mate had enough wit to realise that his new captain must have been very nervous about his navigation to want to know what distance he had covered with such frequency, he gave no sign of it.

'Come below now,' James said to his wife, taking her arm to lead her to the hatch.

'Can I wait to see what they do?' Amy asked, and James, only too pleased she was so interested, guided her to the starboard bulwark.

Amy watched the three men, two of them holding a pole with a loose spool, around which was neatly coiled line with knots at intervals, its outer end tied to a large piece of wood. At the same time as the wood was thrown over the side to hit the water and drift astern, pulling the line from the freely turning spool, the third man, who held a large sandglass, turned it over to start the timing. When the sandglass ran out the seamen immediately stopped the line from running and started to haul it back in, counting the knots.

'You see,' James explained, 'every knot represents a small portion of a sea mile, the sandglass the same portion of an hour, so by knowing what speed I'm doing I can tell what distance I'm covering over the water.'

'How clever!' Amy enthused, grasping it at once. 'How very clever, I'd never have thought of it.'

'Neither would I,' James admitted, 'and if I didn't have that and a compass and knew something about the currents I might be so far up the Charles River that only Indians would find me.'

Woodsmoke fled from the galley stovepipe that rose above the deck as they began to make their way down the companionway ladder.

'I remember now, James!' Amy said, suddenly stopping halfway down, 'I remember.'

'Remember what?'

'Apart from the fact that I love you,' she smiled, 'one nautical mile equals one minute of arc at the equator or along a meridian.'

'Where the devil did you learn that?' asked James, taken aback.

'Mr Hayne told us,' Amy replied, without having to confess that at the time she did not know exactly what a minute of arc was.

It was not the last surprise James was to get on his first day at sea as master. When they finally escaped from the passengers, all of whom wanted their attention, another awaited him after they had reached the privacy of their cabin.

'There's something I haven't had time to unpack yet, James,' said Amy.

James watched in mild curiosity as she opened the battered old sea chest she told him had been given her by Aunt Dorothea and took out two polished wooden cases and a much smaller one. He could hardly believe his eyes. Even before she opened the first he was familiar enough with its appearance to know what was inside. All the same, he found himself speechless as it was revealed in all its new and shining brass glory and at first he could only stare at it. He had known nothing of Amy hurrying up narrow, cobbled Broad Street and round the corner to Mr E. Hawkes, instrument-makers and suppliers, while he had been busy directing the hold stowage on his freight.

'How much is a sextant, chronometer and deck watch?' she enquired on reaching the counter and Mr Hawkes had just gaped at her. Never in all his years of business had a pretty girl come in to ask for such things, and Amy quickly realised his confusion. 'I'm Mrs McBain,' she hastened to tell him, 'wife of Captain James McBain of the *Nantasket*.'

'Ah, Mrs McBain, of course,' Mr Hawkes said, enlightened, and with an appreciative eye thought what a lucky man the captain was. He produced the goods and gave her his prices. Amy looked at them, did a quick sum in her head, said, 'I'll be back, sir, or I hope I will,' and dashed out again in a whirl of skirts, leaving Mr Hawkes gaping for a second time.

'How much, sir?' she said in the jeweller's shop, producing her necklace, and the man to whom business always came before pleasure seemed to take forever to examine it, and in some disdain at that. It was a mistake to tell him, in her eagerness and apprehension, how much she needed. He reluctantly offered just a little more than that while, unknown to Amy, he had valued it to be worth four times as much. But Amy could not have been happier or more satisfied as she hurried back to Hawkes.

'I take it the captain has the Almanacs to go with it,' Hawkes said as his assistant wrapped up her purchases.

'Almanacs?'

'The sextant will be of no use without them, ma'am.'

And those, and the old second-hand sea chest she bought, used up every penny she had left.

In the cabin, James did not have to be told how she had done it.

'You should never have sold your necklace just to do this for me,' he said somewhat angrily, but Amy had foreseen this.

'But they're not for you, James,' she explained, instinctively allowing him to keep his male ego and superiority, 'they're for me.'

'For you?'

'Yes. I want you to teach me how to use them. I want to be useful to you and not spend all my days just talking to women passengers about food and fashions.'

James could be none other than amused by that. It tickled him to think that his wife thought it was all so simple anyone could do it. Good God, navigation was one of the most complicated things on earth. After years of knowing what he was doing, he still found trouble with it. But he could not tell her he found it impossible to take her seriously. Far better to humour her instead.

'You won't mind,' he said to her, his navigation anxieties swiftly receding over the horizon, 'if I borrow them from you now and then?'

'No, of course not, James,' she replied in all seriousness. 'What do you think? All I have is yours, isn't it?'

At dinner, the passengers were entertained by the young Captain McBain and his even younger new wife. Even the English baronet who, during his visit to the New World had acquired a distaste for these brash Americans, could not help but be charmed by the sparkling Mrs McBain while James was just starting to realise what an enormous social asset she was going to be to him. The only sour note on board was a gentlemen who was travelling for the sole purpose of attending a Temperance conference in Liverpool and was determined to lecture on his subject every time anybody raised a glass.

As the wind and sea rose James ordered the royals and topgallant sails to be taken in and was up and down a dozen times during the night to ensure all was well with his ship, but in the morning he was below, bent over his charts, when a distraught and horrified-looking Amy burst into the cabin from an early visit to the deck. 'Come quickly, James,' she cried, 'quickly! Stop them!' and went, James hurrying after her, up the companionway.

Amidships, a seventeen-year-old seaman had his hands tied above his head to the lower shrouds of the main, his torso bare. Blood was trickling from his back. The bosun's mate whose duty it was wielded the lash while Mr Ludham stood by him making the count. As was the procedure, all hands had been called to witness while several of the passengers looked on, too.

'Stop them, James,' Amy urged, and watched James in great anxiety as he walked forward over the rolling deck as if it might have been dry land, but no anger showed in him.

'What happened, Mr Ludham?' he asked.

'This baskethead started a fight and stabbed another with his sea knife, sir,' Ludham replied, and it came as a relief to James that the punishment was genuine since there were 'Bucko Mates' who struck men down with belaying pins or had them lashed simply out of malice or for the sheer pleasure of it. All the same, the time had come to show his crew just what kind of captain he was, and let Amy know, too. He had the man freed and faced him.

'Are you satisfied that your punishment was justified and fair?' he asked him loudly so that all could hear.

'Yes, sir,' the young man confirmed and was sent back to the fo'c'sle. On being assured that the man stabbed was not seriously injured and had been treated, James still contained his anger, but he was not finished with his first mate.

'Be in my cabin in ten minutes, Mr Ludham,' James instructed

30

him and returned aft to take the still-horrified Amy below. It was difficult for him to fully understand Amy's reaction to what was perfectly normal. He himself had felt the lash once in the past and quite undeservedly, but he had made no complaint about it. All the same he wanted to give her all the comfort of which he was capable.

'Without discipline, Amy,' he explained, 'you couldn't run a ship and every seaman who signs on knows what he's in for if he commits a crime. And the men themselves prefer to see the law upheld. Without it, not a man of them would ever feel he could sleep safely in his bunk again, and I know, I've been there. Without it, the fo'c'sle could turn into chaos and the passengers, freight and ship would be in danger.'

But although Amy still saw it as cruelty, she knew she was going to have to come to terms with it while James knew that for her sake he was going to have to keep the lash down to the very minimum. Not long after, he received the mate on his own.

'I don't know what authority other captains have given you, Mr Ludham,' James said severely to him, 'but on my ship I'm the only authority. Do you understand?'

It was clear from the hurt, perplexed look on Ludham's face that he did not. In all his life at sea he had not once disputed the authority of any master.

'What I'm saying,' James was forced to go on, 'is that no man on this vessel is to be punished unless I myself have examined the circumstances and passed sentence or reprieve.'

Ludham's broad, whiskered face cleared at that. He should have known. He was not being keel-hauled after all. It was nothing personal against him, purely a matter of a new captain, new holystone.

'Yes, sir,' he replied quite happily.

'And in future,' James added, 'if there is to be any further such punishment, it's not to be witnessed either by the passengers or Mrs McBain.'

'I'll see to it, Captain,' Ludham assured him.

'Yes, I know, Mr Ludham,' James said, a little sorry at his anger. The man had only been trying to help him and had meant him no harm. Dismissed, Ludham headed back to the deck quite content with young Captain James McBain. Besides, McBain was not one of those college-educated ones but a sailor like himself who knew every block, stay, shroud, halyard, brace, sheet, every knot and splice there was to know.

It was to try to help take Amy's mind off the morning when, later in the day, as the sun appeared James fetched her on deck with the sextant.

'Lesson number one, Mrs McBain,' he told her, and patiently explained what had to be done. Amy was immediately intrigued but after a frustrating hour refused to give it up until she got the hang of it. Braced against the rail, eye glued to the small, telescopic eyepiece, she chased the wobbling sun through the world of filters, double images and mirrors, and lost it and found it and lost it again with the rolling and pitching of the ship.

'That will be enough for today, Amy,' James said, trying to get her to give it up.

'No, it won't, James,' she replied and tried again. James had never been so patient. Seven bells of the afternoon watch rang out on the foremast and the sun was already lowering towards the west, and still Amy would not give up.

'I've got it, I've got it!' she suddenly squealed in excitement, and all on her own brought the round, filtered ball down to sit steadily on the horizon. Then she lowered it to read off the degrees and minutes on the arc as she had been previously shown.

'There, I have shot the sun,' she said with satisfaction, already having picked up the proper seamanlike term for it, 'and now we know where we are.'

James was astonished, not just by her having managed it so quickly but by having done so at all. In the navigation schools that existed in towns along the Eastern Seaboard it took men a long time to learn how to take a sun sight, and standing on dry land. He hardly had the heart to tell her that her achievement was only the beginning, but he knew she would not forgive him if he did not appear to be taking her seriously.

'Well, not quite,' he said. 'You have to have the exact time to the second as you do it, then there's quite a lot of work to be done with those Almanacs.'

'Then we'll do it all properly tomorrow, James,' she said, not at all dismayed, 'and once I know the rest there will be no need for you to bother with it.'

James could not have been more amused by such sweet innocence but thought he had better not laugh and managed to keep a straight face.

'Right,' he agreed, and she looked so adorable to him. He felt he had done an excellent job of taking her mind off the incident that morning. It was how he expected women to be, their interest jumping from one thing to another. There was no question in his own mind that once he showed her all the long, laborious calculations that could take hours in working out a position for the ship she would give up and turn her attention to crochet or stitching like most of the ladies usually did if they were not overtaken by seasickness.

But as wave after wave of the North Atlantic came rolling up from astern to raise the *Nantasket* and surge under her hull to push on ahead it was not the young bride who was being naïve but the captain. For him, the real surprise was still to come.

Chapter Four

They were only five days out of Boston when James came below to find Amy in their cabin, worriedly poring over the chart, surrounded by the Almanacs and the scribblings of many figures. She was holding the dividers in her hand.

'You'll have to help me, James,' she pleaded. 'I've made a mistake somewhere and for the life of me can't find out where I've gone wrong. My position is more than seventy miles from yours and I just can't get it right.'

It was as much to humour her that James had allowed her to continue as she wished and she had been on deck every time the sun appeared. And at night, the moon, too.

'Seventy miles is not at all bad, Amy,' James said, discreetly omitting to mention that near a coast in bad weather in poor visibility it could mean the difference between being safe at sea or wrecked on rocks with the loss of life for all those aboard. And for three whole hours, because he loved her, he patiently helped her to go over and over all her calculations and his own. Then the truth of it struck him.

'God damn my eyes,' he said in disbelief when nothing more could be done, 'it's not you who made the goddamned mistake, it was me. Your position's right and it's mine that's wrong.'

'Are you sure?'

'Of course I'm sure,' he replied, angry with himself.

Amy felt suddenly embarrassed for him. 'Anyone can make a mistake, James,' she offered in an attempt at giving comfort. 'Anyway, I'm tired of it and don't want to do it any more.'

But James was beginning not to be taken in by the look of innocence in her large brown eyes. Before him was positive evidence that his wife had a very unusual, natural talent for what he had always had to struggle with. It had taken him years to reach his level of proficiency and already Amy had shown him up. It was quite incredible. But he was no fool. He had been presented with a heaven-sent opportunity and he was not going to pass it up. It was only a matter of saving a little bit of face as he grasped it.

35

'Now, isn't that the greatest pity,' he said. 'And just as I was thinking about officially making you a member of my crew.'

'Me?' Amy questioned, her eyes even wider with surprise. 'A woman? A member of your crew?'

'Highly irregular, I know,' James said and shrugged. 'Ah, well, never mind, they would probably have laughed at me for it anyway.'

'Now, you wait a moment, James,' Amy demanded as he turned for the door, 'I'm perfectly willing to accept your offer if it's what you want.'

James stopped and turned back to her. 'But I thought you just said you didn't want to do it any more,' he reminded her.

'I have changed my mind,' Amy said. James held her apprehensive eye for a moment then smiled.

'Very well, Mrs McBain,' he said. 'From now on we share this particular duty and I'll inform Mr Ludham to that effect.' And a moment later the navigator was kissing the captain with gratitude and delight.

In truth, although Amy had wanted to be useful to James at sea, that was not why she had bought the sextant in the first place. She had done so simply because she knew James wanted it. It was not until she had raised it to her eye and become aware of the vast expanse of ocean surrounding her that the very idea of being able to tell exactly where the ship was on it drew her like a magnet. It was an almost mystical feeling, as though it was the answer to one of the questions on the mystery of the universe, a link with the sun, the moon and the stars that had some meaning. And it was far from all young Amy McBain wanted to know. How wide was the Gulf Stream? What currents were in it and where? What might the wind be doing elsewhere? How did you know you were steering your exact course when the movement of the ship was constantly swinging the compass all over the place? What was Leeway and how did you calculate it? Why was the Gulf Stream's eastward route the best? And many other mysteries. James was able to answer only a few of her questions, the knowledge handed down by tradition, and, as he told her, only God knew the rest. What she had as yet given no mind to because of her total confidence in her husband was that danger and even death stalked ships at sea.

On deck, James took in the sky. Overhead, mares'-tails gave their sign, a sheet of cirro-stratus in hot pursuit, descending to dark, threatening banks that were almost black on the horizon astern.

'Take in sail down to the tops'ls, Mr Ludham,' he ordered, and

Ludham went for'ard, bawling out his orders to send men scurrying up the ratlines on to the yards. James then ordered the steward to instruct all passengers to stay below but assure them they were safe. In what seemed like no time, the taut shrouds of Russian hemp were wailing in high-pitched protest, drowning out the squealing of the pigs in the barnyard. Three men struggled together with the helm in the failing light. In the quickly rising sea, James was about to order all remaining sail to be taken in and let her run bare when several things happened at once. Amy, who was not a passenger, had started up the companionway. At the same time, James heard the deafening roar astern and saw the gigantic mountain intent on total destruction charging at full speed from behind and already almost on top of them. All he had time to do, like the rest of his crew there, was to make a quick grasp for a firm hold. The ship's stern was too narrow and too slow to rise to the monster's steepness. James just caught sight of Amy as she appeared on deck and the instant of fear on her face at what she saw, but his desperate shout of warning was too late. The great towering crest spitting white spume crashed fifty tons of angry sea down on the afterdeck, lifting her bows from the water, shaking the entire ship like a fragile box and shuddering the masts as if to split them all asunder, obliterating everything and washing one of the men at the wheel to the bottom of the bulwarks. But before he could even scramble to his feet, Ludham was grabbing him by the scruff of the neck, cursing him for his buttery fingers and buttery feet and practically hurling him back towards the helm like a piece of waterlogged rag. Sea still pouring from him, James looked to the main hatch but Amy was no longer there. Yet, for all his fear, he first had to make a quick decision and knew that even with a sea anchor out astern to slow her down, she was going to be out of control.

'Prepare to heave to, Mr Ludham!' he yelled over the roar of the wind to his first mate and dashed towards the main hatch. Never in all his life had he felt such relief at making out Amy at the bottom of the ladder, where she had been swept, seated on the sole of the main cabin which was awash.

'Are you all right?' he asked anxiously, quickly getting down to her and picking her up, but he could not have been more pleased to know that she was not only safe and unhurt, even if she was a little shocked, but that there was still colour in her cheeks and that it was pink, not green.

'Next time you wish to bath me with my clothes on, Captain,' Amy told him, 'you might at least give me time to fetch a bar of soap.'

37

Despite all his other anxieties for his ship, James managed to laugh at that. For him, there had never been such another woman in all Christendom.

'Hang on, I'm going to bring her around,' he said and, much cheered, hurried back up on deck, securing the doors of the hatch behind him. Ludham had all hands standing by. The danger was that in bringing her round into the wind the ship would, for a time, be side-on to the waves and, if another rogue struck, might be put on her side or even capsized. Neither could he afford to look in the slightest doubtful or nervous and weaken the confidence of his crew. Keeping a sharp eye astern, he chose his moment, and with four men to the wheel ordered her hard a'port. The *Nantasket* swung, heeled hard over in the trough, but came around.

'Fore staysail hard a'weather!' he yelled and men quickly hauled their hearts out on the sheet. Then with only that and the reefed-down spanker aft set hard on, the ship rode to the wind, rising to each wave and plunging down into the next, but safe.

For a day and a half the ship was hove-to, but the cook was able to cook and milk was still got from the cow while, despite seas coming over the great wide bows to send water ankle-deep over the deck, the cabin boy was able to bring up the privy buckets and empty them over the side.

'Is this as bad as it can get, James?' Amy wanted to know, a little concerned.

'Well, yes,' James replied and thought he had better temper his lie a little by adding, 'Or almost.'

It was to be over three weeks after setting out from Boston that, in good visibility, and with Amy's careful positioning, James was able to identify the small island of Inishtrahull off the north coast of Ireland, beyond which was Malin Head. For the *Nantasket* it was a respectable time and the passengers were pleased. But Amy was much more than just pleased. Not in all her young life had she felt so much satisfaction, so great a sense of achievement as having navigated to that landmark then seeing it there with her own eyes.

'It's like magic, James,' she said excitedly, but James knew full well it was she who was the magic. Not only did he have a perfect helpmate but a totally confident and competent navigator into the bargain, and he felt that no man on earth could ever have been so fortunate in his life.

Later, as they left Rathlin Island to starboard and headed down the North Channel, reaching on a fresh, westerly breeze, the flag was hoisted on the signal halyard to indicate to pilots they were Liverpool-bound. But it was not until after they had passed the Isle of Man that a Liverpool pilot cutter appeared. A rope ladder was thrown down the side and eventually the pilot was making a skilful leap for it to clamber aboard. In no time, the short, nuggety, whiskered man was to find himself bemused by the captain's pretty young wife questioning him on his knowledge of the Irish Sea and of the tides and currents on that part of the English coast. Not even his own wife had ever asked him such things, but it would have been superfluous to have pointed out to the ship's master what an unusual, engaging and fascinating woman he had in Mrs McBain. The pride in his young spouse was writ large all over the young American captain's face.

'I want her made as shipshape as she was when we slipped from Long Wharf, Mr Ludham,' James said to his first mate, referring of course to his vessel and not to Amy, who looked to be in even better condition than when she left.

No seaman's hands went idle. Scraping, painting, tarring, splicing, stitching, holystoning, the scrubbing down of all bare wood with vinegar, even the hunting down of cockroaches and rats.

Into Liverpool Bay, Amy took in all the procedures with great interest. The coming aboard of the Port Health Officer, the Customs men, an assistant to the Harbour Master with his own signalman. Then she went below to write up all the knowledge she had coaxed from the pilot, so did not see the two newsmen come aboard from a boat, eager for any fresh news from Boston. They were to be disappointed. The passengers were all too keen to get ashore to think of anything else. The English baronet's dislike of all Americans and all things American, except Captain McBain and his charming young wife, was not news. And they had no sympathy with the Temperance campaigner's views, especially the reporter with the large, bulbous, purple nose which had been acquired at great expense over the years. Thirsty, they quickly departed back over the side, into their waiting boat. Otherwise they might have stumbled on the story of the young American woman who had taken up navigation. They would have made it an interesting tale, one likely to have caused a lot of controversy and much heated argument not only around the waterfront but behind the doors of English homes, inspiring many a wife to make favourable and unacceptable comment and anger many a disbelieving husband.

For Amy, her first visit to the Old World was a happy and fascinating one, and with his payment for carrying the mail James had a little money in his pocket, but ten days later, with a full complement of passengers and the hold loaded with freight which was mostly textiles, they were heading out into Liverpool Bay again.

'This is our route,' James pointed out to Amy, running his finger over the charts. Down the Irish Sea to clear the south of Ireland and heading south-west until they picked up the north-east Trade winds, then across towards the West Indies before turning north for the American coast.

They were a hundred and fifty miles south-west of Ireland when the wind died and the sails hung uselessly, flapping only with the movement of the ship in the swell. James paced the quarterdeck impatiently, taking in sky and sea, but it was hard for him to conceal his anxiety. But that was not the reason why, for the very first time, Amy's intuition about the sea surfaced without the asking. Everything appeared perfectly normal. Passengers were strolling the deck, enjoying the sea air.

'Something's going to happen, isn't it?' she said to James, and James was surprised by that as he had already come to the same conclusion.

'What makes you say that?' he asked.

'I don't know, I just feel it.'

'Well, don't worry, Mrs McBain,' James smiled. 'If we're in for a bit of heavy weather we're ready for it.'

But it was soon to prove a lot more than just a bit of heavy weather. The wind began to rise from the west and they were under way again by dusk, heading south. But as darkness fell the wind increased so quickly that even James was almost caught off guard.

'Shorten sail, Mr Ludham,' he ordered with urgency and men scurried up the rigging while passengers were advised to take to their cabins. Without warning, the wind suddenly backed to the south-west and struck full force. Such was its howl that the only way James could make himself heard was to shout into Ludham's ear. Aloft, men were still struggling and fighting to take in sail while the seas which had risen with incredible rapidity became confused, waves trying to overcome each other from different directions. The broad, blunt bows of the *Nantasket* rose to one wave only to smash down as if to bury themselves in another. Water came roaring down the deck as the hull shuddered from stem to stern. There was no question this time of James giving the order to heave-to. He considered himself too close to the south of Ireland and without knowing how bad it was going to get or how long it was going to last there was the danger of being blown back on to a lee shore and shipwrecked on rocks. And he could not turn and run in that direction either. He had no alternative but to force his ship to keep clawing to windward with whatever staysails she could carry. In one great lurch, the wind in the rigging shrieking, the ship went almost on her side and two seamen on deck were swept from their feet by the sea that came aboard and raced their bodies down the inside of the bulwarks almost the full length of the ship before they could get a hold.

Anxious for James, Amy fought her way up the companionway ladder on one side of it, having to use all her strength in the effort. As her head got above the level of the deck, she was amazed by the screaming force and violence of it all. Even partly sheltered she could feel the breath being sucked from her body and when, as she clung on, she stuck her head round to try to see forward, her eyeballs were pressed back into their sockets and she was immediately forced to look away. It might have been a sailor's apocalyptic vision of the ends of hell. In an incessant sheet, spray flew horizontally through the screeching air, carrying millions upon millions of plankton and hurtling them to their deaths against anything in its way, each minuscule particle of life marking its grave in a ghostly light of greenish blue. Yet she could make out men there, thigh-deep in rushing white water as they hauled on a rope, and suddenly she feared for her husband, a fear soon to be fully justified.

'Captain!' she shouted, as yet unable to identify him, but her words were drowned. Neither did she hear the other deadly cry of 'Man overboard!' that was let out forward, or see the man blown from a yard on the foremast. What she saw, with unbelievable horror, was the figure of James suddenly appearing to throw himself over the bulwark into the raging sea, to vanish. How she made it from the hatch to the after rail in a desperate run she never knew but there she stood screaming her head off into the darkness before water swept her off her feet. She only faintly remembered being dragged back to the hatch by two seamen. In shock, she was not aware of Ludham ordering wind to be spilled.

'They'll get the captain, Mrs McBain!' one of her guardians shouted into her face, but that had little meaning either. Indeed, to any experienced seaman who had seen what Amy had, these would have been empty words, and they might as well have pointed out to her that her lost husband must have been insane. You could not simply turn a ship around in a storm as if it were a horse and wagon and then calmly make a search as if you were looking for a lost bracelet in a cornfield. Even if you could, and even in daylight, the chances of finding a tiny thing like a man's head in such a tormented ocean was less than an improbability. In dark it would have been impossible, or at least a miracle. And a lowered boat would quickly have been capsized in such extreme conditions, resulting only in a further loss of life. It was why captains sailed on, leaving hapless sailors to die in their watery graves. A misfortune. A prayer for their souls on the following Sunday then forgotten. It was a risk that went with the job. Some even saw falling from the yards into the sea as a consolation since they considered landing on deck only to live as a helpless cripple to be a worse fate.

'He's dead. My husband's dead,' Amy muttered, but neither of the two seamen detailed to keep her there heard her from the shrieking of the rigging and the roar of the sea. And it was as well they held her as she might well have made another run for the stern and thrown herself into the waves. She did not want to live without James at that moment and since James had gone all she wanted to do was die.

At the bulwark rail aft, it was as much as Ludham and the men with him could do to stay upright. Without a strong hold on at least one hand, either the wind would have blown them over or the force of rushing water which the scuppers were unable to carry away would have taken their legs from under them. Yet they had to do more.

'Easy, God damn you! Easy!' Ludham yelled at them.

Amy had no idea how long she was held there in the depths of her tearless despair at the top of the tilted and heaving companionway ladder. And she might well have died had she known how to will herself to. What she remembered next after what seemed like a lifetime of inconsolable grief was unreal and incomprehensible.

'Look, ma'am, look!' one of the seamen was shouting at her but it had no meaning for her. She felt her body being dragged higher into the hatchway opening and rough hands turning her head and forcing her to see. What she saw was a group of men clinging for their lives at the bulwark almost abeam of the hatch itself. The weather sides of their bodies and heads were outlined in a ghostly glow. Two men were being brought to their feet out of a small, heavy cargo net that had been used to fish them aboard. One of them was conscious, grasping at the other who was limp. But it was in total disbelief she saw that the hatless figure standing upright was that of James. Although it was probably no more than a few seconds they struggled there, the wind picking up the partly freed net to flail it like a whip, to Amy it was as if time had ceased for this illusion of resurrection and might have been framed there in the screaming darkness for all eternity.

'See, it's the captain, ma'am, he's done it!' one of the seamen told her and she stared at the vision of the drowned ghost. Then Ludham and another man were carrying the rescued seaman towards her and manhandling him past her to get him below. Behind came James.

'What in the hell are you doing up here?' he shouted angrily at her. 'Get below!' And unable to separate illusion from reality, she could make no reply. Not even when James turned back and yelled at the crew to have the few staysails hardened up again did she dare to believe that her husband's life had been given back to her. It was not for another half-hour that her senses returned and she wept for joy over the renewal of life. Never before had she been so grateful to God. She was not the only one. Once the water had been pumped out of the seaman's stomach as he hung over the cabin table and recovered, he too said a silent prayer.

For Ludham, the God-sent relief was for quite another reason. When he had seen McBain tie a thin line around himself, secure the other end to a dead-eye on deck near a scupper, and coil the rest up, he felt a powerful relief. He had never seen a ship's master do such a thing before, but he assumed it was for his own safety. And what Ludham lived in constant dread of, ever since he had become a mate, was of a captain dying on him at sea one day and forcing on him the ultimate responsibility. That, he knew, he could never have faced. He did not know that James had readied himself for an altogether different purpose. James had seen men he had known been left to drown before and had vowed to himself that if ever he did become a captain he would do all in his power not to let this happen. So when he saw the figure blown from the foremast he had leapt, able to grab him before the ship sailed on to drag them both astern. He had known the risks. Not only was it possible to drown being dragged through a sea like that but a line light enough to be able to swim with might have snapped with the sudden forces it had to take.

Youth helped Amy bounce back quickly from the nightmare.

'At the height of the storm,' she wrote proudly in the logbook when the storm had abated and all was well, 'Captain James McBain, without any thought for his own life, threw himself in the darkness into the sea and rescued Able-Bodied seaman Jesiah James from drowning.'

'You can't put that,' an embarrassed James protested on seeing it, 'I'm supposed to be writing that. I can't say that about myself.'

'All right,' Amy said defiantly and instead of striking it out signed it 'Navigator'.

Navigator she had certainly become, studying everything that was known about the subject and becoming strangely intuitive about what was not. Passengers were highly entertained to see the young lady in her fine skirts standing at the rail with her sextant and watch or politely asking the mate to have the log put down. And they were charmed by the young captain and his wife since although on deck she always formally addressed her husband as 'Captain' and he her as 'Mrs McBain', their passion for each other could not have escaped the blind.

. Forty days out of Liverpool the lookout for the Semaphore Telegraph Company at Wood's Hole identified the *Nantasket* as she entered Nantucket Sound. The long arms clanged with their signals on the tower and, within a matter of hours, the message was relayed through the system all the way up the New England coast to Boston and on to the tower on the roof of Long Wharf, with a messenger taking it down into the counting house of the owners, Kimball and Jay.

Amy felt herself to be a woman of some achievement when, a couple of days later, after all the usual port procedures, they came slowly into Long Wharf to tie up. Aunt Dorothea was standing there in the summer sunshine and she had so much to tell her. She had no idea at all of the twisted bitterness in her aunt's heart as she stood there smiling and waving at her niece's arrival. It was James she thought was mad.

'You shouldn't have, you shouldn't,' she objected when later ashore he presented her with an expensive necklace that cost almost half his primage. And indeed, for a man who had never had any real money in his life before, it was a touch of madness.

Watching them, Aunt Dorothea knew she would have to be patient. In the meantime she would satisfy herself when the urge came on to find what victims she could in the asylums and, with her new sea connections, be seen devoting herself to yet another charity by collecting donations for the Boston Port Society who were planning to build a new Seaman's Bethel in North Square the following year.

For another fourteen months, Amy and James McBain happily plied the Atlantic between Boston and Liverpool without a single thought that it might not be forever. For Amy, life could not possibly have had more purpose. For James it could never have been more fulfilled. Yet the future promised even more. At Noddle's Island, a much more modern vessel was being built for Kimball & Jay to compete with the growing packet service and James was to be her first master. Even when Amy announced she was going to have a child, it seemed none other than a cause for celebration since James knew it could be born nowhere else but at sea. He would not have been the first captain to have acted as midwife to his own child.

But it was just the opportunity Aunt Dorothea had been waiting for. All she needed for her plan was the help of Dr Amos Drew and she would be able to separate her Amelia from Captain James McBain. She wasted no time in going about it.

Chapter Five

In the warm afternoon sunshine, Miss Dorothea Jackson walked along Boston's Hanover Street past the sailor's church on her way to the home of Dr Amos Drew. Although intensely jealous of the women who wore the latest European fashions, it was not from the lack of a dollar that she herself wore the simplest of old-fashioned clothes, her purely practical, black, lace-up boots pushing their way out from under the hem of her navy-blue dress as she went. One only had to look at her to realise she was a lady serious of purpose, a woman to whom people might freely give their trust. And that was just what she wanted. Several men she passed who recognised the figure raised their hats in respect to her as she went by.

Such was the depths of her cunning that no one alive knew her true nature. Indeed, the only one who might have spoken out against her was not only dead but had hardly been of an age of understanding at the time to do so, since she had been only two and a half years old when her elder sister Dorothea had pushed her into the family pond and kept thrusting a stick at her until she had stopped struggling. For Dorothea there had been good reason. Her young sister was the pretty one and much favoured, the one with the curls that everyone remarked on, the one who deliberately broke all the things she treasured and who demanded, and got, all the attention. It was not really surprising that no suspicion whatsoever was levelled at Dorothea for what was taken to be a tragic accidental drowning. Civilised men and women, and especially parents, simply did not want to believe that any child of so tender an age was capable of murder. The very thought of it would have destroyed all belief in innocence and rejected the word of God Himself. But not only had it been murder, it had been premeditated. From the moment Dorothea had woken on that morning to find her little parasol had been torn and broken by her only sibling whose life she had cursed since the day she had been born she had planned it. And she had taken precautions to make sure her deed had gone unwitnessed. At the time, despite her screams as she ran to her mother at the house, Dorothea had felt an overwhelming satisfaction over what she had done. Moreover, when all the sobs and wailing were over and only silent sorrow was left, Dorothea was restored to her rightful place. It was not until a few years later that she several times felt the terrible urge to confess and more than once had been on the very verge of it, but had somehow overcome it and continued to hug her secret within. And as she grew, Dorothea learned how to conceal many things from the world she felt she wanted to punish. But not her motherhood.

She was eighteen when she had shattered the relative peace of her parents with the announcement in tears to her mother that she was going to have a baby. Suddenly it became a house full of shock, horror and shame.

'Who is he?' her scarlet-faced father demanded to know.

'I can't tell you!' Dorothea cried, 'I can't!'

'You will marry him! And at once!' her father ordered, but no fury, no striking at her was to drag from Dorothea the name of the father of her child. Day after day it went on, hidden behind their doors, and when her breasts began to swell and her mother took to her bed, ill with it, the shame became unbearable. Before neighbours or anyone else could find out, Dorothea was sent, on the pretence of it being a long vacation, to far-off Ohio with secret arrangements made to put her in the care of a doctor there. It was also Mr Jackson's request to this doctor that when the child was born it was to put out to adoption and, to make sure of it, he put up a good sum of money to go with it. The doctor wrote back to Mr Jackson to confirm that his daughter was already four months advanced and that he would see to the adoption.

It was a most stressful time in the Jackson household and Mrs Jackson, a meek woman, found it an unbearable strain having to keep up a cheerful face outside her home and answer enquiries as to how Miss Dorothea was enjoying Ohio.

It was not until another three months had gone by that the Ohio doctor started to become puzzled by his patient's condition and called in an older colleague to give his opinion. Together they examined Dorothea as closely as medical discretion and ethics allowed, which was not very far, not even to the lifting of her nightdress.

'Is it possible?' the doctor asked his senior on his suspicions when they were alone.

'I've not had such a case myself,' the second opinion admitted honestly, 'but I'd say from what I've seen at this stage, if the time elapsed is correct, either it's a very tiny child or it's dead.'

'And if it was dead,' the doctor returned, 'nature would have taken its course and let go of it, would it not?'

'That's been my experience,' his colleague confirmed, but was reluctant to commit himself further. He had seen some strange things happen in his career.

The Ohio doctor waited another month, all the time keeping a close eye on his patient in her birth-bed. Then he called in a midwife he had engaged to stand by for 'Mrs Jackson's' event. The midwife, who was able to make the kind of examination the doctor could not, took little time in making up her mind. She emerged from Dorothea's room looking suitably solemn and closed the door behind her. 'I'm afraid there *is* no child, sir,' she declared to the doctor with confidence. 'The lady is just imagining it and I think in time the swelling of her stomach and breasts will go down.'

Whether or not this was a result of some deep, subconscious desire by Dorothea to replace the child she had destroyed was never to be known. As it was, the Ohio doctor was only surprised by how quickly Miss Jackson was to recover from the shock on being told of her phantom pregnancy, but it was not the end of the matter. Dorothea managed to convince him, much against his better judgement, that in order to avoiding embarrassment all round he should write to her father and inform him that her child had been still-born, an outcome she insisted would satisfy everyone and see the finish of it.

Thus did Dorothea return to Boston the same virgin she had been when she left and although, from then on, it was never mentioned again, either inside the Jackson home or out of it, with not so much as a whispered rumour casting a shadow on the Ohio vacation, there was the fresh ghost of another dead child, this time an illegitimate one, to haunt Mrs Jackson in her sleepless hours.

Aunt Dorothea arrived at the door of Dr Amos Drew and pulled at the polished brass bell knob. Amongst the many things she had learned in life was never to tell a lie if you could find someone else to do it for you. She had known Dr Drew for many years and it was he she used to gain access as a credited charity visitor to her incarcerated female lunatics, as Dr Drew himself liked to be seen as a charitable man and gave his services free to several public institutions, including the Boston Asylum for Indigent Boys on Thompson Island.

Mrs Bellow, short, rotund but fleet of foot, who was Amos Drew's housekeeper, opened the door then stepped aside to let her in. But Miss Jackson did not have to wait long before she was ushered into the doctor's study. Amos Drew stood there, his practised smile just a little too wide, holding out a welcoming, freshly washed hand that smelt slightly of soap. Narrow of face with high, protruding cheekbones and side-whiskers that reached down below his chin, there was a faint air of pomposity about him, even a hint of a man of insight. No one ever seemed to notice that he was, in fact, a man of hindsight, always reserving his words of wisdom and knowledge for after the events.

'Sit down, sit down, Miss Jackson, please,' he said, 'Mrs Bellow will bring us some tea.'

'It could be very wrong of me to bring you my problem, Dr Drew,' Dorothea began as she sat, 'but I feel I have no one else to turn to.'

'Whatever's wrong?' Amos Drew enquired, seeing by her agitation that it had to be something more serious than the troubles of weed-hauling in her well-tended garden.

'I hesitate to tell you,' Dorothea replied, 'because it's not about myself and I don't think I have any right to be interfering. All the same, I can't help but fear for her.'

'Her?'

'Amelia, the dear child, dear child,' and she smiled bravely through her concern. 'Listen to me, there I go. Silly old aunt calling her a child when she's all grown up and a married woman.'

Amos Drew knew all about Amelia. He had attended to her more than once over the years on the occasions she had been staying with her aunt, although the most serious ailment had been chicken pox. And he had known, of course, of her hasty marriage to the young captain.

'And what about Amelia, Miss Jackson?'

'She's going to have a child, Doctor,' Dorothea told him and he could not understand her anxiety. The only surprise, considering the time she had been married, was that she did not already have one.

'Is that not to be expected?'

'Yes, of course,' Dorothea explained, 'but it seems she's quite determined on giving birth at sea and I can't bring myself to tell her what I know. Her mother and all her mother's sisters in the South – they all had the greatest trouble with their firstborn and it was only with God's infinite mercy they survived. You as a doctor probably know what causes such a thing, I don't. But I do know this: if Mrs Hall or any of her sisters had tried to give birth at sea without all the proper care and attention they needed they would not be alive today. And it's not only for Amelia's sake I worry. Can you imagine the tragedy it would be for that young captain to have both his wife and child die in his arms on board his ship?'

Amos Drew had no idea whatsoever what condition might have

caused Amy's mother and sisters to have such troubles but it was not at all unusual for medical problems to run in families, as Dorothea well knew too.

'I see,' he said and, putting his fingers together, considered it. 'And Amelia doesn't know of this?'

'Oh, no,' Dorothea said, 'and she must never be told or the worry of it might even make it worse for her.'

'Then you must somehow try to convince her to have her child here in Boston,' he suggested, 'and also perhaps see to it that she takes plenty of rest.'

'She would never listen to me, Doctor,' Dorothea told him. 'The sea's already in her blood. She thinks of nothing else. And I'm only an ageing aunt who knows nothing about such things. But if the advice came from you she would listen. I know she would. She must be stopped from committing this folly.'

'I see,' Amos Drew said again and sought a way out of what was being put on him, but he was given little time to find one.

For a long time Dorothea had wondered why a likeable man such as Amos Drew had reached the age of forty without showing any interest in ladies. There had been plenty of attractive women over the years who had certainly shown an interest in *him*. And desperate to push her cause, she suddenly decided to make a wild, outrageous guess of hope.

'I know it's presumptious of me to ask such a thing of you,' she appealed, 'but I'm thinking only of trying to save the life of a poor innocent girl and her unborn child, and I think she's as deserving of God's mercy and our help as all the others we give to . . .'

'Yes, I'm sure of it, Miss Jackson,' Amos Drew hastily tried to interrupt, 'but I don't see quite what . . .'

'Surely . . .' Dorothea went on, cutting short his reluctance – and struck . . . 'more so than those indigent boys to whom you give your services freely. I don't wish to seem unkind but, pity them as we might, they still have to show they've reformed from their life of vandalism and whatever other unspeakable crimes they've committed.'

Amos Drew might have been frozen to the spot at that and it was to his great credit that he did not so much as flinch. There had been two occasions years before when he had lost his control and had sexual relations with two different, only too willing boys at the home. And although he had bought them expensive gifts and they had sworn to God never to tell, for a very long time he had lived in absolute terror of being found out, often waking in the middle of the night in sweats about it. It would have meant total ruination for him and, no matter where he had tried to escape to, the hounds of shame and disgrace would have hunted him down. But as the years had passed his daily fears had eased. Now, all his terror had returned. He felt confused. It seemed inconceivable that the kindly and angelic Miss Dorothea Jackson was trying to blackmail him but it was what he strongly sensed. Her remark could not have been more pointed. He had no idea what she knew or did not know but amidst the terrible fear that had risen in him he knew that he could not afford to take the slightest risk. It was perhaps as well that only moments later Mrs Bellow appeared with the tea tray or he might well have visibly shaken. The interruption gave him time to compose himself. After kindly thanking his housekeeper, he turned to Dorothea again with a smile.

'You're right, of course, Miss Jackson,' he agreed. 'We must do all we can to help the young lady.'

Although it had only been a guess on Dorothea's part, she knew at once by his change of attitude that she had touched him close to the nerve, and was even a little surprised by her good luck.

'That is very, very kind of you, Doctor,' she smiled in return. 'God will thank you and reward you for it. There must be a great satisfaction for you in knowing you can save lives.'

And they sipped their tea.

Dorothea made sure that the opportunity presented itself to Dr Drew by having him invited as an official guest to the launching of Kimball and Jay's new packet the *Atheneum* at Noddle's Island shortly after. It was well attended not only by the shipyard workers and their families, sparmakers, sailmakers, and all the other craftsmen involved but a large section of the public. Anything that added to the prosperity of Boston was always an event. But if Kimball and Jay were the owners there was no prouder man there than her master, Captain James McBain.

'She's the finest ship ever built, Amy,' he had said, not for the first time. 'Just look at her.' And Amy had glowed with happiness for him. He was so impatient to get his hands on her and, indeed, Amy herself could hardly wait to navigate her. The ship was very modern but not only because the bows were a fraction sharper and her stern a little broader. Instead of being between decks, for greater comfort the passenger accommodation was constructed above with a forty-five-foot-long cabin containing eleven staterooms, each six feet square. Not only that but a section of deck abaft the mainmast was covered over for passenger use while a closed-in bathing room had been thought of. To starboard on the quarter were cubicles with the privy buckets and opposite to port the barnyard.

'*Luxury State Room travel to Liverpool*!' Kimball and Jay had acclaimed in leaflets spread all over town and beyond. '*The new and highly luxurious* Atheneum *sailing mid-September. Mattresses, bedding, wines and all other provisions included free! $140.00.*'

But sadly, as the amply proportioned and much-adorned Mrs Kimball officially named her after the preacher had said his piece and the hammerblows of the team of men rang out along her keel to send her sliding down with gathering speed towards the water that would give her life, there was one voice that remained silent amidst the cheering and flag-waving: Mr Ludham's. He had always found it difficult to accept changes, and did not like this ship a bit.

'I'm sorry, Captain,' he had told James much earlier with respect, 'but I can have no hold with such a vessel. I couldn't work men with damn houses cluttering up her decks and don't see how they's goin' to do it. A ship like that'll cause nothing but complaint an' bring nothing but trouble. If you don't put it against me, sir, I'd rather stay with the *Nantasket*. I knows her well and won't mind doin' the West Indies run for her new owners if her captain will sign me on.'

James was very sorry, too. He had come to like the man but Ludham had been adamant and all he could do was give him the highest recommendation to the new master of the old ship. Little did he know that, in time, he was going to regret it.

'Ah, Mrs McBain, what a delightful occasion,' Dr Amos Drew greeted Amy the moment he saw James being hustled off by Mr Kimball to have a drink with some important gentlemen.

'Isn't she the finest packet there ever was, Dr Drew?' Amy said.

'Indeed, indeed,' Dr Drew replied, 'and I believe, if I'm not offending you by mentioning it, it's not the only good news you have.'

'Not offended at all, sir,' Amy replied, knowing immediately what he was referring to. It was no secret.

'I take it you won't be sailing out with the *Atheneum*, then?'

'Oh, yes,' Amy told him, 'I wouldn't dream of doing anything else,' and saw the look of concern that came over his face.

'Is that wise?' he questioned.

'Why shouldn't it be?' she asked.

'No reason I know of,' Amos Drew returned, 'but if you're determined to risk such a thing perhaps you should come to see me before you go.'

'But I feel perfectly healthy, Dr Drew, apart from what's only to be expected,' Amy told him.

'I was only suggesting it as a precaution. Wouldn't want anything to go seriously wrong, would we?'

Amy was disturbed by that. His tone suggested that his practised medical eye could see something wrong with her she was not herself aware of. She had always been a little in awe of the cleverness of doctors and she trusted Amos Drew. Ever since she had been a child he had been there on and off as part of the backdrop to her life. As the day progressed her concern for herself grew, but she did not mean to worry James with it when she mentioned it to him later that night.

'What in the hell did he mean?' James wanted to know.

'James, it's probably because he still sees me as a little girl and unable to take care of myself,' Amy replied but did not sound convincing.

Intent on looking into it, it was a worried James, with a hundred and one other things to do in preparing his ship for sea, who pulled at Dr Drew's bell the next day and was shown in.

'My wife seems to think you're concerned about her health, Doctor,' he said without wasting any time. 'Is there any reason for it?'

Amos Drew felt distinctly uneasy facing the young captain and might have questioned the ethics of what he was doing had not his fear of being unmasked overcome any qualms.

'Captain McBain,' he said, gathering what medical authority about him he could muster, 'I'm very sorry to say this but there could well be.'

'What exactly do you mean, sir?' James asked, more worried for Amy than ever.

'There are things I find difficult to explain to you medically, Captain, and I doubt if you'd understand if I tried, any more than you could explain to me in a few words how you sailed a ship. But I knew the Halls and I happen to know that there has been great trouble in the family with the carrying and bearing of their first-born. You must not, of course, let her know of it. I've seen excessive anxiety bring on miscarriages in women which in itself can be a cause of toxaemia and I'm sure you know what that means.'

'What are you telling me?' James wanted to know.

'I'm telling you, Captain McBain, that if your wife goes back to sea and doesn't get the attention she might need – and indeed might need all the way along from now – there is a chance you may lose both her and the child. I'm sorry to be so forthright but I'm sure you're the kind of man who prefers it that way. So I just want to make clear that if you take Mrs McBain away on your fine, new ship I cannot be held responsible. I can only give my advice. The decision as to what to do is, of course, entirely your own.'

James would no more have questioned the word of a learned doctor than, as a cabin boy, he would have questioned the order of a ship's master. The information staggered him. He was totally appalled by the thought of Amy's life being in danger because of their child. It was a notion that never once had so much as crossed his mind.

'You must on no account tell your wife what I've told you,' he heard Amos Drew add.

And an unhappy doctor Amos Drew was. Essentially a gentle and rather ineffectual man, he could see for himself the damage he had just done to the young captain and hated himself for it. He knew it was very wrong of him to have acted purely on hearsay without having done any checking, but he had done so and even more weight had been added to his already heavy conscience. More, he had made a prognosis, something he spent his life avoiding, and if it turned out to be incorrect and Mrs McBain had a perfectly normal delivery it might reflect on his medical ability. He felt even worse as James thanked him, and after the captain had left he went to the white china bowl of water and washed his hands.

Chapter Six

Rain did not deter the enthusiasm of the assembly as it waved and cheered the departure of the *Atheneum* on her maiden voyage. On other ships tied up and at anchor, bosuns' mates blew their farewells on their copper foghorns. The new vessel, laden with currant jelly, shaving soap, rubber shoes, cow horn, ham, cheap cheese, sassafras and corn, was hauled out into Ship Channel and turned her bows east to raise sail, her master Captain James McBain trying not to look back towards the shore.

On the wharf the deserted Amy stood in tears and the arm of Aunt Dorothea that had gone around her was of little comfort. Nothing she had said, no arguments she had put up, no promises she had made, no pleading and no prayer had been able to change James's mind. If she had not been told the truth, or rather the lie about her childbearing prospects, and knew nothing about it, every other excuse under the sun had been used for leaving her ashore. The possibility of a lack of iron in her blood, her occasional morning sickness that no Atlantic tempest had been able to drag from her, James's insistence that if she were to take ill in a storm he would not be able to take care of her, his first duty being to see to the safety of his ship and all others aboard her.

It had been far from easy for James to do what he had done, even though he knew he had no choice in the matter. But at least he had had the support of Amos Drew and Aunt Dorothea in whom he was obliged to confide.

'Oh dear, oh dear, the poor girl,' Dorothea had cried with an agonised wringing of her skinny hands when he had explained it to her. 'And I didn't know. Oh, the poor girl.'

'If I might impose on your kindness and ask you to take care of her while I'm away I'd be greatly indebted to you, Miss Jackson,' James had said, and had no suspicion whatsoever that it had been Miss Jackson who had brought his happiness and security crashing down around him.

As he headed out into the Atlantic with his passengers and freight, the sense of being alone again made him more and more angry at having to be separated from Amy even if, as he then believed, it was only temporary. And for the first time, he soundly cursed the child, as yet unborn, who had caused it. There was anger too at Mr Ludham having been right. More and more complaints could be heard from the crew who were having trouble working the running rigging as he demanded because of the superstructures on deck. But Captain James McBain was having none of it. He ordered that the next man heard using it as an excuse for tardiness would have money taken from his pay. And there were other changes in James without Amy.

As the wind rose higher and higher, he stood by the helmsman watching his course and six hours later with the seas risen too he was still there, drenched to the skin with rain and spray. And an increasingly worried mate kept looking at him until he could no longer contain himself.

'The main topgallant is labouring to split its seams, sir!' he shouted at him over the wind. 'We have to take in!'

'It holds full, mister!' James shouted angrily back at him. 'You will let it stand!'

Never did a new packet have such a baptism and the mate looked in fear and awe as the *Atheneum* raced on her reach over the waves and with two men to the wheel heeled over to an alarming forty degrees, her lee bulwarks almost under and the lower yards carrying full sail sweeping perilously close to the tops of the white-crested waves, flying spindrift. Neither deck officers nor the men who sailed before the mast could understand it. The whole of the Boston waterfront had it that Captain McBain was the fairest, most reasonable and happiest ship's master there was. But a curious thing began to happen to James as he forced his ship to the very edge of her limits. The exhilaration of it helped to ease the pain of his loss and he kept on pushing hard to keep it that way.

'Jesus goddamned Christ,' the foremast hand swore in the fo'c'sle to the off watch. 'We got ourselves a "Driver" here an' no son-of-a-bitch warned us. If you don't look smart an' get up to sogering it's goin' to be belayin's-pin soup he's goin' to be feedin' you for goddamned breakfast.'

Soup, or rather broth, was also what Miss Dorothea Jackson had very much in mind back in Boston, particularly as Dr Amos Drew recommended it as a daily diet for Mrs McBain's health. But in fear of her plot being uncovered she gave thought to the water which would go into it. It might just cover her tracks. If she could make her Amelia even just a little ill, neither Amos Drew nor the captain nor anyone else could ever suspect the truth, and keeping Amelia ashore would appear to have been perfectly justified.

Dorothea remembered the rumours of a few years before surrounding the pond near the shot tower across the other side of town in a poor section. Some of the women who lived close and who drew their water from it claimed it to be the cause of sickness, although none of them had been able to point to an actual death. All the same, a health officer inspected the pond, had his dog drink its water for a week to no ill effect, declared it safe and dismissed the talk as another superstition. But the women were far from satisfied and chose to draw their water from elsewhere from then on, swearing that health officer or no health officer it *was* bad.

The shot tower where gunshot was manufactured was a tall, four-sided tower, tapering upwards and clad in clapboard. At its top, molten lead was poured through small apertures, the droplets falling down through the air inside, forming perfect little balls as they went before ending with a sizzle in the large tank of water at the bottom. When enough shot had been made the water was drained to the earth outside from where it seeped back into the pond and the shot in the tank was gathered up. Then with more water pumped back in, the process began again.

'Here's a whole five cents,' Dorothea beamed to the boy she found to fetch it, 'and you'll not tell a soul how I manage to grow roses longer into the season than anyone else. You hear that?'

'Yes, ma'am,' the ragged boy answered obediently and hurried off with the can and his fortune, cunningly avoiding the temptation of boasting about his good luck in case they tried to cut in on his highly profitable business with Miss Jackson, particularly as it was to go on.

At least once a day the unhappy Amy supped the broth Aunt Dorothea so kindly made specially for her, but trying to keep her confined to her bed as Amos Drew strongly advised was another matter.

'I simply can't lie here all day every day doing nothing,' she said defiantly and got up, praying for the time to pass quickly so that her child could be born and she could return to James on board. In her efforts to shorten the weeks she wrote letters to acquaintances she had met in Liverpool and on voyages, always careful to keep them bright and cheerful. And she arranged to have brought to her every book on navigation that could be found.

'It says here,' she pointed out to Aunt Dorothea, 'that vessels must stay well clear of Cape São Roque on their way to Rio.'

'Then I'm sure they do, Amelia,' Dorothea replied, not having the slightest idea where that was and interested only in seeing some signs of pallor in her.

'But it doesn't say why,' Amy complained, 'whether from shoals, calms, storms, adverse winds and currents or what.' In all, she was very dissatisfied with the books since none of them told her what she wanted to know and she felt that if she could be of even more help to James when she returned to sea, he might never be so cruel to her again in leaving her behind.

'You are a silly dear,' Dorothea told her as she gave her an auntly kiss, only to see that even close up her skin was still of good colour, 'and you'd better take care or you'll make yourself ill worrying about such silly things. You leave all that to the sailors. What you have to think about is yourself and your child and take more fluids like Dr Drew said.' And to that end she filled Amy's water jug too with the water the boy secretly fetched. It made her apprehensive to see little change in Amy's health but, in hope, she persevered.

If James, who worried much about his wife, ever wished he had her back with him it was now, as he was not at all confident about his position. The *Atheneum* was shrouded in fog and barely making way with every sail aloft, many of them unable to hold any wind at all, hanging limply and dripping. The lookouts on each mast could see no further than the deck beneath them. The course was due east but just as the master had total faith in doctors so did the passengers have faith in captains, and in the cabin they played cards, chatted and drank their free wine. No one knew they were headed directly for the rocks and as the leadline could not reach the seabed, the mate felt a false sense of security.

'Can you smell land, Mr Watson?' James asked him.

'No, sir, not yet,' Watson replied.

There were times when James could smell land as far as twenty miles away after a long time at sea but between the fog and the scent of broiling mutton that drifted from the stovepipe of the galley it was impossible. For days he had seen neither sun nor moon to help him, not that the help might have been accurate. Without Amy he had fallen back on his old ways, setting courses as was traditional practice for the crossing, only to find with the sextant now and then that he had again covered many unnecessary miles – assuming his calculations had been correct, or near enough. By his estimate he should have been approaching the north of Ireland with Inishtrahull and Malin Head far to starboard. So it was at the starboard rail he stood, eyes pinched as he tried to pierce the fog. Again, the bosun blew on the brass foghorn to warn any other shipping but the sound moaned out eerily into the surrounds where it was soon soaked up to die.

The *Atheneum* ghosted on towards the rocks without so much as the cry of a fog-bound seagull to give them away.

'One and a half knots, sir!' the log man called to the mate as they crept on towards disaster.

James was never to know exactly what happened or give any plausible explanation for it. Suddenly, in the silence, without any such expectation or other warning, the voice of Amy was talking to him in his head. 'Course north, James,' she said with the greatest urgency, 'course north. North.'

'New course north, mister!' James heard himself shouting at his mate and jumped to the helm himself to take over the steering. As the mate barked his orders and the bosun raised his whistle to blow it, the seamen sprang into action, wrenching out their belaying pins. It was not so easy as it sounded because the ship did not have enough way up to bring her around. James roared and cursed directly at this crew from the wheel and passengers came out on deck to see what was causing the sudden commotion.

'What's happening?' a gentleman asked the bosun who was himself taken by surprise at the suddenness of the attempted manoeuvre.

'Nothin', sir,' the bosun replied. 'The captain's decided to change course, that's all.'

'Oh, I see,' said the gentleman and asked his companions to return with him to their game, quite unaware that within a short time he might be asked to swim for his life or drown.

It took all of half an hour for James using all his skill with helm and sail to bring her round and hardly had he done so when all at the one time the log man was calling eight fathoms and the men aloft were simultaneously calling their warning. James heard it, too. The unmistakable sound of the Atlantic swell smashing on unseen rocks, and he was shouting desperately for quick adjustments to take her higher to what drifting wind there was. For the next two hours he held his composure but had he been a nailbiter there would have been little of them left. And as the fog lifted enough for them to see, the sight of black rocks was less than a mile away.

'Holy Christ,' the mate muttered in overwhelming relief and although he was fully appreciative of Captain McBain having saved them, as were the seamen to a man, he never did find out how he knew to alter course in the nick of time since James could not even explain it to himself. But there was no question that had he not done what he had at that moment, the rocks it would certainly have been.

After sailing over three thousand miles, the significance of making an error of only forty miles south was evident. And James was only too conscious that even had his life been saved on wrecking his new ship on her maiden voyage, he surely would have lost his captaincy. He sensed strongly that the spirit of Amy was with him and in that certainty felt she was all right and being well cared for.

In better visibility and with soundings being taken constantly, the *Atheneum,* in a breeze that veered and filled in from the north, fetched up nor'-east within sight of the rugged coast of Donegal for another day and a half before she was able to start rounding her proper landfall and ease sail to run for the North Channel. But not once in all that time did he leave the side of the various helmsmen except to urinate. And once more he drove her for every fraction of a knot he could get out of her, the crew showing more willing to cope with the obstructions in their way. It was all due to his compulsion and not his other abilities that he completed the passage to Liverpool in only twenty-seven days and, if it was not a record, it was better than average and everyone was pleased with him. In port came another warning.

'You know, Captain McBain,' one of the senior men at the agents for Kimball and Jay told him, 'with all the new packets you're building over there, we foresee a limit on what you can bring us from Boston. It's not going to be easy to keep on finding buyers for more sassafras, corn husks, cow horns, rubber shoes and the like. Passengers and cotton and tobacco, yes, but it's New York that's controlling these and that's where most of the business will be coming from in the future.'

James paid little heed at the time. He had enough on his mind as it was and did not see it as his own concern. His two main ambitions were to have Amy back with him and make his reputation as a captain.

Ten days later, again carrying mostly textiles, the cabin packed with as many passengers as could be squeezed in, James headed the *Atheneum* south for Madeira to complete his cargo with Madeira wine. Praying that he might not have to sail around for days to find the tiny specks, he allowed his mate to do the navigating. Apart from two frustrating days becalmed, only a day was lost in searching for the islands, a capful of cloud over them eventually giving them away. That accomplished, fresh fruit as well as the sweet-smelling wine hauled up over the side from small boats bobbing in warm sunshine over a couple of days, he weighed anchor. This time it was the thought of getting back to Boston and Amy as quickly as possible that made him drive the ship on for all she was worth, and well he had got to know that very edge of her limits without breaking spars or topmasts. But on the route he took he did not know how lucky he was not to become becalmed again since he was much too far north for the steady Trade winds and crossed an area of the Atlantic that was normally full of windless holes. As it was, Mr Kimball and Mr Jay were very happy with him when on 14th December he was reported by the signal station at Marshfield to have passed through Nantucket Sound.

It was agony for him to nurse his patience through all the port procedures, but eventually he was there, all his gifts for his wife and Aunt Dorothea gathered up, the *Atheneum* hauled into her berth until her bowsprit protruded proudly right over the wharf itself. James was astonished to see Amy standing there in the care of her anxious-looking aunt, but chains would not have held the determined, pregnant young woman from seeing his arrival home and it was only moments later he found himself facing her.

'I told her she should not have done this, James,' Aunt Dorothea said, 'but she refused to listen and there was nothing I could do.'

Amy looked a little pale and shy, afraid that James's first words might be to scold her for her disobedience. But James could not say a word; so overwhelmed with emotion was he at seeing her that he knew if he tried to speak his voice would break and he might instantly burst into tears. And Amy, feeling it, thought that, at any moment, she too might burst into an uncontrollable flood. It was almost as if they were meeting for the first time and falling in mindless and heedless love all over again. She was even more beautiful than his imagination had pictured her in his days at sea and he, to her, had become even more handsome than the memories in her room. Without either of them having spoken a word, his arms were around her and hers around him, hugging each other with their unborn child between them. James was quite unaware of the hatred Dorothea Jackson felt for him at that moment, and her voice did not betray her. Indeed she sounded light-hearted and joking as she clicked her tongue then said, 'Everyone's looking at you, you know, as if they've never seen such a thing before. Well, let them look if they have to but wouldn't we all be better off if you had your reunion in front of a good warm fire instead of standing here freezing?'

Although James made sure to thank Aunt Dorothea profusely for taking such good care of his wife, for all the rest of that day and all of next, James and Amy could hardly take their eyes off each other for a moment.

'It's the God's honest truth,' he ended when he told her of what had happened when he had almost gone on the rocks of Western Ireland, and Amy stared at him in wide-eyed astonishment. Although there had been several times she had felt he might be in danger she could not remember giving him any such instruction.

'Maybe it was in a dream and I can't recall it,' she said, but she was delighted and flattered to believe she had saved him.

They were the happiest of days, during which Dorothea was clever enough to make it obvious that she was deliberately staying out of their way as much as possible. For that, she collected even more appreciation for her thoughtfulness and kindness. And if James had to go to the wharf many times to attend to his ship's business, he wasted no time about it, returning to Amy at the cottage as quickly as possible. It was not until Christmas Eve with black-hatted sailors and whores already making merry all over Broad and Purchase Streets instead of being in church that, down in the counting house, he was given the disturbing news.

'We're a bit short on cargo this trip, Jim,' the wharfinger told him. 'Mr Kimball wants you to go south first to Savannah and complete your loading with cotton.'

'I'm not sure the *Atheneum*'s shallow enough draughted to get over the bar at Savannah,' James pointed out to him. 'She's not a cotton packet with a flat bottom built for it.'

The wharfinger knew perfectly well that McBain's worry was more for his wife than getting over the bar but did not say so. 'We're sure you can do it, Jim,' he said reassuringly.

'And what about the diversion for the passengers?' James tried to argue.

'We're contacting them and doubt if any of them will have any objections.'

'Well, I know what I would do if I wanted to get to Liverpool in a hurry,' James told him in some annoyance. 'I'd get a schooner down to New York and catch a packet going direct from there.'

'James,' the wharfinger said patiently, 'there's nothing else we can do. It's Savannah first or we can't be profitable.'

James hurried to the Exchange where the merchants met every day to discuss business and waited to see Kimball and Jay but although they apologised to him for the last-minute change in arrangements, it made no difference. What it meant was that James was going to be away from Boston much longer than he expected and because of what Dr Drew had intimated to him he felt desperate to be back in time for the birth. Once more he was faced with an impossible choice. If he backed out it would be like telling the

64

owners, who had given him his chance, to go to hell and stick the *Atheneum* up their counting house. And at such a late stage they might not find it easy to find another master. It was also likely that all the merchants would get together at their 'Change and make sure he never took another ship out of Boston.

'Don't you dare even think of such a thing, James,' Amy told him firmly when he put it to her. 'For heaven's sake you're a captain with a captain's responsibilities and I'm going to be perfectly all right. And even if the winds are unkind to you, why, won't I be ready and waiting with a little bundle to come straight back on board? In fact I'd come back aboard right now if only you'd let me.'

'No,' James got in quickly to stop her, paused and raised a hand of surrender. 'All right, all right. You stay here and I go. As your aunt might say, the Lord must be testing us for some good reason,' and patting her gently on the stomach, added, 'and it better be a goddamn good one.'

With snowflakes, church bells and rum-mill hangovers all along the waterfront, Christmas was soon over. And on New Year's Day, Amy, once more broken-hearted at the parting, did her best to wave at the sailing of the *Atheneum* while not long after, with every inch of canvas he could carry, James was pushing her out through the icy waters of Boston harbour to head for Savannah as fast as he could go. Again he cursed the unborn child, not only because it had caused this separation but because it might bring harm to his wife.

Amy drank her broth and the water from her pitcher but it appeared to be doing her little harm, and every day on Dorothea's table she spread out old charts and, with purely speculative calculations of winds and currents, tried to estimate the position where he might be. But she sensed no danger, either for him or for herself. And all the time, Dorothea Jackson surreptitiously watched her closely for signs of some illness that did not appear. But since she cunningly reasoned that perhaps it was only in winter that the water from the pond by the shot tower was affected, she continued with it in hope.

James was doing his own calculations and had worked out that with good luck and a few gales behind him between Savannah and Liverpool, and fair Trade winds on the return, he still had every chance of getting back to Boston in time. So it was in the greatest frustration that when he eventually arrived off Savannah he was met by a pilot cutter and told that with his draught he would have to lie off at sea for a few days and wait for a higher tide before trying to cross the bar.

'The hell I will,' James said and ordered the jolly boat over to go ahead, and with the leadline, find the deepest part. It took several hours but the deepest water turned out to be almost the same as his draught. Small boats came out from all over the place when they realised what this captain was going to try to do, and they looked on in astonishment. The madman took his ship some distance back out to sea, brought her around and with all sail set, himself at the helm, shouting orders directly to the crew, gathered way and with all the speed he could make charged the spot. For a few moments as the bows reached it, she looked as if she might make it. Then the keel scraped and suddenly, only moments later, she shuddered fast aground, throwing a few passengers who were not holding on face-forward to the deck. But it was the captain who was most indignant.

'Damn and curse you!' he roared angrily at the unhearing bar, and he was far from finished with it. Still with all sails set, he had two kedge anchors on heavy warps taken out on the boats and put to the seabed over half a cable ahead. 'Backs to it!' he shouted, calling for more effort from the sweating, bare-torsoed seamen as they tried to winch and haul her over the mud with sheer brute force. That it was to no effect made no difference. The captain did not give up. At each high water during daylight and dark he kept on trying. Then, two desperate days later, a cheer went up as the keel was cleared, and the bemused pilot guided the *Atheneum* into port.

'Who is this Captain McBain?' all the white men around the waterfront wanted to know. Never before had they seen a vessel in such an unholy rush. But had they been told it was due to anxiety about his pregnant wife they would not have believed it. Three waiting days on, every hour of which was maddening for James, they were to find out more about him.

'If these men were free and paid for their labour they'd be a damned sight more willing!' he shouted in angry frustration down from his rail at the white man in charge of the black slaves who were taking their time loading the bales of cotton.

'Get back to the Pest House where you belong, you stinkin' Yankee chinch!' an anonymous white voice yelled back at him from somewhere in the shade.

But despite every effort James made, his draught deeper than ever, it was to be yet another four days before he was just able to scrape over the bar to get out again, by which time he hated Savannah for more than just the slavery.

Yet when the buds on the trees of New England looked ready to

66

burst and spread their shades of green and Amy went into labour there was no news of the *Atheneum*.

'Oh, my dear, my dear,' Aunt Dorothea sympathised as Amy writhed with the excruciating pains over two days.

'The child isn't helping,' the midwife declared and an anxious Dr Drew engaged another to help her, at the same time feeling a little satisfaction in knowing that he had been perfectly right in paying heed to Miss Jackson's warning. It was after the third day of labour that the two midwives decided between them to forcibly extract the child, even if it did do some damage to the young woman. Her own life was more important to them, and Amy, having reached total exhaustion, could do no more.

At first they thought there was little hope of saving the weak and sickly baby but eventually, strung up by its heels and smacked over and over, they got a small, pitiful cry.

'It's a boy, my dear dear Amelia,' Amy remembered her aunt say as she bent over her.

'James,' Amy murmured and was immediately asleep, her face almost as pale as death.

It was two weeks later when James returned from Liverpool to be met on the wharf with the news that a son had been born to him, and he rushed to the cottage, urging his cab driver all the time to take his horse on faster.

Not only Aunt Dorothea was standing there greeting him but Dr Amos Drew. Amy was sitting up and did her best to smile but it only took him a few moments to realise that the tiny, sickly creature who was still hardly alive, and who needed special attention from Dr Drew and others to keep it that way, could not be taken to sea. Amy knew it too, but neither were aware of the full extent of the damage Aunt Dorothea had done with her water from the shot tower. Indeed, they were never to know that Dorothea had done anything at all other than provide shelter, friendship, kindness and comfort. For Dorothea there was great relief in feeling safe again since the outcome was almost exactly as she had falsely predicted to Amos Drew, although in truth she was not quite sure whether or not it was her broth that had caused it since nothing was known about lead poisoning or its effects. The cause no longer mattered. The result was not only that Amy could never have another child, but the one born to her needed her care and kept Amy with her. It was to be some good time before even Dr Drew began to suspect that the child was not only weak of body but backward of mind, too.

'I'm sorry, James,' Amy apologised in tears when they were alone.

'Quiet, quiet, quiet,' James said tenderly, kneeling by her to kiss her. 'It will be all right.'

But as Captain James McBain sailed out of Boston harbour it was in greater loneliness and anger than ever. This time he cursed to the depths of hell the son that had been born to him and who, at Amy's insistence, was to be baptised James.

Chapter Seven

Before James McBain junior was a year old, James took a house in Boston, a narrow, two-storey brick residence with a stoop to the entrance. But it was not for want of accommodation. As everyone was made to know, Miss Dorothea Jackson was only too willing to continue to provide that. Rather was it born of the need to provide a personal meeting place, and since James was rarely to be in it, that was really only what it was. A link that somehow helped to bind them together in their separation. There, on his all too short visits between the long voyages, could be kept the memories of what had been. Here it was that, every now and then, the strangers came briefly together to rediscover each other, creating fantasies in each other's arms of what still might be, then parted. And here it was that Amy saw the James she had always known, jealously reserving for him all the moments she had to give by having the sickly child taken out of his way when he was there and temporarily put in the care of her kindly aunt and a nursing woman. So although James never once neglected his duty of bringing gifts for his son, he had almost no contact with him.

It was merchants and their wharfingers and the crews of ships who saw the changes in the young captain who had quickly established himself as a driver. Although he had never been considered a frivolous and light-hearted man, he had been a happy one, one who had already attained his ambitions and appeared content with them. That was no longer true. There was a dourness about him and if his acquaintances were many, his friends were few. And neither to them nor to the many passengers with whom he socially mixed, from poets to princes, did the lonely man ever mention the son who had caused so much pain. Away from Amy his vessel was his bride, the sails her gown, and he threw himself with full force into the business of the sea. If becalmed on a Sunday he would stand bare-headed on deck, Bible in hand, read the service then demand from passengers and crew alike that they bow their heads for two silent minutes and pray for wind rather than the souls of the dead.

'A hundred dollars?' Mr Kimball said in surprise at McBain's request for a bonus on his return from a voyage.

'No less, gentlemen,' James told them. 'I've done my calculations and believe it is my due.'

'We'll have to think about that, Jim,' Mr Jay considered. 'We've no obligation to pay anything, you know.'

'They you'll have to get yourself another master,' James said firmly, and Kimball and Jay, although they did not like it, knew they could do no better and paid. Thus did James fight for every red cent of bonus he could get out of his employers, for if his navigation left a lot to be desired, he still made fast times. He also alienated a lot of other captains and mates by vociferously supporting the introduction of a Federal Statute prescribing punishment for any deck officers who, simply out of malice, hatred or revenge, beat or wounded a member of their crew. But if that led seamen to sign on with McBain in the knowledge they were not serving on a blood ship, they were to find there were other drawbacks. The next man Captain McBain risked his life for by plucking him from the sea in a mid-Atlantic gale was not quite so thankful when his saviour then imposed a fine of fifteen dollars on him for his carelessness in losing his footing aloft in the first place. It was not surprising that 'Chargin' Jim' was the original nickname he was given behind his back, particularly after, at full speed, he attacked the bar away down at Mobile in the same way he had at Savannah, this time more successfully, then refused to pay the pilot more than half his fee for his ill-advice to wait three days for higher water.

'What bothers you, Captain?' asked a travelling professor of philosophy who found little else to do but stroke his long beard and carefully study his cabin companions for signs of disturbance in them.

'What bothers me, sir,' James answered politely enough, 'is President Jackson, poor sea cooks, and getting you as safely and quickly as I can to your destination.' And that was as far as the professor got in his attempt at invading the master's privacy. But he was not the only one. Men in general became cautious of Captain McBain and no doubt because he stayed so apart and was different there were those who feared him. Certainly he often put more than forty knots up his crews when, fighting to weather, he laid his ship almost on her side.

'Damn it to hell, hove to, mister!' he thundered at the mate when the main topmast came crashing down into the angry sea over the lee rail in a tangle of rigging and he sprang to take the wheel himself. It was not for long and not for comfort. He personally directed the bosun and carpenter as if every life depended on it, and men struggled with knives, blocks and tackle both on deck and aloft to make repairs and fit a new one. And the second it was done, only five hours later, he was putting the helm over to fresh orders and racing off again into the night, every bit as dangerously as before.

It was worse for Amy when it began to become evident that the child, apart from being weak and sickly, was also mentally retarded and could not ever be taken to sea. More than once she was racked by guilt in wishing that James McBain junior, to whom she had given the name Jayjay, had died at birth. Try as she might, she could not get the baby to respond either to herself or to anything else.

'There must be something you can do!' she said in desperation to Dr Amos Drew, but all he could do was sadly shake his head.

'I'm very, very sorry, Mrs McBain,' he told her, 'but there's nothing. It's a misfortune we have to bear.' That *he* had to bear? He had to bear none of it. Once he was on the verge of suggesting that the child be put in a small, private asylum he knew of, but he sensed that the distraught mother might have physically attacked him for such an idea and suspected that Miss Jackson would have had none of it either.

'Look what I've got you, Jayjay,' Amy said in her upstairs room as she lowered a tabby kitten into the cot in the hope that it might provide stimulation, but her child did not even attempt to put his tiny hand to it. 'We'll call it Captain,' she went on. 'Isn't that a fine name for it?'

There followed the spaniel pup called Bosun but if both cat and dog showed an interest in the fragile life with the blank expression it was all one-sided. For someone who once claimed not to have enough patience to teach anything to her young sisters, Amy McBain showed a futile excess of it. Almost all day she spoke to the child, cut out paper figures for him, read him stories, even books on navigation for want of anything else. And all the while, Aunt Dorothea hovered in the background and Captain ate the Bosun's food and the Bosun ate the Captain's.

'God has protected the child from all the worries of life,' was the way Miss Dorothea Jackson put it to her other ladies of charity and they thought it a very charitable way of putting it. But Amy did not see him as being so favoured.

'You've ruined our lives and you give me nothing in return!' she exploded in awful, angry frustration right into the child's face at the end of another, totally unproductive day. Then, suddenly, she became aware of his eyes that were almost as blue as his father's looking directly back into hers. In them, for the first time, there was a reaction, a recognition, but it was far from a happy one. What she saw there was deep pain, accusation, and a terrible struggle taking place. And when he dropped his gaze, she fell to her knees, buried her head in her hands and wept bitterly in shame. She did not know how long she had been there like that when rescue appeared in the shape of the nursing woman bearing the medicine Dr Drew had prescribed for the weak and sickly child.

'You try to do too much, Mrs McBain,' the woman chided her kindly but Amy hardly heard her.

'He knows me,' Amy tried to tell her. 'He knows me and he knows I'm trying to help him. I'm sure of it.'

'Yes, yes, yes, I'm sure of it, too, Mrs McBain,' the woman said, believing not a word of it, 'but I think a little walk in the open would do you the world of good.'

It was with a fresh resolve to do more that Amy emerged from that experience. She vowed never to reject him again. And if she did not at first realise that she had become firmly caught between the love for her husband and the growing love for her helpless son, with little hope of ever making both compatible and bringing them together, she threw all the energies into helping both.

'It is sad to see,' the neighbours whispered to each other as the pretty young Mrs McBain spent almost all the child's waking hours picking him up and putting him down, all the time talking to him. And since James McBain junior was unable to sit up like a normal child, Amy tied him up in that position and, in a clear voice, read to his drooping head anything she could lay her hands on. Everything from Shakespeare to cat and dog hairs went into the seemingly mindless ears of James McBain junior.

'Everyone is wrong but only you and I know it, Jayjay,' Amy told him as if he understood everything she said and she did not care if it was only vague noises and not words she got back. Neither did she care about the glances of pity as she carried him to the street to point out the horses and wagons and what goods they were carrying. Slung on her hip, she took him to see the new naval drydock built all of granite, and to the new wharves with all the ships. And she stopped with him before the Post Office.

'One flight of stairs up there is Topliffe's News Room,' she explained quietly, although his eyes were almost buried in her dress. 'Every morning the merchants go up there to find out what has been happening in the world while they've been asleep. Up there are papers and messages and lists of ships coming and going, including your father's. Maybe one day you'd like to become a member of Topliffe's.'

It was hardly surprising that while those who knew them saw Miss Dorothea Jackson as a caring and kindly aunt of sound mind, it was her so-called niece who seemed to be losing hers. Only when the captain came home on his brief visits did she regain some semblance of the shining bride who had once attracted so much attention.

'Bobo,' James junior said when he was twenty months old, clearly meaning Bosun who followed them around everywhere, inside and out, but if Amy was the only one to hear that first clear word he uttered, it sent her into a paroxysm of delight. So much so that within the hour, almost everyone she knew in Boston had been made aware of the unbelievable news that James McBain junior had spoken the name of their dog. If it impressed no one, they did not say so.

'You must praise the dear child for it,' Dorothea Jackson warned them. 'His mother expects it.'

But there were also the days in which the child appeared to regress to the stage of giving up life altogether when Dr Drew had to be fetched in a hurry.

Yet even Dorothea who was to be found as often in the McBain house as she was in her cottage was to be taken by surprise. She had just returned there one day after one of her satisfying visits to an asylum. She could hear her Amelia's voice talking upstairs as usual as she removed her coat and, since it was a day off for the nursing woman, prepared to make afternoon tea.

'I'm in, Amelia!' she called up. 'I'm here!'

Hardly had she spoken when she heard what amounted to a scream come from upstairs.

'Aunt Dorothea! Quickly! Come quickly!'

Quickly lifting the hem of her dark skirt above her black boots she hurried up, not knowing what to expect but anxious since she did not want to see this child die. Not even Amy knew what a growing attachment Aunt Dorothea had for James McBain junior since she had been clever enough to conceal any more than might have been expected from such a caring lady. Grave of face she arrived panting in the child's room. And there she stopped, staring in amazement, the proudest mother in all Christendom standing a little way off, looking on. For the first time ever, James McBain junior was actually standing upright on his own two feet, one hand firmly flat on the seat of a chair for support. There was even the hint of a smile on his lips and beside his skinny legs stood the Bosun, wagging its tail. Only the tabby Captain represented what might have been the attitude of the rest of the world since they would hardly have considered it an achievement for a two-year-old.

Curled up on another chair, its eyes opened by all the commotion and seeing nothing of interest, it closed them again.

'Oh, you dear, dear boy!' Dorothea exclaimed with such emotion that she almost gave her feelings away. 'Oh, you dear, dear clever boy!'

And so that the clever boy's triumph might not fall to the floor in disgrace, Amy rushed to him and swept him up into her arms, kissed him and said, 'I told you you'd be strong, didn't I? And you're going to be even stronger. As strong as anyone.' But if that seemed a vain prediction, at that moment she believed it. Indeed, she could hardly wait to tell Amos Drew of the progress she had made.

Dr Amos Drew smiled kindly at her. He was very sorry he had made his prediction that nothing could be done with the child. It was about the only one he had ever made in his professional life and he should have known better. If the improvement in the child was small, it was still an improvement and he sought to recoup his status and honour.

'It was my belief from the beginning, of course, Mrs McBain,' he said, 'that the child might show some more awareness, but I didn't want to raise your hopes too high. Indeed, I still don't want to do so now but there is no doubt you have done a wonderful job with the boy. Wonderful.'

'I've done very little, Dr Drew,' Amy returned modestly. 'It's Jayjay who's done all the fighting. He has the spirit for it and I can see it in him. But what I want to know is, do you think he can ever improve enough for me to take him safely to sea?'

Amos Drew looked distinctly disturbed by that. One prediction in his life was mistake enough. And the young woman's obsession with returning to the sea simply to be with her husband more was somehow abnormal to him, while taking such a child with her was positively indecent. One heavy throw of his body against a bulk-head in a storm was likely to break all his fragile bones. Besides, if he was any judge, the very sight of a wave was likely to turn the sickly boy greener than a field of alfalfa. It was hard enough to keep food down in his stomach when he was still. But he had no intention of expressing any of that. Anything he advised could turn out to be wrong.

'That is impossible to say, Mrs McBain,' he intoned, 'because what you're really asking of me under the circumstances is not so much my medical opinion but rather a declaration of my faith and I'm not really qualified for that.'

With Amos Drew reluctant to commit himself further, it was as much encouragement as Amy could get.

'We're alone, Jayjay,' Amy said to her sleeping son on her return home, 'but alone we will show them.'

In the counting house of Kimball and Jay, other acts of faith were being followed.

'We must build another packet,' Mr Kimball said to Mr Jay across the large desk where they sat every day facing each other.

'Of shallower draught,' Mr Jay agreed.

'More passenger accommodation,' Mr Kimball added.

'More cotton,' Mr Jay contributed further.

'McBain as master?' queried Mr Kimball.

'None better,' Mr Jay concurred.

They had very good reason for that. James, despite hounding them for larger bonuses and driving hard bargains, had made more profit for them than any other captain they had employed before and their only concern was losing him. It was why they also agreed between them that they would give James the honour of naming their new vessel, a decision based on the theory that it would be harder for the captain to desert a ship he had named himself. That she was already building was the first news James got on his next arrival back in Boston and by the time he reached home, where he was expected, his head was full of it.

'You'll not believe the progress he's made, James,' Amy could hardly wait to tell him regarding the child as they held each other tightly. 'He says words now and everything. You must see him for yourself. You must.'

'Not today, there's plenty of time,' James replied and before she knew it he was rushing her off to a yard on the North River. There, two large draught horses harnessed in traces were being made to haul on a heavy rope of the primitive wooden crane as another giant rib was raised into position and temporarily secured. All around, men were busy hammering, sawing and adzing. Holding Amy's hand James eagerly helped her over all the obstructions in the way and up the steps to the builder's loft. There, a small team of men were marking out on the floor the full-scale patterns of more of her timbers. Although James had not seen the builder, a Mr Cranford, before, Cranford knew immediately who he was and came forward, holding out his hand. James proudly introduced his wife but was impatient to study the half-model from which all was devised and which lay on a bench. Cranford gave it to him and Amy was only too aware of the light in James's eyes as he held it. With his fingers he stroked along its smooth, curvaceous lines then handed it to Amy as if it might have been some precious, fragile jewel, expecting her to admire it. Amy held it, appearing to study it, feeling unreasonably and passionately jealous of it. Desperate to find some criticism of the lady, and having read books about the building of ships, amongst all the others, to her retarded son during the long periods of James's absences, she found one.

'Very pretty,' she said. 'But although I have to admit I know very little about such things, doesn't she have a rather flat bottom?'

Cranford stared at the woman in astonishment and James, too, was taken by surprise at Amy's knowledge, since although the feature was deliberate, what she had pointed out was only too true.

'That, Mrs McBain,' Cranford felt obliged to explain as he quickly regained his composure, 'is to give her shallower draught so as to get easy over the bars at Savannah and Mobile, but she should be fast all the same.'

'I have no doubt of it, sir,' Amy replied, handing the model back to him while James, a little embarrassed, thanked Cranford for his kindness and time and hurried Amy out of there before she could find any more faults with what was a ship designer's dream. But although he was perfectly aware of some irritation in her he thought it better to ignore it and let it ease off. It did not. As he stopped in the yard to look up at those first dozen ribs of the new creation he was to master, he got carried away.

'Flat-floored or not, Amy,' he said, 'she's still going to be the most beautiful thing ever to come out of Boston.'

'If I thought for a minute, James McBain,' Amy told him as she turned on him, 'that your promiscuity with ships extended into other areas, I'd kill you.' But as James glared briefly back into her beautiful, serious face she wished that she might have swallowed her accusing words since it had never once crossed her mind that he might be unfaithful to her and it was only his attraction to the new ship she was jealous of. Then, to her relief, he smiled.

'And you so clever,' he said. 'Don't you know there's never a minute at sea when you're not in my mind? Don't you realise how much I miss you not being with me? Don't you know there could never be another woman in the world who breathes for me?'

'Yes, I'm sorry, I know, I know!' Amy cried, throwing herself emotionally into his arms for him to hold her. It was not until they both became aware that all the hammering and sawing had stopped and the workmen were staring at them in their embrace in wonder and amusement that they untwined themselves and moved off.

It was not difficult for James to guess that it was the child who was the cause of Amy's disturbance but he said not a word of it, while Amy knew instinctively that to present James junior now to show off his improvement would only have destroyed the days of carefree happiness left to them. But the night before James was to sail away again, as he prepared to switch roles once more to the strict, driving master of a trans-Atlantic packet, his sense of duty at last prevailed upon him. Besides, he knew full well that it was going to make Amy happier.

'You said I should see the boy,' he said to her. 'If he's well enough I should be able to find enough time in the morning.' And although Amy did all she could to suppress her excitement it was obvious enough to him.

Thus the following morning was James junior hurried from the cottage by Aunt Dorothea and the nursing woman who, after handing him back into the care of his mother, discreetly found other things to do around the house. Shortly after, Amy stood holding the child's hand as she helped him to stand beside her, doing all she could to hide her pride in him. Facing them was James, tall land hat in hand, ready to leave. After an awkward pause, it was duty alone that forced him to crouch to his idiot child but the tinge of sympathy he felt for him he quickly cast aside. This was the being who had caused so much pain, who had robbed him of his wife, who was the cause of all his long days, weeks, months and years of miserable loneliness, who had destroyed fulfilment and who made Amy suffer. This was the curse on him and if it was impossible to hate someone who had no power to retaliate or fight back, he came close to it. No signal went out from father and none was returned by son. If James junior was aware of anything it was only of an unwanted stranger and if he felt frightened by him he did not show that either.

'I have brought you things from England,' his father said to him, obliged to speak for Amy's sake, 'but your mother will give them to you.'

And duty done he straightened. And yet again, only a few hours later, Amy stood on the shore with tears in her eyes as she watched the *Atheneum* raise full sail out on the harbour and, slightly heeled, speed off down Ship Channel, bound first for Mobile then Liverpool. Then, while still nursing her loss of the one, returned with her love to the other. And the leaves of New England that had turned on their full glory of reds and golds and browns began to fall.

Chapter Eight

The biggest, most drunken, female-deprived sailor in Boston would have thought twice about approaching Miss Fanny Blossom. As a woman she was huge, as a keeper in this particular asylum, formidable. Under her ruddy cheeks, a long apron stretched stiffly over her big unyielding bosom, and stuck in the leather belt around her waist was a stout stick. As she led Miss Jackson down a dark, smelly corridor, she bore a ring of large keys in one hand and a three-legged stool in the other.

'It's a while since we've seen you here, Miss Jackson,' Miss Blossom said as they went.

'I've had to visit other places,' Dorothea explained, 'and apart from all the other charity work I've had to do, I've been kept very busy having to help raise my niece's little boy. That's been a great trial for me.'

'Yes, so I've heard,' Miss Blossom returned, at least up to date with her gossip.

'But he's the most wonderful child and he gives me great joy,' Dorothea added hurriedly.

'That's nice for you,' Miss Blossom said.

Miss Blossom had known Miss Dorothea Jackson over years from her periodic visits and if she saw them as pointless, especially as her lunatics never seemed to appreciate them, it was not her place or her business to question what her superiors and doctors regarded as charitable work. Her job was to supervise her charges and keep them in order and she was not alone in believing she did it well. She stopped in front of an iron door and searched for the right key.

'We've got this one as timid as a lamb now,' she told Dorothea, 'but we have to keep her separate since others attack her for stealing from them. She's a magpie. Put anything down, especially if it's got colour in it, and she'll have it under her skirt before you can blink an eye. I don't know what you've brought for her but if it's shiny she'll love it. Just watch her.'

'Don't worry, I'll take good care,' Dorothea assured her and the door was opened to reveal a woman of uncertain age with matted

79

hair, crouched in a corner by a filthy bench that was secured to the dirty brick wall. Her clothes were no more than rags and the stench of insanity that mingled with the smell of urine made the air foul, but Dorothea was well used to all that. Indeed, to all who knew her, she had always been accorded the credit of a minor saint for going into such places. In the cell, Miss Blossom put down the stool for the visitor since there was nowhere else clean to sit.

'If you need me, just call, I won't be far away,' she said, and leaving the door wide open, made her way back up the corridor.

Dorothea sat on the stool, clutching her large purse in which was her bait, studying her victim as if sympathetically for a few moments. As always, the first thing she had to do was to discover the woman's greatest weakness, although she had already been given the most helpful clue.

'And how are you today?' She smiled at the crouched figure as if she had met her before, and the woman smiled weakly and nervously back at her. That was a good start.

'I'm not going to hurt you, you know,' Dorothea went on, gradually gaining the woman's confidence. 'I'm here to help you and give you things. Now why don't you sit up so we can talk properly? You want to talk to me, don't you?'

The woman was not at all sure but Dorothea encouraged her by dipping into her purse, pulling out a cheap, bright red bookmark and, leaning forward, putting it down on the bench out of her reach. Moments later the woman was seated up there and the bookmark had disappeared.

'What's your name?' Dorothea asked.

'I'm a flower,' the woman said.

'What kind of flower?' Dorothea wanted to know.

'I'm a flower,' the woman repeated.

'But what kind of flower?' Dorothea persisted. 'A daisy? A rose?' And as she went through a whole list of flowers, it became clear by the increasing anxiety and frustration on the woman's face that she did not know and did not have enough wit to either make a guess or tell a lie.

Already Dorothea had her mark and it had been so easy. For a time she kept on pushing the woman about it and said eventually, 'If you can tell me what kind of flower you are I'll give you something wonderful.'

'I'm a flower,' the woman continued to repeat.

Then, from out of her purse, Dorothea slowly pulled what was a most colourful piece of fine English china. A lady dressed in bright blue with bonnet and tiny bucket, seated side-saddle on a large, long-horned goat of shining gold and white. Captain James McBain had come in very handy in bringing such gifts to Aunt Dorothea for her charity work and both he and Amy imagined that she made the very best use of them.

'Isn't it beautiful?' she smiled and watched the woman gape at it in covetousness.

As always before, Dorothea had found an impossible task for her victim to perform. In the past it had been everything from knitting difficult stitches to the repetition of some long, little-known psalm read only once to them. This time it was the simple naming of a flower.

'You tell me the name and I'll give this to you,' Dorothea told her and watched the desperate and futile struggle taking place in the woman's mad eyes.

'I'm a flower,' she said yet again and stretched out a pleading hand towards the glittering gift she was so sure was hers.

'I'll ask you just once more,' Dorothea smiled, savouring every last moment of the strong satisfaction it gave her to torture in the safety of such a place. It did not matter that she could not explain the craving for it that rose in her at intervals. It was like a drug to her that was necessary to ease the pain of her existence. Slowly she rose, teasing with the forbidden fruit, watching the outstretched dirty fingers that so desired it. Furtively, she glanced quickly outside to make sure no one was near, then moved a few feet closer to the woman.

'Give me, give me,' the woman pleaded.

'You didn't give me the name,' Dorothea said to her quietly and, as the woman got up and moved to her as if to snatch the colourful lady on the goat from her, Dorothea lifted her arm and suddenly threw the treasure down with force on to the stone flagging at her feet where it shattered into little pieces. The woman stared for a moment, then fell to her knees, her nails scrabbling in the remnants as if expecting the undamaged whole to be still there amongst them.

'Dahlia,' she tried to say through her tears.

Miss Blossom, having heard the crash, came running, stick in hand, and pulled up at the cell. Quickly surveying the scene she immediately made her usual assumption and hurrying to the woman raised her stick to beat her.

'You ungrateful sow!' she shouted angrily at the wretch, who threw herself back to her corner to cower there with her hands over her head.

'No, no, no!' Dorothea cried as she clutched with both hands at the stout arm. 'You mustn't! She didn't mean it! She dropped it by accident!'

81

So, with Dorothea imposing restraint, the poor woman was only struck twice and Miss Blossom calmed herself.

'I don't know why you bother, Miss Jackson,' she panted. 'They do this all the time to you and it's all you'll ever get from them for your kindness. I know them.'

'It doesn't matter, doesn't matter,' Dorothea hastened to assure her. 'It really doesn't. The important thing is to try.'

It was astonishing that for all the time Dorothea had been doing this no one ever questioned why it was that everything she brought to these lunatic women was either ripped to pieces, broken beyond repair or smashed to smithereens. To Miss Blossom and others like her, the only mad ones there were those who were locked up for it and no suspicion whatsoever had yet fallen on the kindly Miss Dorothea Jackson. Indeed, Miss Blossom apologised several times for the bad behaviour of her charge as she locked the iron door again and led her back up the dark corridor, three-legged stool once more in hand.

As Dorothea emerged from the front entrance into a light fall of snow, she was momentarily startled by the sight of Amos Drew arriving in his tall hat, long winter overcoat of the finest cloth buttoned high around his neck and leather bag in hand. It was rare for her to run into him on her charitable expeditions and the unexpectedness of it so close to her having just taken another taste of revenge on the world could have been more than a coincidence. In truth she did not trust him any more.

'How delightful to see you here, Miss Jackson!' he exclaimed cheerfully and the immediate threat she had felt vanished.

'Dr Drew,' she returned with surprise.

'If I'd known you were coming to this place today I could have brought you in my carriage,' Amos Drew said politely, 'and I'd take you back if you'd care to wait although I may be some long time.'

'Oh, no, no, no, thank you, you're very kind, very kind,' Dorothea said and leaned a little towards his ear. 'It's such a sad place to have to wait.'

'Yes, I agree,' Dr Drew replied.

'They may have been used up for this world,' Dorothea continued confidentially to the side of his head, 'but no matter what people think they are not animals. Not animals.'

'No indeed,' Dr Drew agreed further, 'but it's only a few kind and caring people like yourself who see it that way.'

'I don't think Miss Blossom here sees me as being any benefit to them,' Dorothea went on.

'But of course you are, Miss Jackson. Good Lord, you're the only visitor from the outside world most of them ever get to see and talk to.'

'I only try to do my best,' Dorothea said.

That Dorothea appeared to Amos Drew to be slightly elated as she spoke he found rather curious and strange. He had often enough heard her tell other people how distressing it was for her to visit such places and his own sensibilities were always so assaulted by it that he could not wait to get home to scrub himself down from head to toe in a tub of hot water. There were women he knew who would have wept after coming out of there, even those who might have vomited. But if Miss Jackson gave him the strong impression that she had been uplifted by the experience, he had no intention of either remarking on it or making an enquiry. Ever since Dorothea had made her pointed, if disguised, accusation about his care for indigent boys, he had become increasingly uneasy about her and was very careful what he said to her. Although she was the last person in the world to be suspected as an originator of malicious rumour he was taking no chances. Even the slightest murmur of his secretly nursed guilt could have ruined him.

'You're an example to the community, Miss Jackson,' he smiled, 'and I have no doubt you'll eventually be well rewarded for it.'

'You're too kind and I don't deserve it, Dr Drew,' Dorothea smiled back, 'and I mustn't hold you up any longer from your work.'

Amos Drew politely raised his hat to her departure then continued on in to dispense his own small contribution to charity.

'I see Miss Jackson was just here,' he said to Miss Blossom shortly afterwards but if he expected any explanation for the raising of Dorothea's spirits, he was not to get it.

'A fine lady, Doctor,' was all he got in return and she said not a word of how her lunatics behaved in return for the lady's kindness since she saw it as a poor reflection on her own control of them. So, for the time being, Amos Drew had to be content with being left none the wiser about the woman he had known for so long but whom he was now vaguely beginning to suspect, although of what, apart from that one incident, he had not the slightest idea. But he would not have slept a minute easy in his bed and would probably have moved immediately to New York had he known that Miss Jackson's talents did, in fact, extend to the spreading of rumour, so cleverly sown, usually from a distance, that many a happy couple in Boston were never to know who was responsible for the dissension and distrust that entered their lives with stories of disaffection and accusations of adultery.

It was almost dark when Dorothea reached Amy's house and, with the light snow now driven by high, blustery winds, it had become bitter out. Inside, Amy had it glowing cheerfully with lamps and fires.

'There will be no cold pity come through *this* door,' she had previously announced. 'It's not welcome here and I'll have none of it.' But it was more for the sake of James McBain junior than herself that she kept the entire house so bright and warm, especially as even the slightest chill was likely to bring on more dangerous sickness and fevers in him. And if there had been days when Amy wished, for no specific reason she could give herself, that she saw less of Aunt Dorothea, the thought only made her feel guilty. She had come to accept that her aunt was much more in her house than she ever was at the cottage and she welcomed her return, particularly as she had something to tell her.

'Here, let me take your coat,' she said to her first, 'and get your frozen bones by the fire there. If you ask me, I think it's carrying charity a bit too far for people to expect you to go out in weather like this.'

'As may be, as may be,' the charitable Dorothea replied, 'but it's warm the soul before the flesh, you know, as the good Reverend Dykes always says.'

'Now there's a coincidence for you if you like, Aunt Dorothea,' Amy told her eagerly, 'because I've been thinking something similar all day. It came to me as I looked out the window and saw children running about and laughing. They wouldn't have cared if the frost had bitten off their noses and I remembered I was the same. Even at sea on the *Nantasket* I barely felt the cold because my mind was so happy and warm. So, do you realise just how bored and cold Jayjay must feel being shut up in this house with only adults for company?'

'You're not going to take him out in winter?' Dorothea said with some alarm.

'No,' Amy went on, 'but I can bring other children in to play with him. That's exactly what he needs, more even than me. Watching them, listening to their thoughts, participating in their imaginations. Theirs is a different world to ours and they will help draw him out. I know they will.'

'And where are you going to get them from?' Dorothea wanted to know.

'I've already written to half a dozen people I know who have small children,' Amy replied, 'and explained that if they could bring them here for only an hour in a week it would be a great help.'

But if Amy's confidence in James McBain junior was

unshakeable, her faith in other people was naive. One after the other, mothers replied with their range of excuses as to why it was impossible for them to comply. Nowhere amongst them, of course, was the slightest hint that, in truth, they were all repelled by the very idea of their children playing with one who was subnormal. They did not have to. Amy knew it and was deeply hurt by the rejections of her child. But she also began to realise that it was deep-seated superstition she was up against; the instinctive, primitive fear of the darkness and the unknown.

'Do they think he's a leper or will give them smallpox?' she said angrily to the nurse but although the woman could feel her pain there was nothing she could find to say that might comfort her. All the same, neither she nor Aunt Dorothea were surprised to find that far from submitting to her son's exile, it only made the young Mrs McBain more determined than ever.

'Don't you worry, Jayjay,' she told him as she tried to force him to walk across his room with an unconcerned Bosun and Captain curled by the warmth of the hearth. 'I'll get you a crew of playmates, you see if I don't.' And James McBain junior fell over to be gently raised to his feet again, Amy absolutely sure she could see a glimmer of determination on his own small face as, again, he staggered hesitantly on.

Using what connections she had, including those of Aunt Dorothea, Amy wasted no time in going about getting herself invitations to social functions, something she had previously avoided for the sake of giving her son all her attention. The problem was that going alone as a married woman with her husband away at sea would have been asking for trouble. Thus, once more, she seated herself in the study of Dr Amos Drew.

'I know this may seem very impertinent of me, Dr Drew,' she said boldly, 'but I thought as a medical man you might understand that a little outing might do my own health the world of good. I've come to ask you if it's possible for you to oblige me by escorting me to the Boston Port Society Ball next week.'

For a few moments, the soap-scented Amos Drew stared down at her in surprise. He had been expecting nothing else but to extricate himself yet again from making any prediction whatsoever on as much as a day in the future life of James McBain junior.

'Oh, dear, I see I'm out of place again, you must forgive me,' Amy apologised in disappointment and began to rise.

'No, no, no, no,' Amos Drew hastened to assure her, easing her back down into her seat with his long fingers on her shoulder. 'You're perfectly in place, Mrs McBain.'

For Amos Drew who was quickly recollecting his thoughts it seemed a perfect opportunity. To escort such a pretty young lady could only help to allay any suspicions anyone might have about his sexual inclinations, especially if he indicated it was giving him pride and pleasure. To such functions he always went and returned alone. All that worried him was what had motivated her to ask such a thing of him. Amy sensed that and was quick to ease his mind.

'You see, I simply can't risk my reputation by going alone, can I?' she explained. 'And there are people I'd like to meet to talk to about their own young children. But I can only go with someone like yourself whose own reputation is beyond doubt.'

Amos Drew clasped his hands together across his stomach and gave one of his rare, genuine smiles at that.

'Mrs McBain,' he said, 'nothing would give me greater pleasure than to be your escort.'

Amy spared no expense in shopping for the finest evening dress in emerald-green silk she could find and when the day came washed her hair and rinsed it with an infusion of rosemary. Finally dressed, she stood in all her shining glory and the nursing woman gazed on her almost in awe.

'You look beautiful beyond compare, Mrs McBain!' she exclaimed. 'Simply beautiful!'

'That's the whole idea,' Amy returned with pleasure and neither she nor her help had the faintest idea that Aunt Dorothea was burning to the depths of her soul with envy for there she also stood smiling with admiration. She herself did not go to such functions fearing that to do so might in some way unmask her disguise of the purely practical, sober, kindly, charitable, unfrivolous woman she had taken such trouble and care to build. But since the proceeds for many of these occasions were distributed for worthy causes, she was always to be found at the head of the line to pay for a ticket which she then returned, knowing that the gesture would be recorded in her name as a donation.

'Quite exquisite, Amelia,' she offered. 'Quite exquisite.'

When the pair of black horses steaming into the frosted night air arrived pulling the carriage, Amy lifted the hem of her gown in both hands, ran upstairs to kiss her sleeping child, ran down again, threw her heavy cloak over her shoulders and dashed fussily out of the door to go off with Dr Amos Drew to the ball.

The string orchestra was playing and many people were already there as Amy was formally ushered in, and the effect was electrifying. Almost all conversation stopped as the heads of young men and elderly alike turned like puppets in their stiff white collars. But although Amy felt excited herself at being there amongst all the colour and glamour she restrained her usual impulsiveness and did not show it. A most dignified, sophisticated lady she wanted to appear to them. And if she was fluttering and bouncing and hopping all about inside like the sixteen-year-old she once was, she stepped forward into the ballroom with the control and grace that might have been expected from a visiting European princess, but without the air of superiority.

'Well, damn my eyes,' a bearded gentleman amongst a group of men wanted to know quietly from another, 'is that a walking portrait Drew's brought with him or is she real?'

'I think that's the wife of Captain James McBain,' he heard another younger man tell him softly, 'the one with Kimball and Jay they call Charging Jim.'

'Lucky Jim more like it,' another businessman murmured from between the long side-whiskers that curled all the way to his chin. 'If she was mine, you wouldn't find me out at sea. No, sir, I'm damned if you would.'

But normal conversation quickly broke out again over the sound of the music for the sake of good manners, even if minds and eyes did continue to follow her everywhere she went. Many of the women, too, were intrigued with the elegant lady in the green dress and only the most insecure amongst them did their best to ignore her presence. Amos Drew, looking very pleased, made quite a number of introductions but it was to be half an hour later that Amy's first opportunity came. And, as with all the others, it was clear to see that Mr Hinton Garrison was thoroughly charmed by her. Even her large eyes, he felt, were smiling with warmth and affection. After a few opening words on the fine occasion and the benefit it would bring to the underprivileged, Hinton Garrison said, 'It seems a pity that Boston society doesn't see more of you, Mrs McBain.'

'My child keeps me busy, I'm afraid,' Amy told him, 'otherwise I might well get out more.'

'One child?' Hinton Garrison said. 'Surely that's not a hindrance. Why, I have three. Aged two, three and four, and I don't find them any inhibition to my social engagements,' and he turned to his wife. 'Do I, Sophia?'

'Not at all, Hinton,' Sophia obediently agreed.

'Ah, but happily you're more fortunate with them, I'd guess. You see my own little boy is . . . how can I put it? Of restricted ability.'

Amos Drew felt highly relieved that she had not put the responsibility on himself for describing the child's condition.

'Oh, I am sorry, madam,' Hinton Garrison said.

'No, no, no,' Amy told him. 'No need to be sorry. He's perfectly all right. Ten fingers, ten toes and everything else as it should be. It's just that he's a little mentally slow although he's improving all the time and I'm quite sure he'll finish up as bright as anyone.'

'Mrs McBain has done the most wonderful job with him,' Dr Drew felt obliged to comment, even if he did privately believe that James McBain junior had gone about as far as he was ever going to go. 'Quite remarkable.'

'The only sorrow,' Amy went on, 'is that he needs the company of other children now and again to encourage him further, but that's impossible.'

'Why impossible?' Hinton wanted to know.

'Well, we don't yet live in an age of enlightenment, sir,' Amy explained, 'and a gentleman like yourself and a lady like Mrs Garrison might find this hard to believe, but although he is the sweetest and, as Dr Drew can tell you, probably the most harmless child on earth, I think other mothers see him as some kind of monster who's going to eat their own children up. I understand it, of course, it's perfectly natural.'

Hinton Garrison who liked to consider himself as enlightened as any man in Boston looked shocked and affronted on behalf of this charming and beautiful young woman whose aunt was so well known for her own charitable dispensations.

'I don't think it's natural at all, madam,' he declared, springing to her aid, and turned to Amos Drew. 'Do you think it's natural, Doctor?'

'Nature is a curious thing, sir,' Amos Drew replied, not wishing to commit himself.

'I think it's a disgrace to our community,' Hinton Garrison went on, taking Amos Drew's remark as confirmation, and turned to his wife again. 'Isn't that a disgrace, Sophia?'

Sophia was not at all sure whether it was or not but was in no position to say so and had no option but to meekly nod her assent.

When Amy finally left the ball with a pleased Amos Drew, it was with mixed feelings. On the one hand she had succeeded in what she had set out to do. On the other she felt she had betrayed the honest integrity of her womanhood by taking such unfair advantage of men like Mr Hinton Garrison. But, for the sake of her son, she was prepared to suffer the guilt of that.

Thus it was that a few days later, at the insistence of her husband, a reluctant Mrs Garrison was driven through the snow in the family carriage with her three children and deposited at Amy's door.

Already she was dreading every minute of the hour she would have to spend there and had found it very difficult to warn her offspring what to expect without frightening them to death.

Amy, who had been worrying all morning in case the woman changed her mind, threw her arms around her like a sister in her welcome. That was the first surprise. The second was that the house was not at all gloomy and distressing as she had imagined but had an atmosphere of open, warm friendliness about it. The third was that when she first set eyes on James McBain junior he looked not at all to her like a monster. More than that, he smiled engagingly up at her with a look that was enough to melt the snow. Within ten minutes the sworn resolution she had made to herself to keep her brood tight about her protective skirts while she was there had gone right out the window.

'Ga,' said James junior as he tried to push the Bosun aside from interfering with the rest of his crew and they competed with each other to show him how to build his nest of colourful wooden boxes into a tower.

It was closer to two hours later when Sophia Garrison left with her clutch, happily promising to come back the following week. From then, a close friendship began to flower between her and Amy and it was not long after, to the sheer delight of both of them, that James junior, at almost three years of age, rose to his feet on his own and walked unaided after his playmates.

'I'd be very careful with these Garrison people if I were you, my dear Amelia,' Dorothea tried to warn her.

'Why?' Amy asked in surprise.

'They have a lot of old money and a lot of power and influence,' Dorothea explained. 'If for any reason you were to fall out with them they could do a lot of harm to James's career.'

Amy was taken aback by that. It was the first time ever she had seen a flash of jealousy in her aunt but she understood it and instantly excused it.

'Don't worry,' she said, giving Dorothea a quick peck on the cheek. 'No one is going to fall out.'

'Oh dear, oh dear, I'm being a silly old aunt again,' Dorothea apologised with a nervous smile. 'Perfectly silly.'

No one knew where it had come from but the gossip about Hinton Garrison's infidelity came as a shock to Sophia and it was to Amy she hurried for comfort.

'Calm down, calm down, Sophia, I order it,' she said to the distraught woman. 'It's all utter nonsense and you should know it. Look at you. You're a pretty woman and I've seen for myself how your husband regards you. It's ridiculous for anyone to suggest he would want anyone else or that he would do such a thing to you. And, for heaven's sake, how could he? You're with him almost all the time, aren't you? Besides, you yourself would be the very first to know if anything was wrong, and you don't, do you? You must ignore this and cast any doubts from your mind. And you must realise that there are people in this world who actually get pleasure from seeing people like yourself brought down. It's what they want, don't you see? Let their black tongues drop off if they like but don't you dare be affected by it.'

It took a little more than that but it was very much due to Amy that Sophia overcame her distress, but not for a moment did Amy ever imagine that, in the years to come, she would be reminded of her words. For Dorothea Jackson some appeasement for her frustration in not being able to destroy the friendship came only when, once more, the hard-driving Captain James McBain returned from the sea to resume briefly his treasured role of husband and lover. And be loved. For ten whole days Dorothea was in possession of James junior at her cottage. And whether the child understood it or not, while the nursing woman was momentarily absent, it gave her the greatest satisfaction to whisper clearly into his ear.

'It's a great pity your mother can cast you so easily aside like a rag when it suits her,' she told him, 'and the man who's supposed to be your father wants nothing to do with you. But don't you fear. Aunt Dorothea will take good care of you.'

Chapter Nine

A bright spring morning sun had risen over the Boston wharves and as men pushed barrows and horses hauled carts and wagons over the cobblestones, the scents of produce from all around the world mingled sweetly and spicily in the air. And since Kimball and Jay had just sold the *Atheneum* to another shipping operator involved in the Baltic trade and got a good price for her they should have been happy men. They were not.

'It's nothing less than downright, goddamned embarrassing,' Mr Kimball declared to Mr Jay over their desk in the counting house at Long Wharf, it also being the day before their new ship was to be launched.

'Mrs Jay doesn't like it either,' Mr Jay said.

'If I'd known it was going to be like this I'd never have done it,' Kimball went on.

'Neither would I,' Mr Jay agreed.

'Unheard of,' Mr Kimball suggested.

'Unprecedented,' Mr Jay returned.

'The best vessel ever built in Boston,' Mr Kimball pointed out.

'Probably in America,' Mr Jay pointed further.

'God in heaven. Eight hundred tons burthen of her.'

'Mainmast a hundred and thirty feet high,' Mr Jay added.

The reason for their upset was that their new vessel, their new pride and joy was still nameless. Having given the privilege to Captain James McBain and being men of their words they now very much regretted it. Normally a ship was named the moment her keel was laid or even before, but not this one. Every time Captain James McBain had returned from Liverpool, it was the first thing Mr Kimball had wanted to know, going so far as to thump his fat fist on his desk, alarming Mr Jay.

'Damn it, James, you have to name her,' he demanded. 'And now!'

'You must, James,' Mr Jay got in.

'We're never done here being hounded by people asking,' Mr Kimball had continued. 'Four times Mr Jay here and his wife have suffered the discourtesy of having their carriage stopped on their afternoon drive by newspaper men.'

He should have known that the man who charged through Atlantic gales as if they were no more than stiff breezes, who charged bars and everyone else was not to be so easily pressed himself.

'I'm very sorry about that, Mr Jay,' James apologised to him before addressing Mr Kimball again, 'and to you, sir. But I have a list I'm considering and will decide in due course.'

In desperation, Mr Kimball had tried his hand at making guesses in the hope of seeing a flicker. '*Blue Star*?' he said, '*Moonraker*?' and continued through a whole list. '*Flying Cloud*?' he ended and James's face did flicker.

'Now there's a fine name, Mr Kimball,' he said.

'The *Flying Cloud*?' Mr Kimball said, full of hope. 'Is that it?'

'I will certainly add it to what I have,' James replied but otherwise stuck to his guns, not even prepared to hand over a copy of his supposed list.

'What *is* she to be called?' Amy also wanted to know, quite unaware that he himself had been given the honour. 'Everyone asks me and I can't tell them.' But James could not tell her either.

It became a joke and the newspaper men did their best with it.

'The new packet "no-name" at present building at Mr A. Cranford's yard for Messrs Kimball and Jay,' one reported, 'is undoubtedly a fine vessel of magnificent proportions and is to be finished to the highest of standards with such crafted refinements as polished mahogany trim and brass capstan heads. It therefore seems a great sorrow to our maritime community and the general public at large that she continues to remain nameless.'

Mr Kimball continued sitting at his desk, looking glumly at Mr Jay who looked glumly back. At six thirty that very morning, after a sleepless night, an anguished Mr Kimball had sent his carriage to the house of Captain McBain and had him fetched to the counting house.

'This has gone too far, James,' he announced as James entered. 'With the launching advertised for tomorrow and so many important people invited, it's far too late to cancel it or delay it. You have left me with no alternative but to name her myself.'

If James was shaken by that after all the trouble he had gone to he showed not a bit of it.

'And I, Mr Kimball, will be left with no alternative but to ask you to find her another master. New York beckons me in any case.'

'Goddamnit!' Kimball swore as he thumped his desk so hard this time that his inkwell bounced, spilling ink. 'We cannot launch a ship without a name!'

'I'll have a name for her tomorrow,' James said. 'That I promise.'

'Tomorrow, tomorrow?' Kimball exclaimed in despair. 'It will be too late by tomorrow! The name will have to go on today – if it isn't too late already!'

'Either you trust me to name her in time or you don't,' James said captainlike, 'and I ask you for your decision on it now. Right now, Mr Kimball.'

'Oh, my God,' Kimball muttered, putting his defeated head into his hands. And that was more or less the way Mr Jay had found him when he came into the counting house at precisely 7.15 as he did every morning, leaving precisely at 12.50 to go to the meeting at the Exchange and complete his working day.

Driven in Mr Kimball's carriage, James returned feeling rather pleased with himself. He would have been very sorry to lose his appointment as first master of the new ship. All the same, his threat of taking himself off to New York had been no bluff. New York attracted him. As he had once been warned in Liverpool, he could see that more and more it was New York that was dominating trade. Boston might have been the centre of American aristocracy and intellectualism but New York was where the new money grew. And money was another element that could help compensate for his loss of Amy and his loneliness at sea. All that had stopped him making the move was the thought of the upheaval it might afford Amy herself.

'What did he want?' Amy enquired of Mr Kimball's early call the moment James was in the door.

'He still can't decide on the name,' James explained.

'He must be mad,' Amy said.

'I reckon that would be a fair and honest description of his condition,' James acknowledged, 'and it wouldn't surprise me in the least if he keeps everyone up all night trying to help him.'

That was his excuse to be absent but it was well after dark when he left, not for the counting house as Amy believed but for Mr Cranford's yard as he had previously arranged. Once there, he had Cranford assemble the men he had retained to work through the night and they gathered, lit by torches, looking up at the tall-hatted figure of Captain James McBain as he stood, legs apart, atop a pile of timbers.

'The name of this new vessel has been finally decided,' he told them as if he were planted on his quarterdeck reading his crew the riot act, 'and I give you this warning. If any man here has the tongue of a parrot you had better cut it out now because if any one of you as much as breathes this name to another soul before the launching tomorrow I will personally seek him out, have him brought aboard, and lashed and keel-hauled within an hour of her touching the water. That is not a threat but a solemn promise. Do you understand?'

The group of men gaped at him in astonishment. Not one was left in any doubt by the captain's manner of delivery that he meant every word he said.

'I said, do you understand?' James repeated and they all began to nod and murmur their assent, even if they did not understand the reason for it. And none felt courageous enough to enquire.

The work of getting the name on bows and stern began, but it was not all. Under James's direction through Mr Cranford, the figure-head already in place was removed and the other that James had ordered from a figurehead carver at his own expense arrived through the night cradled in a horse-drawn cart.

'It's beautiful, Captain,' Cranford said, seeing it for the first time.

'Not at all like the real thing, of course, Mr Cranford,' James replied, 'but the best that could be done.'

As most of Boston slept behind the empty streets and the arms of the semaphores at their stations hung limply down, in Cranford's yard torches flamed and flickered and lamplights swung while every now and then the bright moon slipped from between clouds to sheet the river beyond in a pearly glow.

'It's going to be another fine day,' James judged, glancing up.

At the model bench in the pattern loft, well lit and alone, an engraver with special cutting tools skilfully carved the letters deep into the shining new bell.

It was four in the morning when Amy who had stayed up with fire and stove kept going heard James's footsteps and hurried to put the kettle on.

'Well?' she wanted to know after he had kissed her.

'I love you,' James replied.

'I don't mean that. I mean the name.'

'I don't know, they're still arguing,' James said, 'but I refused to stay any longer. You're more important to me.'

Amy, although she thought the whole thing utterly ridiculous, was forced to be satisfied and like everyone else who put on their finery for the occasion had no idea what to expect.

When a deeply anxious Mr Kimball turned up at Cranford's yard for the launching, he was amazed. Although long before high tide the place was packed, with hardly a square foot left to stand on. It seemed as if half of Boston was there with streamers to wave and even the roof of Mr Cranford's yard was crowded with the more athletic who had climbed up there for a better view. A large band was already playing to keep them all amused while they waited.

'Make way there for Mr and Mrs Kimball!' a yard worker implored as he tried to clear a path for them through the crush. But at the mention of the name, newspaper men cut swathes towards him.

'Mr Kimball!' one shouted at him over several heads and the noise of the crowd, 'I represent the *New York Herald*! May I have a word with you, sir?'

'It's Mr Kimball!' shouted members of the public, having picked up the name. 'Mr Kimball! That one there! There!'

'Is Mrs Jay going to unveil her before the launch or not, sir?' another newsman wanted to know and Kimball gazed at his ship in even more amazement. Unveil was the right word. The figurehead and name, port, starboard and stern, had been covered over with sail canvas sheets with lines attached so they could be lifted and hauled inboard. Standing beneath each was a guard to make sure that no one could get close enough to lift them and try to peek underneath. Even the bell hanging on the fare mast had been stitched up in canvas. It then began to dawn on Mr Kimball that he had never attracted so much attention in his life before nor had Kimball and Jay ever been given such valuable free publicity and he began to feel exceedingly pleased with himself, even more so when an Admiral of the US Navy extended his hand to him with 'Congratulations, sir. With all this mystery you have created a ship that must surely be remembered.'

'There is nothing I can tell you yet,' Kimball smiled, brushing people off. And indeed there was not.

Mr Jay was similarly surprised on his arrival.

'You didn't tell me it was going to be like this?' Mrs Jay said, and he heard her clearly enough for although she was only a tiny woman she had a voice as strong as a horn.

Kimball looked cheerful as he mingled with all the important guests in the shelter of the building as they happily sipped their drinks and munched on seafood snacks. They had never seen such goings-on over the launching of a ship. It was only as time passed that Kimball became anxious again. Two things were still missing: Captain McBain and the name of the ship. Mrs Jay whose honour it was to be had her speech well prepared but still did not know the most important thing of all.

'Go and find him,' Kimball ordered his wharfinger who wore his finest top hat. It was some long time before the wharfinger escaped from the sea of bodies back into shelter.

'I can't see him, Mr Kimball,' the wharfinger reported, 'but I can tell you this. Jim's done you a favour. I already have more bookings to sail on our new ship than I can handle. There are people out there clamouring for berths to Liverpool, no matter what diversions she has to take on the way. You won't have to spend a penny on advertising now.'

'Is that so?' Kimball beamed.

Only James guessed that the yard might be packed to the gunwales. And in order to avoid what was bound to be much confusion, he deliberately delayed his own arrival. He had also planned to be in a prime position for the event and that, as far as he was concerned, was on the foredeck of the ship itself, together with Amy and her friends the Garrisons. Hinton Garrison was pleased to meet Captain McBain since, although he knew nothing about sailing, he had it in mind to have himself built a private yacht and needed the advice and counselling of someone like the master. For Sophia, the invitation was a different matter.

'I can't,' she had said at first as the whole idea of it frightened her.

'It's nothing, Sophia,' Amy told her.

'Nothing?' Sophia returned, 'Standing on the deck of a big ship slipping precariously down over land with nothing to keep it from falling over; then, if it ever gets that far, plunging backwards into the river? You call that nothing?'

'It is not going to fall over, Sophia,' Amy assured her, amused, but it took much more reassurance than that to get her friend to change her mind, and she was still nervous when they eventually got to the yard, not helped by the unexpected scene that met them.

'Good Lord, what's all this?' Hinton Garrison said.

'This,' James told him, 'is a demonstration of the power of human curiosity.'

Amy, too, looked in astonishment but there was little time or opportunity for enlightenment.

'Get these ladies and this gentleman up on deck,' James ordered one of the yard workers and the man immediately started pushing and calling for way as he led Hinton Garrison, Sophia and Amy in the direction of the starboard side of the ship. There, an enormous ladder had been lowered into position by the wooden derrick.

'I can't go up there!' Sophia protested.

James forced his way into the building to the great relief of the Kimballs and the Jays.

'Thank God,' Mr Kimball greeted him, 'It's only an hour to full flood tide.'

96

'There's no need to wait for that,' James told him. 'Mr Cranford assures me she'll have a full fathom clear as it is. And since not another man, woman or child is going to squeeze into this yard there's no point in delaying it.' With that he took an envelope out of his pocket. 'That's the name, Mrs Jay,' he said, handing it to her.

'James,' Kimball said, 'I would like to know . . .' but James had already turned and was making his way out again. They focused their attention on the small figure of Mrs Jay who was opening the envelope.

'What is it, what is it?' they almost panted and Mrs Jay looked back at them and, seeing their faces, suddenly decided to enter into the spirit of the mysterious occasion.

'That is for me to announce with my speech,' Mrs Jay said and they could hardly believe her.

'Give it to me, Mary,' Mr Jay asked of her.

'No, Horace,' Mrs Jay replied and quickly stuffed the paper into her purse before anyone could snatch it.

When James reached the bottom of the ladder, Sophia Garrison was still only halfway up and, eyes tightly closed, looked as if she might stay there forever. Above her, Hinton was doing his best to encourage her to continue. Below, Amy was crushing her new hat as flat as a pancake as she stuck her head into Sophia's bottom both in order to keep her there and help her up.

'There's nothing to be frightened off, Sophia. Now open your eyes again and take another step but don't look down.'

Had it not been for James ordering a man on deck to lower a line for Amy to tie around Sophia and keep it taut to give her more confidence, it is doubtful whether Sophia would ever have made it on to the deck. And the crowd, with little else to entertain them, loved every minute of it. But Sophia had well recovered her dignity by the time Mrs Jay appeared up on the rostrum. Indeed, she felt somewhat enlivened by having successfully survived the dangerous experience and only wished her children had been there to witness her bravery.

The Kimballs and the Jays led their special guests up on to a rostrum facing the bows and the band broke into a fanfare to bring the noisy crowd to a hushed and expectant silence. Men took off their hats as the pastor read his lesson, offered prayers for all men of the sea and stepped back. Mrs Jay's small figure stepped forward. The woman was not a fool. She could feel the growing impatience that bordered on hysteria and decided to forget her own little speech, sensing that it might only detract from her moment of glory.

'Ladies and gentlemen!' her voice boomed out, surprising everyone with its power. 'I shall hold you in suspense no longer!' And she hesitated, to savour her last few seconds with not as much as a murmur to be heard. 'I name this ship *Amelia*!'

If she added 'God bless her and all who sail in her' it was drowned. Suddenly everything was happening at once. '*Amelia*!' cried the crowd in one great roar, not so much for the name itself as for the fact that it had been named at all. The covering canvas was whipped up to reveal at the bows an exquisite figurehead with dark hair and large, brown eyes, adorned in sweeping robes of green, gold and white, the mystic guide who would lead this vessel through rain and mist and calms and storm and clearly recognisable as Amy McBain. At the same time, on James's signal, the Stars and Stripes broke out at the top of the mainmast to flutter in the breeze while far below at the keel men swung their hammers with blow after blow on shores and spurns to release her from the land.

As the band struggled hopelessly to make itself heard again amidst all the cheers and frantic waving of flags and streamers, and the *Amelia* began to slip towards the river forcing a short squeak of panic from the lips of Sophia, Amy stood speechless. She could hardly have failed to hear the name but for the first few moments, such was the unexpectedness of it, it meant nothing. Then, as the shock of surprise washed over her, she thought it might have been some mistake or referred to some other Amelia. Even as the truth began to sink in, it was more like some dream than reality, an illusion heightened by the sea of faces with waves of arms flying a white spume of streamers that, beyond the bowsprit, was beginning to recede. It was not until the ship was about to hit the water as she felt James's hand grip at her arm in case she should fall that the full realisation of what had happened began to surface from the whirlpool of her mind.

'Help,' squeaked Sophia, eyes tightly closed, as Hinton held firmly both on to her and the starboard rail, but Amy was unaware of her.

'You did this, didn't you?' she accused James, still looking half dazed, but James only grinned.

'It had to be something,' he replied, and the *Amelia* plunged into the river with a great splash, swept out into it, righted to her unladen trim and was born. Men ran everywhere along her decks with lines and warps to halt her way and temporarily secure her with the help of small craft.

Sophia bobbed up again as quickly as a cork. 'Amy! Amy!' she cried, rushing to throw her arms around her friend in congratulations. 'And you didn't say a word!'

'Wait till you see the figurehead, Mrs Garrison,' James told her and Amy herself rushed to clamber over the bowsprit and, before anyone could stop her, end hanging almost upside down so that she could see it. Even from that angle it was instantly recognisable.

'It's me, it's me!' she almost screamed in delight, and looked to be in danger of falling into the river. The Garrisons were most alarmed as they watched James haul her back to safety.

Not for a moment was Amy deceived by James's explanation of the ship's name being a last-minute afterthought. To start with, there had been that strange man who, all through the winter months, had kept coming to her door to try to sell her firewood when she already had enough. He had not looked at all like a woodcutter. Now she knew he had been a figurehead carver studying her features. And there were all the other little odd things. Looking back, it became all too obvious. For almost a year James had planned to give her this one day of honour, pleasure and surprise and she was deeply affected by the gift. And if it had not been his original intention, James was quick to take advantage of the other benefits it brought.

'What can I say, James?' Mr Kimball voiced warmly, offering his hand at the very first opportunity. 'You gave us all the most pleasurable day and have done more for our new packet than a whole callithump of boardmen, signwriters and printers. It wouldn't surprise me at all if we could sell the *Amelia* for much more than it cost us. It is much appreciated and on behalf of Mr Jay and myself I would just like to say that it was wrong of us to doubt you.'

Before he had even finished, it was primage that sprang immediately to James's mind, the percentage of passenger fares and cargo profits on which packet captains relied for most of their money. Mentally, he tightened the braces on his yards.

'Appreciation in itself is worthy but hard to live on, Mr Kimball,' he replied. 'I'd much prefer it if you could do something more practical by raising my primage from six per cent to seven. Then I'd be in the fortunate position of being able to return your appreciation. With interest.'

Much of the shine removed itself from Kimball's face and he wavered. How times changed. This was the same young man he had felt was about to embrace him when told of being given his first command and he studied him for a moment. He had little respect for a man who had no respect for money. All the same, with less good wine in him, he would never have mentioned that the new ship might be worth more than it cost them because of all the attention the captain had got it. He should have been more alert. McBain was far from being in need and was making more and more money all the time. The problem was replacing him with another 'driver' as good.

'I can't hold out much hope of that, but I'll speak with Mr Jay about it,' he said.

'When you do,' James suggested, quietly unfurling his main top royal, 'you might remind him that a Blackballer, Red Star or Blue Swallowtail master going direct from New York and back gets in almost two round trips to my one with all the diversions for loading I have to take.'

James got his seven per cent and was pleased to get it but before many months were out his gratitude, in tragic circumstances, was to be shown to someone else.

As the *Amelia* sailed out into the Atlantic, bound first for Mobile, her shrouds and stays strained to their limit as against a south-westerly gale, Captain James McBain drove her hell for leather south, the image of Amy on the bluff bows rising to the waves and diving down again.

Once more Amy switched her love and attention to the further development of her backward son, stimulating him with everything she could think of, even several times bringing in a fiddler from the streets to play to him. But she felt herself more divided than she had ever been. Much of the time only half of her was there, the rest aboard the *Amelia*. She would have given anything to return to the sea with Jayjay by her side and resumed the life which had become no more than a treasured memory, a dream, but he was much too delicate for that and every infection he picked up threatened to take him away. She found herself spreading charts on the floor and making a useless attempt to involve him with plotting estimated positions of where his father might be. Now that he could walk and the winter was over, she was able to take his hand for outings, but always she drifted towards the shore or to the wharves, the scene of so many tearful partings.

'You're away again, Amy,' Sophia smilingly reminded her as they sat watching the children play in James junior's room.

'Oh, I'm sorry, Sophia, I'm sorry,' Amy apologised, springing at once out of her reverie. 'I'll make us tea in a minute.'

Louisa's children had just made another tower when, suddenly, Jayjay swept out a hand in a flash of rage and sent it crashing. 'Bad man!' he said as he did so. Both Amy and Sophia were taken completely by surprise. They had not seen anger in the child before but although any display of emotion in him was to be welcomed, their reaction was overtaken when he then bursting into screaming tears and Amy swept him up into her arms, Sophia, her children, Bosun, and Captain, awoken from his sleep, all looking on in curiosity.

'Hush, hush, hush,' Amy comforted as she cradled him, 'what bad man? There's no bad man here. Look. There's just us. Hush now, hush. There's nothing to be afraid of.'

'It's probably some vendor who calls he's frightened of,' Sophia suggested. 'Maybe he thought he heard his knock on the door.'

'Probably,' Amy agreed as she continued to try to quieten the howls. 'I've never seen him like that before.'

It simply did not enter either Amy's or Sophia's head that the bad man who had so swiftly broken into James junior's mind without warning was not a vendor or some evil-looking man he had seen in the street but one he hardly saw at all: the one in the tall hat and dark suit, Captain James McBain, his own father. And as the performance was not to be repeated, neither the angry words nor the ensuing howls, the incident was happily accepted as a show of spirit, whatever accounted for it, and that was none other than a sign of more progress. There was certainly no cause whatsoever to connect it in any way with Aunt Dorothea.

At sea, James was pleased by the speed he was making. Only the flying jib boom cracked under the strain and he quickly had that replaced without losing an inch. Downwind, he discovered, she was much faster, too, and he reached Mobile two days ahead of his estimate, once more frightened the pilot by running at the bar under full sail and made yet more enemies by loudly expressing his views on slavery. But it was more by good luck than his skill at navigation that he sighted Cape Clear at the southern tip of Ireland on 14th June 1837.

'She is indeed a fine ship,' the agents for Kimball and Jay in Liverpool said as, finally in dock there a few days later, James proudly showed them over the *Amelia*.

It was on the afternoon of the twentieth after the cargo of cotton bales had been discharged and the new loading was almost complete that James noticed that the English wharfies had drifted off. He hurried ashore and strode across the dock into the counting house.

'What in the hell is going on with my loading?' he demanded of the agents, all of whom stood with funereal faces.

'It is a time of mourning, Captain,' one of them explained. 'We've just heard the King died this morning.'

James looked at them. Damn the King. The whole goddamned world knew he was ill. It was not unexpected.

'How long is this mourning going to last?' he asked.

'At least today and tomorrow,' he was told.

'My full complement of passengers is already aboard,' he pointed out.

'We're sorry, Captain, it can't be helped.'

'I offer my sympathies in your loss, sirs,' James said politely and strode out. The agents were wrong if they thought it could not be helped. Back aboard he shouted for his first mate who came hurrying.

'We complete the loading ourselves, Mister,' he said to him. 'Get both watches to work.'

It was not that James was anti-British. If the restrictive trade practices of their Navigation Act riled him, there was much he admired in them. It was simply that he did not consider the death of a king a good enough excuse for holding him up. But neither was he neglectful of his duty. As his own seamen took up the rest of the loading, in the main saloon above decks he conducted a special service for the passengers in memory of King William the Fourth. And as most of them were English, they greatly appreciated it, several of the women weeping into their handkerchiefs. Little did James know that soon he would be shedding a tear of his own for quite another death.

By the evening of the following day, the loading was complete, hatch on the cargo hold secured.

'We sail in an hour,' James instructed his mate as he kept one eye on the breeze and the other on the water rising to full flood tide.

'We won't have a pilot, Captain,' his mate reminded him.

'Damn the pilot, Mister,' James replied curtly. 'I can make my way out of here with no arms, no legs and my eyes shut.'

As they waited, news reached them that the young Princess, niece to William, successor to the throne, had been declared from St James's Palace in London that day to be Queen Alexandrina Victoria. So, two heavily bumped channel buoys and a near grounding later against the awkward, westering light, it was of Queen Alexandrina the passengers spoke so fondly as, in some relief, James got his ship clear to the bay and out into the Irish Sea. For once, fully laden, he was going to be able to make a direct crossing back to Boston instead of making another diversion far to the south. And that took him all the sooner back to Amy.

When the *Amelia* eventually came within sight of the Boston Light having made good time, the news schooner swept up abeam and James shouted his news down to them through his loudhailer.

'We heard that from New York three days ago!' a voice came back.

James was gravely annoyed by that. It meant that a New York packet which had probably left London after his departure from Liverpool had beaten him to it. Worse, he was well out of date with the news, for the schooner was able to tell him that the new Queen of England was to be known only as Victoria, and not Alexandrina. As far as James was concerned at that moment, it was damn the New York packet for robbing him of his headline and the hell with the English Queen who did not seem to know what her goddamned name was supposed to be.

After the usual port formalities, the *Amelia*, all sails furled neatly to their yards, was eventually hauled into her berth at the wharf, the figurehead under the bowsprit stripped of streaks of colour from face, hair and robes by the Atlantic waves.

James looked down and was taken by surprise to see Amy at the front of the usual welcoming crowd of friends and sightseers. The forlorn figure gave much the same impression as her wooden image and he could tell straight away that something was seriously wrong. Making his way through passengers eager to disembark, he was first down the gangway to get to her.

'What is it, what is it?' he wanted to know as he reached her.

'The *Nantasket*, James,' Amy told him. 'She went down. Mr Ludham. He's lost.'

That news had been sorrowful to Amy not only because of the man she had once known who had so readily accepted her position as navigator, despite her gender. Nor was it solely for the idyllic happiness that ship had given her. It was also a painful reminder of the vulnerability of James himself who was forever at the mercy of the sea. She could have endured drowning with him but the thought of being left without him was unbearable to her.

It did not take long for James to get the story. The *Nantasket* had been caught out in a hurricane in the West Indies. The mizzen mast had crashed to the deck and crushed the life out of her captain, a master James did not know, the vessel shortly after being blown on to a reef where, pounded by gigantic waves and screaming winds, she had broken up, together with her boats, and gone down in what had seemed only minutes. Ludham, in disregard of his own life, spent the night swimming amidst the chaos, somehow finding floundering men in the darkness and the impossible conditions and heaving them up on to pieces of wildly tossing wreckage, to cling for their lives. Eight he had saved like that before, at dawn, his strength must have finally given out. One saw him overwhelmed by a wave and disappear, not to rise again. All the survivors told of his courage and he was given almost half a column in the *Maritime Gazette* as well as reports in the local newspapers. And that posthumous praise, which would soon be forgotten, was all the reward Mr Ludham would get.

Captain James McBain was not a man to cry over the loss of another sailor at sea. He wiped his tear away with the back of his hand, disciplined the choking of his throat and set to making enquiries around the waterfront about Ludham's family. He was surprised to learn from a bosun that there was a Mrs Ludham somewhere since Ludham had never mentioned a wife. From a ship's carpenter he was to discover why. He was not legally married to the woman who lived in Salem. James made no moral judgement on that. It somehow seemed in keeping with Mr Ludham that he had avoided the responsibility of being a lawfully wedded husband.

'I must go up and see her,' James told Amy and the following morning he made his way up to Salem. It had been some time since he had thought of Ludham but he did so now and he missed him. Not until after they had parted had he come to fully appreciate the mate's qualities. He had belonged to that rare species of men who were totally dependable, totally loyal, who took orders without question and lost no time in seeing them carried out, yet who were fully aware of their own limitations and stuck to them. There was no side to them, no deviousness, no dishonesty. For little more in wages than an able seaman they provided the strong, indispensable right arm to a captain's head.

Directed to the house of the late Mr Ludham at Salem, James approached it. The washing on the line was frayed and the half-dozen children eyeing him with a mixture of curiosity, shyness and suspicion were poorly dressed. Although, apart from giving his condolences, this was what he had come to find out, he felt a twinge of regret at having made the journey. The emotion he felt for Ludham's death was overtaken by another. Too much the house reminded him of the small, impoverished home in Quincy where he had been raised and had so long left behind as a faded and unwanted memory. The woman who came to the open door wore a dowdy dress and although not much more than thirty had a harrowed face. He introduced himself and was invited in. The bare, wooden floor was unpolished but scrubbed, and the sparse furniture was clearly home-made.

'I'm deeply sorry about what happened to your husband,

ma'am,' James said, according her full status. 'He was a fine man, an excellent sailor and the best first mate I've had.'

'Thank you, sir,' the woman replied. 'Mr Ludham talked about you a lot when he was home.'

'Kindly, I hope,' James said.

'Oh yes, Captain McBain. And he always said he'd made a bad mistake in leaving you, sir.'

'I didn't know that,' James returned, realising that if he had made more of an effort to keep him he might perhaps still be alive. But he could hardly blame himself for that. It had been Ludham's own choice. In any case, it was not what was uppermost in his mind. Instead, it was the memory of his own childhood, his father's sudden death, and his mother quickly finding another man to support her rather than face a future in the 'House of Industry' as the Poor House was so euphemistically called. That, as it turned out, had only been exchanging one hell for another. He wanted to be out of Ludham's house and away from there as quickly as possible.

'I'll arrange for you to have three hundred and fifty dollars to help, ma'am,' he told her and the woman's worn face gaped at him. That was hardly surprising. It was almost as much as Ludham earned in two years.

'Please don't be offended or embarrassed,' James went on. 'No one but ourselves need know about it. It's my own memorial to Mr Ludham and you're the rightful inheritor.'

'Three hundred and fifty dollars, sir?' the woman managed to get out, not at all sure if she had heard right.

James confirmed it and a few moments later the woman, still flabbergasted, not knowing what to say or how to thank him properly, could only listen as Captain McBain made excuses for being in a hurry and watch as he quickly put his tall hat to his head and made his way back out through the open door past the children who were all gathered there looking in.

'God will bless and favour you, sir!' the woman called at last but if the captain who was well on his way heard her, he did not acknowledge it. James did in fact hear but did not want to look back. God favouring him? That was not goddamned likely. All he had done he had done on his own without any help. The only time God had favoured him was in giving him Amy and He had wasted no time in taking her away from him again. It was in that state of mind that he vowed to himself that never would he become just another of those old captains retired to Summer Street, forgotten mariners eking out their genteel existence, slowly dying in the present and living in the past. Worse, leaving Amy as a widow there, taking in paying guests to supplement her income. No, by God, Captain James McBain would be more than that. The goddamned world would hear of him before he was through.

The evening summer sun was well down as he returned to Boston but he did not even tell Amy of the money he had given to Ludham's woman. Unlike Aunt Dorothea and her charitable ladies, he considered that taking credit for charity only served to rob the receiver of dignity and corrupt the giver. It was no one else's damned business. What he did have to impart to Amy after reassuring her that Mrs Ludham had already gotten over much of her grief and was a woman who would be able to manage was quite another matter.

'I give myself another year with Kimball and Jay,' he told her, 'two at the very most. Then we're moving to New York.'

It was no great surprise to Amy. He had talked more and more of New York on his visits home but she had deliberately not broached the subject of how that might affect the child.

When Dorothea Jackson heard the news she was at first disturbed, but quickly recovered. No matter what happened, she had no intention of letting go of the McBains. More important now, only she understood her determination never to have James junior taken away from her.

Once more, on the morning of James's departure, his son was brought before him to be shown off by his proud and loving mother. James junior stood on his own, a shaft of sunlight falling at his feet.

'Go on, Jayjay,' Amy coaxed and encouraged, 'say something to your father.' But James junior remained steadfastly silent. Amy was disappointed by that and excused it simply as shyness.

James looked down at the small figure standing there. He was not aware that behind the limpid, innocent blue eyes in that expressionless face there had already been sown the seeds of an implacable enmity.

Chapter Ten

Amy could not have been prouder of the miracle in the little sailor's suit of black pumps, white trousers, red check shirt, navy pea jacket, black silk scarf and stiffened, shiny black canvas hat with its trailing black ribbon that dawdled between herself and Aunt Dorothea down busy Wall Street in the New York spring of 1841. Just turned seven years of age, no one could have guessed that Jamie McBain, as they had recently begun to call him, was the same severely retarded child who had been known as Jayjay.

Sophia Garrison, too, saw it as a miracle and considered herself lucky to have been witness to it in the time she had known Amy.

'If you saw him now, you'd not believe it, Doctor,' she had told Amos Drew with great enthusiasm after another visit down to see her friend. 'You'd simply not believe it.'

'I'm absolutely delighted for her, Mrs Garrison,' Amos Drew had replied with a wide smile, 'although many might remember me saying at the very beginning it was possible. A very unusual case, of course, and remarkable that the child survived at all. It goes to show what, between God's will, a mother's perseverance and the right medical attention, can be achieved. But I did say.'

Neither Amos Drew nor anyone else knew that it was as much due to the often mysteriously selective healing powers of nature as to Amy's unremitting struggle to reach into his mind that was responsible for the eventual emergence of normality.

Down Wall Street, the miniature mariner dragged his feet. Although he had lived in New York for three years he was beginning to take a much greater interest in his surroundings. Not so much in the busy traffic of public stages, two wheeled hansoms, wagons and trucks but in the sidewalk activities. The black man cutting firewood from logs that had been dumped there for the purpose. The many stands offering everything from pies to oysters. The vendor boy carrying a large basket of freshly baked tea rusks crying, 'Ruk ruk, ruk – tea ruk!' The travelling cobbler, his pole festooned with a variety of footwear as he walked by with it aloft. The little sailor stopped and turned to gaze at him.

'Come along, Jamie, come along,' Amy encouraged, reaching out her hand towards him. 'If you can't keep up I'll have to lift you, you know. And whatever will people say if they saw me having to carry an able-bodied seaman down the street?'

Deliberately, Jamie continued to dawdle. It was the only protest he could think of to make against the way he was dressed. But as he had given no indication to his mother, Amy did not know how much the child disliked his get-up and saw it only as connecting him more closely with the man who came and went and who was supposed to be his father.

The chimes of St Paul's rang out midday as Amy reached the step of A E Mann, watchmakers and suppliers of navigational instruments, and it was clear she intended going in.

'Oh, not again, Amelia,' Dorothea said.

'But it's three months since I had a look, Aunt Dorothea,' Amy replied.

Her appreciation of Aunt Dorothea's companionship had worn thinner since taking up residence in New York. It was not the same as Boston where Dorothea had been able to retreat with the child to her cottage every time the signal station heralded the return of James. In New York, both Jamie and Aunt Dorothea were there with them in the same house. Furthermore, each time James came home, the child was almost guaranteed to go down with some ailment, forcing Amy to divide her love and attention between father and son at the same time to the complete satisfaction of neither. So often, feeling that she had failed her husband and destroyed his all-too-brief moments of security and happiness, she had gone to her room after he had sailed away again and wept in what she thought was privacy. But James McBain junior had long since been aware of it and, in his mind, his mother's tears and his father's visits had become inextricably linked, a condition subtly and secretly confirmed to him by Aunt Dorothea.

Several times Amy had tried to explain to Sophia how she felt disturbed by Aunt Dorothea but it was hard for her to rationalise.

'Then you must tell her to go back to Boston,' Sophia had advised.

'How can I?' Amy had said. 'She's shown me nothing but kindness ever since I was a child. Sometimes I feel cruel and ungrateful at not being able to love her as much as I used to. I don't know, maybe it is I who's at fault. Apart from us, all she has is her charitable work.'

It was not for want of Sophia's understanding and comforting that Amy found it impossible to suggest to her aunt that she should go, but impossible it was. There was no reason she could give her. Not one.

As Amy entered the watchmaker's Mr Mann, who had an eye for more than a well-made clock, positively beamed at her appearance, at the same time removing his glasses from the end of his nose to expose his face without blemish.

'Ah, good afternoon to you, Mrs McBain,' he welcomed, 'and to you, too, Miss Jackson,' and he feigned the greatest expression of surprise as he gazed on Jamie. 'And what have we here?' he went on. 'Damn my eyes if we don't have a crew. Haul hard on yer tops'l lifts there, my lad, an' it's Cape Stiff ahead and you're Hawaii bound.'

Jamie lowered his head and cast his eyes to the floor to hide his pout of disgust. No one yet knew of these stirrings of resentment in him against ships and the sea: not even in his own mind properly formed or reasoned, simply felt. But, as only a few moments later Mr Mann produced a beautifully polished box, put it on the counter and opened the lid, he became aware of his mother looking down on it with great admiration in her large eyes, and the wave passed and he became curious. Aunt Dorothea sat on a chair pretending to be interested in other things as she gazed about her, but Amy lifted Jamie up to sit on the counter by the box.

'Look, Jamie, look,' she said. Inside, set on double gimbals which were concealed was a chronometer heavily rimmed by what might have been shining gold. 'You see?' Amy went on, lifting the box and tilting it both back and forth and sideways. 'It doesn't matter which way I put it, the clock stays still.'

For Jamie there was a fascination in that and he put out his hand to touch it and make it swing. There was mystery there.

'It's a two-day, Mrs McBain,' Mr Mann explained, 'and not only is the second-hand dial of the finest to half a second but that other one there is an entirely new invention. When fully wound that hand goes up to there. Then it goes backwards around the dial over the the two days to warn you when it needs rewinding.'

'It's wonderful,' Amy said. 'It used to worry me that I might forget, even if I did get into the habit of winding every eight bells of the middle watch. At times when a lot of things are happening it could be so easy to forget. Then you're lost.'

'Indeed, indeed, Mrs McBain,' agreed Mr Mann.

Jamie put his fingers to the edge of the chronometer again to watch it swing and quickly come to rest. Mr Mann smiled at him.

'Your famous father would love to have that, wouldn't he, my lad?' he said.

And suddenly James McBain junior had lost all interest in the mysteries of the floating clock. 'I want to go to the cookie shop,' he replied.

But calling Captain McBain famous was still something of an exaggeration except perhaps in Amy's eyes.

It had been far from easy for James when he had first come to New York three years before and it had taken no time at all to quash his enthusiasm and ego. The name he had made for himself in Boston was nothing here.

'Captain who again did you say?' asked the first shipowner he succeeded in meeting.

'Nothing here for you at the moment, Captain,' said another, 'but if you like you can leave your name and address with our wharfinger.'

All along the East River there were captains with established reputations. All of them known 'drivers'. They had to be. Competition on the passenger packet was as keen as a seaman's knife. If you could not make good times on your passages you were quickly discarded.

It was a much dispirited James who walked the length of South Street past the lofty array of masts and bowsprits, who wore down boot leather from Coffee House Slip at the lower end of Wall Street to going down every other street that led to a wharf, slip and counting house. Moreover, the timing of his arrival had been bad. Shortly after, the steamship *Great Western* had arrived from England, belching black smoke as her huge paddles churned the water. It was only to be expected that men who had all their money invested in sail would be anxious.

With money running low, it was in desperation that James took the captaincy of a brig belonging to L Johannsen to take a general cargo to the Baltic and return with Swedish steel. He felt lowered and not a little humiliated by that and Amy had been in agony for him. It was to be the only vessel in his entire life that was not more beautiful than the last. But once he had cleared Sandy Hook and the Floating Light, he perked up considerably, his determination returning.

'All sail, Mister,' he ordered and the mate had stared at him. It was starting to blow close to a gale.

'What?' he questioned.

'You heard me, damn you, I said all sail!' James commanded, and at first everyone thought he was mad. Well, if he was not exactly that, he was angry. Never had the old brig gone so fast before as she bashed her way through the waves across the Atlantic, creaking and shuddering.

It was with astonishment that Mr Johannsen heard from the sempahore signal station on Navesink Highlands overlooking

110

Sandy Hook that his vessel had returned. It was two weeks faster than she had ever managed the round trip before. For that, Captain James McBain got his first mention along the East River. The next was not long in coming. James took the brig out again, this time bound for England with grain to return with rails for the ever-expanding railroad around New York. In the Western Approaches to the English Channel the foremast topgallant blew out and James considered the seamen too slow for his liking in their efforts to tame the madly whipping torn canvas that could cut a man's face open and tear out his fingernails. In disbelief the rest of the crew saw McBain scurry aloft where, taking over, all the while bawling at them against the wind, he gave them a very quick lesson on how best to handle it, get it off and bend on a new sail. No captain ever went for'ard, never mind up the mast. When he returned to the deck, the mate was standing legs apart, gaping at him.

'Carry on, mister,' was all McBain said and went below to his tiny cabin to wipe the blood off his face.

Although James had still not mastered the art of navigation as opposed to the technicalities of it and was often to be found with his fingers crossed in the hope of seeing a pilot cutter come over the horizon, he did it again. Ten days before he could reasonably have been expected, he was back in New York for a good bonus. But it was to be more than just that. The crew told stories in the groggeries about this tough, strange man and the more they drank the wilder their tales got. Within twenty-four hours his name had been mentioned in almost every bar along the entire waterfront and two days later, to Amy's relief and delight, James was offered the New York–London packet belonging to the independent operators, Merriman and Rudd, on a primage of five per cent. He could not wait to show her over it.

'Well?' Amy enquired after the tour of inspection. The pride in his latest sea bride was unmistakable, but with life having changed so much the better for him she felt in a playful, teasing mood.

'Well what?' James asked.

'Is she the finest ship you're ever had or not?' Amy wanted to know and James, never a man to hesitate, hesitated.

'No, no, no, no, not at all,' he said. 'The *Amelia* was undoubtedly the finest. No doubt at all.'

'You don't have to lie, you know,' Amy smiled, unable to keep him in discomfort any longer, 'I don't care, I really don't.'

'You don't?' James said in surprise and some relief.

'No, silly,' Amy told him and threw her arms around him for him to hold her. 'It was only a name and what's in a name? This *is* the finest ship you've ever had.'

'In my heart I'll think of her as the *Amelia*, too,' he promised quietly into her ear.

With his new packet, James not only kept up with the Black-ballers, Red Stars and Swallowtails but gave them a run for their money. Within a year he moved from the small house in Stanton Street that ran down to a shipyard on the East River to a bigger and better one with a stoop off Wall Street that had been rebuilt since the Great Fire of Wall Street a few years before.

But James's life became more divided than just between ship and shore, between the ocean and Amy. On board there were also two Jameses. In the main saloon he was the affable, increasingly accomplished host who could mix comfortably with the famous, infamous and never-been-heard-ofs alike. They had all paid their fares. Many were the ladies who found him wittier, more charming and desirable than their husbands, while women travelling alone would sometimes make extraordinary excuses to try to lure him to their staterooms.

'I'd be much obliged,' he would request of his first mate on such occasions, 'if you'd go to Miss Whitefield's cabin and extend my sincerest apologies for not being able to see her personally. Tell her my duties prevent me. Assure the lady that the ship is not in danger of sinking. Put her at ease, Mister. Make her comfortable.'

Sometimes he was curious as to how his mate achieved that but he never asked.

On deck it was, 'Goddamn you to hell, mister', as his eyes glowed with fire at seeing as little as a poorly coiled tail of a sheet or brace, never mind a sail not trimmed to its maximum efficiency. Hard men jumped at his appearance in case he found them at fault. Yardarm furlers and argumentative mates lasted only one voyage with him. Yet if a seaman took badly sick, McBain, like all the best captains, had him removed from the fo'c'sle to his own cabin and with the help of that other ship's bible, *Dr Lowe's Sailor's Guide to Health*, did what he could for him.

No one saw the James who was often to be found alone in the middle of the night, gazing over the stern at the wake, staring at his own emptiness. But he became well known the length of the East River and men recognised the 'driver' in his tall hat and dark suit as he passed.

On a morning after James had just returned from London, the air was warm, the sun shining. Having finished his business he was striding along South Street towards Maiden Lane to look for a cab when for no apparent reason he happened to glance up and something strangely familiar suddenly caught his eye. He stopped, stepped back to see better and was transfixed in utter amazement. He thought he must be imagining it. For a full half-minute further, carts and barrows forced to avoid him, his eyes stayed glued to it, but it did not change or go away. Four storeys up on the five-storey building, it was writ large on a huge, freshly painted board – *KIMBALL & JAY* and underneath, in smaller letters, *Shipowners and Merchants*. He hurried inside and up the stairs of the counting house, not knowing what to expect, and burst in unannounced. It was a slip in time and he felt a flush of emotion and nostalgic pleasure at the sight. Mr Kimball and Mr Jay were seated facing each other across a large desk as if they had been transported there from Boston by some wave of a magic wand without so much as getting up off the seats of their trousers. They did now.

'James, James!' they both cried on seeing him, simultaneously rising to their feet, and after shaking hands with him, offered him a chair. Mr Kimball missed the days he had spent haggling over money with the captain while Mrs Jay had nagged her husband endlessly over his stupidity on not being able to keep McBain.

'I had no idea,' James got out as Kimball and Jay repositioned themselves.

'It wasn't exactly a sudden decision,' Mr Kimball explained.

'Not at all,' Mr Jay squeezed in.

'For some time we've been thinking if we didn't alter course we might end exporting ice like young Freddie Tudor,' Kimball went on.

'To Jamaica and such places to cool their drinks,' Mr Jay elucidated.

'What about the *Amelia*?' James asked.

'She's here,' Kimball told him, 'having a refit at a yard at the foot of Fifth Street.'

'Seventh,' Mr Jay corrected.

'Fifth and Seventh then,' Kimball compromised. 'She'll be all cargo now.'

'No passengers,' Mr Jay added.

James was amused to be reacquainted with the double act but there was more to come. A few minutes later, the young, whiskered Captain Eastlake walked in, stopped and froze. James had met him when he had handed over the *Amelia* to him in Boston three years before. He saw Eastlake's eyes firing hostility into the room in the few seconds he stood there, then watched him pull himself to his full height, looking at no one and nothing.

'God Almighty!' he suddenly bellowed. 'I've run aground again!'

and, turning on his heel, he stomped straight out again, flying whiskers bristling. After a pause, James could not restrain his laughter. 'That *was* Captain Eastlake, wasn't it?' he enquired.

'Yes,' Kimball confirmed, 'but it seems this is not the happiest of days for him. Something has upset him.'

'He can be a little eccentric on occasion,' Mr Jay apologised for him further.

'He is a good captain,' Kimball said. 'The only problem is he's inclined to drink a bit too much now and then.'

'But he has signed the pledge three times,' Mr Jay contributed.

James had to smile at that, too. At least it was better than having signed it twelve times. But it was as much of an explanation for Eastlake's hilarious entrance and exit he was going to get. Eastlake could have told him there was nothing funny about it and that he and he alone had been the cause of it. Ever since he had become master in Boston he had had to suffer the ghost of his predecessor as the monkey on his back. Everything he did was compared with McBain. The times he had made on his passages, the way he ran his ship, the way he handled business with the agents in Liverpool. Every goddamned thing. It had got so that hearing the very mention of the name was like being bashed around the ears with a belaying pin. And it had been too much for him after only days in New York to walk into his employers' office and see him sitting there.

Eventually, James headed for home and for Amy, who he knew would be there waiting for him. But as he went he dismissed Eastlake and briefly contemplated instead the lives of Mr Kimball and Mr Jay without a thought that they might ever influence his future again. In their counting house, although Kimball was the more dominant of the two, they had always been the closest of partners, buddies even. But when their business day was over that was the end of it. Neither had ever been known to visit the other's home nor had the Kimballs and Jays eaten at the same table. Their private lives were as totally separate as complete strangers' and the two pairs were seen rubbing shoulders only at the launching of their new ships. It somehow reminded him of his own life, except that his time at home was only an interlude and at the business where he spent most of his hours, days, weeks, months and years he had no such human partner with whom to communicate or confide in. He had to rely for support on the substitutes. The driving of himself, his crew and his vessel. On clearer nights, the visions of wealth and fame glittered in the stars, sometimes seeming so far away, at others so close he felt he wanted to reach out with his hand to touch.

He arrived at his door to see Amy running to meet him, in

competition with the barking Bosun, she letting out her usual little shriek of excitement, her arms thrown around him before he scarcely had time to take off his hat. He held her tightly for a long, long time, his weathered cheek buried down in the softness of her hair. Neither were aware of being watched some distance off through a partly open door. There, in a room off the hallway, Aunt Dorothea in black dress was looking on, James McBain junior in small brown suit, hair brushed back, standing by her side.

'If you don't already know,' they heard the captain say as the tail-wagging Bosun clawed desperately at his trouser leg for attention, 'guess who's moved down from Boston?'

'Who? Who?' they heard mother and niece ask, so curious to know from him, so happy where she stood.

Jamie burned at yet another return of his father, sweeping his mother away from him, but the envy was no less in Dorothea Jackson.

'Kimball and Jay.'

'No!'

'Large as life. I just saw them.'

Jamie felt a tap of comfort and sympathy on his shoulder, could have burst out crying and, lip trembling, glanced briefly up at her. Aunt Dorothea was smiling in a language he was just beginning to understand. 'Do not give them the satisfaction of knowing what they're doing to you,' she was saying without uttering a sound.

Dorothea had been finding it increasingly difficult to hide her bitter jealousy of Amelia. Despite all her niece's past trials she had grown even more beautiful. She could wear what colourful dresses she liked. She was socially sought after and often invited by fashionable wives to have lunch with them at Delmonico's on Broadway. She had everything. James was not only regarded as being amongst the cream of New York captains but with his primage grown to seven per cent was making more and more money. No longer was Dorothea getting the same satisfaction from visits to asylums.

'All right, all right,' the captain was heard to say as he rubbed the appreciative Bosun around the head.

Dorothea knew what she was going to do. It might take some time. There were several things to be taken into consideration. Caution and patience were called for. Even if it took a year. Even two. But she knew what she was going to do. Separate the child from his mother and keep him for herself.

Chapter Eleven

The wheels of the Garrison carriage crunched over ice as it made its way to Central Wharf in Boston. Inside, Hinton looked worriedly at his agitated wife.

'I'm still not sure I should be letting you go alone in weather like this,' he said.

'But I must go, mustn't I?' Sophia, now the mother of five, pointed out. 'I must.'

'If you gave me enough time to rearrange my business affairs I'd go with you,' Hinton offered.

'I can't wait, Hinton,' Sophia replied. 'You know that.'

That had been her reaction the moment she heard. It had come so unexpectedly. The acquaintance she had run into while shopping had been expecting more details from Mrs Garrison and had been most surprised to find she had not heard. So many other people around knew and Mrs Garrison was known to be a close friend of Mrs McBain's. Sophia was shocked. She had had no letter from Amy about it. Nothing. And she had wasted no time in booking herself on a schooner to New York.

It was an anxious Hinton who saw his wife off but he knew he could not stop her. 'You take care, you hear me?' he instructed. 'And don't attempt to walk on deck. Stay below for the whole voyage. You hear what I'm telling you?'

'Yes, yes, I will,' Sophia replied, hardly taking in a word of it.

Although the passage down on a good westerly breeze took under three days, to Sophia it seemed an eternity. She knew exactly what Amy must have been going through. It was not until she gingerly made her way down a gangway on to the frozen, packed earth of a New York slip that the terrible thought struck her. What if people had managed to keep it from Amy and she had not heard? What would she do then? She could not possibly tell her herself. But Amy knew her only too well. She would be able to see from her face that something was badly wrong. She was bound to. Hinton had always said she could not fool a gatepost. Oh, my God. The best thing to do was talk to Aunt Dorothea first and find out.

In a state of distress and confusion she alighted from the cab, walked to the door and pulled at the bell. A few moments later she was looking at the woman servant who recognised her immediately and stepped aside to let her in, but Sophia continued to stand at the top of the stoop.

'I'd like to talk to Miss Jackson first,' she said almost in a whisper.

'She's not in, ma'am,' the servant replied, 'but Mrs McBain is.'

'Oh,' Sophia said in as much confusion as ever.

The woman stood there holding the door open for her.

'I . . . ah . . . I came down from Boston,' she said.

'Yes, ma'am,' the woman replied. 'Ain't you comin' in?'

Sophia had no alternative but to step inside. But the moment she stood in the hallway, the door closed behind her, the confusion went. It was all too clear. The chill air she had let in did nothing to alleviate the atmosphere that was laden with silent gloom. There was no Bosun at her feet. Gone was the cheerful brightness Amy somehow always managed to create around her. It was like a house in mourning. Amy had heard all right and when she appeared her face confirmed it. It bore all the marks of deeply wounded misery but she was trying hard to bear up and raise a welcome smile for her friend. There was no relief for Sophia in knowing that she would not have to be devious, and that she had been right to come. And there was no need for Amy to be told that the news was around in Boston, too. For a moment they looked at each other.

'Oh, Amy,' Sophia said, and they fell into each other's arms, tears squeezing from both of them.

Shortly afterwards in the living room, Sophia glanced at the fire. It looked half dead too and she quickly threw a log on it to spark it up while Amy regained control of her emotions.

'It's wonderful to see you, Sophia,' she said. 'It really is.'

'When did all this start?' Sophia wanted to know.

'I first heard about a week ago, two days after he sailed,' Amy replied.

'Only a week ago?' Sophia exclaimed in surprise at the speed with which she herself had been told. 'My God, who needs semaphore stations?'

'I know,' Amy agreed.

'Do you know who she is, this woman?' Sophia enquired.

'No,' Amy returned. 'I only know she's a titled English lady.'

'Has he ever mentioned her?'

'No, he'd never do a thing like that.'

After all Amy had done for her husband, it seemed inconceivable

118

to Sophia that James was ready to desert her. But it was claimed that the English lady was not only eager to marry Captain McBain if he could get rid of his wife but sail with him.

'What does your aunt say?' Sophia asked.

'She says I'm being stupid and must ignore it,' Amy said, 'but that's only what I'd expect her to say.'

'But she's right, Amy, she's right,' Sophia insisted. 'Don't you remember telling me the same thing when there were rumours about Hinton once? And you were right then, weren't you? Well, now I'm saying the same thing to you. You'll forget it, Amy. It's malicious gossip and nothing else.'

'Why would anyone spread such a thing if it weren't true?' Amy pointed out.

'How do I know? Why people do such things is a complete mystery but they do and you know it. Why did they do it to me?'

'You don't understand, Sophia, this is different, don't you see? It makes sense. James spends as much time in London as he does here, if not more. All the time at sea he's mixing with all kinds of people. This is less of a home to him than his cabin and he gets invited out to all kinds of places in England. My stupidity has been in never letting it cross my mind that such a thing could happen.'

'You also told me a woman would always know,' Sophia reminded her. 'Do you know?'

'Yes, I know,' Amy said sadly.

'How do you know?'

'I don't know, I just do.'

'How? What did he do? What did you find? A letter?'

'No,' Amy admitted.

'Have you been through his chest?' Sophia demanded to know.

'What?' Amy said in surprise.

'Searched through his things,' Sophia went on, 'for a lace handkerchief, a lock of hair, or something of the like. I did with Hinton's before you made me see sense.'

'I wouldn't do that, Sophia,' Amy said.

'Well, I'll do it for you,' Sophia offered, 'and I'll bet you I'll find nothing.'

'It would make no difference,' Amy replied.

Sophia, undeterred, planted herself in an armchair, sat back and crossed her arms in defiance. 'Amy,' she said, 'I'm not moving from New York until you've gathered your wits together again. Get a knife and cut off all those wagging tongues if it makes you feel better but you have to put all this behind you. If you know it's true, I know it isn't.'

In truth, Sophia did not know at all, but was doing her level best to do for her friend what Amy had done for her. Even if it was true there was always a chance of the whole thing blowing over. What she did not fully realise was that Amy had already been over everything a hundred times in her own mind and that every question had already found an answer.

'Please don't think I have any intention of letting her have him,' Amy said.

'You've still given me no proof there actually is a her,' Sophia argued, but Amy had already sorted that one out, too. How could anyone in New York actually point her out when she was more than three thousand miles away across the ocean?

'I still love him as much as I've always done,' Amy continued, 'and she's not going to push me out of the way without a fight. But I'm not going to confront him with it either when he gets back. I believe he still loves me but I'm not going to put him in the position of being forced to make a sudden choice between us. There will be no asking him for a denial or confession. I couldn't do that. It's not in my nature.'

'When you're thinking more clearly,' Sophia interposed, 'you'll realise there's no need to.'

'I'll simply behave as if I've heard nothing,' Amy went on.

'Good,' Sophia got in, thinking she was getting somewhere.

'That nothing has happened,' Amy added. 'What he needs is more time with me to even things up and I'm going to see that he gets it. My mind's made up on that.'

'What do you mean?' Sophia asked, puzzled and full of curiosity.

'I'm going back to sea with him,' Amy said.

Sophia unfolded her arms and sat up. 'You're what?' she questioned, and although Amy had been perfectly coherent throughout it all, she could feel all the pain that had brought her to such a decision. It was not only her husband and herself who had to be considered but her child. Convinced by common sense alone that what was rumoured was true, Amy was faced with a struggle for survival. A matter of life and death. Abandoning her own love for James was to ask her to stop breathing. Allowing him to abandon his love for her without her raising a drowning hand was unthinkable. There had always been a strong streak of romanticism in James, but he had invariably been a man of duty and honour, living by his own code. If that had cracked, it was up to her to heal him and restore him. To whom did she really belong? James or Jamie? How many times had she tried without success to share her love between the two all at the one time? There was no question of taking Jamie aboard with her. Apart from the fact that at eight and a half he was still prone to whatever infections were going around and, in the opinion of the New York doctor who attended him, had to be kept well clear of deadly diseases like ship's fever which would have finished him, James had recently made a decision of his own concerning his son.

It had been on a day when, not for the first time, James, trying to salve his conscience for so resenting the child, had taken a reluctant Jamie alone on an outing.

'Try to keep abeam, my boy,' James said as he strode across Wall Street.

'Yes, sir,' Jamie mumbled, afraid of him.

Many men acknowledged his father with a 'Mornin', Captain', and ignored him. It was altogether different when he was out with his mother.

'Dirty thing, steam,' James said as he took him on the Brooklyn ferry which looked more like a skimming dish with paddles. 'You know how it works, my boy?'

'No, sir,' Jamie replied, knowing perfectly well, Amy having carefully explained it all to him before.

'That makes two of us, then,' James informed him and Jamie ached to go home. A short trip on the railroad that Jamie had made many times before was no better. Jamie felt a little sick but was afraid to say so. James felt awkward. With no memory of his own childhood to speak of and unable to handle children, he too wanted to be home. And Amy knew in disappointment the moment they walked in the door it had been another failure. It was that same evening that James took his son aside to have a serious talk with him. Jamie had sat obediently on a chair, his father remaining on his feet.

'Your mother has done wonders for you,' James told him, 'and I hope you appreciate it. You have much to thank her for. But it's time you were educated properly to take that extra burden from her. You'll have the advantages I didn't have. You'll learn Latin and Greek and literature and music. I've associated with a lot of people who've had that privilege and I know the benefits of it. If you use them in the right way they can bring you wealth and social recognition. Which profession attracts you the most?'

Jamie looked at the captain's boots. They were powerful and black and shiny. He hated them and had no strength to combat the man who stood in them. He made no reply.

'Law?' James prompted, tolerantly suppressing his irritation at his son's silence. 'Medicine? A man of letters?' He left out the

121

Church because of bias, and the Army because the boy could never be physically fit enough for it.

'I don't know, sir,' Jamie answered nervously, which at least was the truth.

'I'll be making enquiries on the best schools available for you around New York and will be taking sound advice on the matter,' James told him.

It was following this insistence by James that his son make a serious start that Dorothea knew her time had come. Until then she had feared that, despite medical advice, Amelia might behave foolishly and take her child to sea with her if the need arose. That danger had now been removed. And Dorothea knew her Amelia and knew how she would react. She had also long since observed that the height of scandal was in direct proportion to the importance of the person subjected to it. Hardly had James left his wharf on the East River bound for London when the mysterious whispering campaign began and in no time was not only hot gossip but 'fact' amongst the ladies at their lunches and in coffee shops.

Sophia poked at the fire to raise more flame. Racked by all the torment in her friend she had never felt so helpless in her life. Truth or lies, she knew she was never going to convince her or shift her. Amy had much more spirit and determination than she had. She was only grateful it was not she who had been asked to make a decision between abandoning her husband and abandoning her child in the hope of keeping both, since that was what it amounted to. All she could do to help was provide evidence that there *was* no such lady and, truth or lies, that was an impossibility.

'What of Jamie, then?' she asked and could feel the tearing of Amy's heart, though she replied reasonably enough.

'It's really quite simple,' Amy said. 'I suppose he might be upset at first but he'll recover from that. He's a sensible boy. It's not as if we won't be seeing each other. He'll go to the kind of school his father wants for him and be back here in the afternoons, and I'll be coming back here all the time. While I'm away Aunt Dorothea will take very good care of him.'

Neither was to know it was more than that Aunt Dorothea had planned for herself. In the meantime, Sophia stayed five days in New York, able only to give comfort to her friend. Amy needed that and it helped her to recompose herself. Not that Jamie was fooled. He knew only too well that something was wrong and knew, too, without anyone having told him anything, that the captain was to blame for it.

'I may have to go away for a little while, Jamie,' Amy told him eventually and saw his stricken face.

122

'What for?' he asked. 'Where to?'

'Now you needn't look so upset.' Amy assured him, doing her best to seem cheerful. 'It's not going to be for that long. I'll be back. But I have to go to London.'

'What for?' Jamie asked again, fighting back tears, and she knelt to him and held him and hugged him. For almost nine years she had nursed him and nurtured him and forced him and held him and not for a whole day in all that time had she been away from him.

'Believe me, if I could explain it to you I would,' she told him, 'but you're still too young to understand. Once I told you you'd be stronger than anyone and I want you to be strong now. You must trust me. You do trust me, don't you?' And she knelt back, still holding him to look into his face, so innocent, so unknowing, so hurting. But although he had no idea of what was happening he strove to return his mother's faith and nodded for her.

In the English Channel, the innocent cause of it all slowed his vessel for not a moment longer than necessary. No sooner had the pilot leapt for the dangling rope ladder than Captain James McBain was calling for all sail to be filled again, leaving the pilot cutter quickly astern. It had been so long since he had felt Amy's spirit aboard, guiding him to landmarks and through fogs, he had almost forgotten about it. Speed and never letting a breath of wind go to waste was what had been his success.

During the followings weeks, Amy prepared more than her mind. She engaged tradesmen to do all that needed doing to the house to make it perfect. She had a dressmaker make the most appealing dress she could devise. She took care of her fine skin. Brushed her hair a hundred times a day until it shone like light. Bought new underclothes and new linen. Reacquainted herself with every aspect of navigation, cloud formation and forecasting she had ever learned. 'When the wind shifts against the sun,' she remembered as she touched her toes to trim her waist, 'trust it not, for back it will run.' Yet all the time she lived in fear that it might have been for nothing and that James would make some excuse for not being able to take her.

For Jamie, who was supervised by Amy every morning with lessons in preparation for formal schooling, the time passed more slowly. So slowly, in fact, that in some vague way he began to believe that his mother's going away was no longer going to happen. As the captain in the shape of the cat curled at night, purring on his bed, he thought that perhaps the other captain had drowned this time and would not be seen again.

Aunt Dorothea waited patiently, keeping discreetly in the background as much as possible, considerate, helpful and kindly.

The captain in the tall hat did return again, to be welcomed in the way he had always been. Never could he remember Amy looking more beautiful but that was no reason to think anything might be wrong. Besides, it always took him a day to fully readjust to their reunion, and Amy gave him time for that. But as he sat that night in his bedroom undressing, he could not take his eyes off her and Amy was aware of it. All day she had been inspecting him for any differences in him that would betray the existence of the London lady.

'I wonder if I could ever be any good at navigation again,' she said as if pondering on it as she slipped out of her dress.

'I don't see why not,' James said, his boots removed and pushed under the chair, but if he appeared calm his heart was pounding with arousal and what Amy had said meant nothing to him.

'It gave me the greatest sense of satisfaction,' Amy said, and her hair released, it tumbled to her shoulders like a sea of silk.

'Yes, I know,' James said automatically as Amy, delicately and unhurriedly, undid her bodice.

'You remember the nights we stood looking at the stars as we made our way towards those tiny specks of the Madeiras?' she said, and sensuously her breasts were gradually revealed to glow warmly by the lights of lamp and fire before, in modesty, she turned partly away.

'Yes,' James replied without even being aware he had spoken.

'I'd so like to do all that again,' Amy said, partly turning back to him as she pulled gently at the bowed tapes that held her lace-trimmed underskirts to her waist but this time James seemed not to have heard. It was not words that had hypnotised him and if there were any stars around they were shooting like red-hot embers through his being.

Amy said no more and shortly after slipped into bed, her hair spreading itself on the pillow to frame the beauty of her slightly apprehensive face. James looked at her for a moment, blew out the lamp and got in beside her, a soft flickering on the ceiling reflected from the grate. He was like a youth. Tentative, not fully confident, but aflame in a world of promise. He put out an arm and tenderly pulled her towards him, his passion still contained but screaming at the floodgates. Then her submissive body was against him, her arms tightly around him. James scaled the heights of heaven and eventually exploded through it with a cry.

When he woke two hours later, which was the longest he ever slept at one time, the ship was not moving. He might have leapt out of his bunk at that had he not quickly become aware that his head was resting partly on Amy's shoulder and that her arm was hooked around his head and he had not been dreaming. Not wanting to disturb or wake her, he lay with his eyes open but there was nothing to see. Then, suddenly, the words he had not heard properly came back to him. What did she mean by talking about navigation and saying she would like to do it all again? It did not quite make sense and there seemed no reason for it, yet he sensed there was more to it and became intensely curious. Why had she said such things? Amy stirred.

'Are you awake?' he said very quietly.

'Mmmmm,' Amy murmured, 'a little.'

'What did you mean when you said you'd like to do it all again?' he asked, still quietly. 'Do what?'

'Go back to sea with you, if you'd have me,' Amy said as if only half afloat and about to submerge again. 'Even this very next voyage,' and she turned on her side away from him with another little 'Mmmmm', appearing to have gone right off again.

James could not believe what he had heard. 'Amy?' he questioned but there was no reply and he was left with it to sink in. Sweet Jesus, had he heard right? Was she just talking in her sleep? As he did not sleep another wink for the rest of the night, he had plenty of time to think about it, and by morning had so convinced himself that all his heavens had come at once that he could hardly bear it. So much so that he began to fear that if he questioned her too much about it, it might suddenly all dissolve.

'You did mean what you said last night?' was the total extent of his enquiries when she was fully awake.

'Of course I did, silly,' Amy replied, studying him closely again for a glimpse of Lady Dilemma.

Two days later, Aunt Dorothea could see there was no turning back for them. The matter was all settled. As he made arrangements, the captain walked about as if his feet were in cloud while Amy could not have been happier at being given the chance to see off her London challenger. Dorothea hated having thrown them together again but that was no longer her priority. She put the final fuse to her powder. She appeared to be in some distress when she informed both of them, 'I'm very sorry. Very sorry. I don't want to upset anyone. But I've been thinking about it and the idea of staying here on my own terrifies me. I can't do it, just can't. I simply must go back to my cottage in Boston.'

Amy stared at her in shock, 'You can't, Aunt Dorothea,' she protested since the implication was clear. If Dorothea could not stay in New York, neither could Jamie. And if that happened, her child would not be easily available to her. She looked to James for help, not realising that he was far too afraid of losing her to make much of an effort, start a row and have everything fall to pieces. Dorothea thought she might have him as an ally.

'You must seriously reconsider, Aunt Dorothea,' he said, but Dorothea was to remain adamant.

'It would be better for Jamie, too, Amelia,' she pointed out. 'He could go to that private day school with the Garrison boys and have friends he knew. They're learning Latin and Greek there, I heard Sophia say so. And if I took ill or anything there would be Sophia at hand.'

'That makes sense, Amy,' James said. 'It *would* be much better for him.'

Amy sensed she had lost before they had gone much further and, despite the fresh stab wound of pain she felt in being further separated from her son than she had intended, tried to tell herself it would be better for him because of the Garrisons.

Eventually she was aboard, doing her best to hide her weeping as the ship was hauled out from the wharf on the East River and she waved. But it was not because he could not see her that Jamie did not wave back. With Aunt Dorothea holding his hand in the midst of the farewelling crowd, tears were streaming down his face. But in the centre of his grief was the powerful desire to exact retribution on the evil captain for having stolen his mother, an act more brutal in the face of his helplessness.

And a few days later, Aunt Dorothea, with the utmost satisfaction, departed for Boston with her child.

Chapter Twelve

As the ship tied up at the London docks, Amy scanned every female figure amongst the waiting crowd, searching for one that might be unaccompanied. That she could not see one in the smoky air did not mean that she was not there or did not exist. Amy would not have been there if she had believed that. And when James went down the gangplank in his shore clothes, satchel of papers in hand, she followed his tall hat through the people like a hawk, all the time expecting her to suddenly appear and approach him. But the innocent James reached the door of the warehouse and agents' counting house without having been stopped or hailed by anyone.

It had been a new experience for her getting here. It was quite a different James to the one she had known at sea before. Certainly she knew he had made a reputation as a 'driver' but she had not expected him to push his vessel to what at first seemed to her the very extremes of danger. And every time he set foot on deck, the crew on watch jumped to stand by sheets and braces as if they expected to be horsewhipped. She kept searching the dockside in some anxiety, but it was she who was approached and was unaware of the first mate having sidled up to her by the rail until he spoke.

'You got us here in very good time, ma'am,' he said. 'The captain never mentioned that it was an expert navigator he kept hidden away at home.'

'Thank you,' Amy replied, continuing to keep one eye on the dockside.

'No, it's us who has to thank you, Mrs McBain.'

'Us?' Amy said absent-mindedly, still preoccupied with the shore. Surely the woman would not have been so bold as to wait for him there in the counting house right in front of the agents. No lady could have been so bare-faced.

'The whole crew, ma'am,' Rivers explained and hesitated. 'And I ain't sure if it's rightly my place to say this, ma'am.'

Amy's heart dropped. He was going to tell her about the lady and inform her where she was. The mate had hesitated again, not sure if he was being too forward.

'Say it, Mr Rivers,' she said, bracing herself, eyes on the dock.

'Well, it's just you've made the captain into a different man, ma'am, and I guess the crew would want me to tell you how much they appreciate it.'

Amy's head turned to him. 'What do you mean?' she asked, a little confused.

'As you'd know, ma'am,' Rivers told her, 'there's blood ships, slow ships, fast ships and happy ships. And that don't depend on the discipline on deck or the rig or the sail aloft. It depends on what kind of heart's beatin' in her. Till you came aboard this was a fast ship, ma'am. Now her heart is warmed and she's a happy fast ship. And I'm sure the captain himself knows better than anyone that a happy fast ship can outrun a fast one any day.'

Amy looked at him in astonishment. Although her mind had had to make a leap she understood what Rivers had said to her. It had not occurred to her that she had brought about any such change in James and it was just the tonic she needed at that moment.

'I'd rather you didn't tell the captain I told you,' Rivers added a little anxiously. 'I know he's a private man and I respect that,' and he turned to go for'ard.

'Mr Rivers,' Amy said, stopping him, 'thank you very much.'

'A pleasure, ma'am,' Rivers replied and carried on, soon barking at a seaman to make one of the mooring lines more secure. Amy suddenly felt much more secure too. She had clearly won the important first round and could not have been more grateful to Rivers for letting her know it.

Without the mysterious lady having put in an appearance, due no doubt, as Amy saw it, to the presence of the captain's wife, it was to be an even happier fast ship that set out on its westward voyage. All the way down the English Channel the wind was from the north, putting them on a fast reach, and it stayed like that until they were out into the Atlantic when it began to veer, then back, in a regular rhythm.

'I think we should go further north,' Amy advised James.

'What, and risk losing this great advantage we have? Only once in my life before have I had it this good.'

'It could be better north,' Amy persisted, 'with stronger winds.'

'What makes you think that?' James wanted to know.

'I just feel it,' Amy said.

But it was only because he so much wanted to please her and give her every opportunity that he ordered a change of course.

'I don't believe it,' he said in amazement when the wind gradually veered and strengthened until twenty-four hours later they were running with full sail before an easterly gale. Considering the prevailing winds at that latitude were almost always westerly it was incredible. Day after day it went on.

'Do you believe in the will of God, Mr Rivers?' James asked his first mate in restrained excitement as they stood on deck, the ship thundering, surging and streaking over the sea.

'Yes, sir, I do,' Rivers replied, 'and in your navigator, too.'

And both turned to look at Amy, hair blowing in the wind, who stood braced at the port rail, sextant raised, waiting for the moment the sun appeared between clouds again, the bosun by her side ready with deck watch and notebook.

The easterly took them more than halfway across the ocean on Amy's course before it eased off and after a day of calm started filling in from the south-west. James, not exactly a man to display his emotions by jumping up and down for joy, was almost ecstatic when the Floating Light off Sandy Hook came up dead ahead.

'By God, we've done it, Amy,' he kept saying, hardly able to stand still for a moment, and Amy had never felt so delighted for him, at the same time sensing that she had won round two against the London lady.

'The London packet *Amphitrite*, owned by Messrs Merriman and Rudd and mastered by Captain James McBain, yesterday smashed the westward record from London by no less than *five days*!' ran the *New York Herald* the next morning and went on to give a full account of it to the public. Merriman and Rudd hurriedly arranged a celebration and, surrounded by admirers, James soaked up the attention like a sponge and got a little drunk. 'My navigator did it,' he said to all.

Captain Eastlake who had just signed the Temperance pledge for the sixth time and who was desperate to master one of the new packets which were getting bigger and bigger all the time was furious. He immediately wrote a letter to the *Herald* pointing out that Captain McBain's record must be discounted and struck out since it was achieved only under freak conditions that might not arise again in a hundred years and that any captain with a ship of similar burthen could have done the same.

The saved days meant much more for Amy than a record. It allowed her time to get up to Boston to see Jamie for a couple of days and get back to New York in time for the next sailing. And despite the many invitations he had from members of the Exchange and business organisations who wanted to hear his account at first hand, James chose to go with her.

'It's my duty to see his school and judge how he is getting on at

129

it,' he said, but the truth was different. He was in fear that something he could not foresee might happen to hold Amy there and that he would lose her again.

Aunt Dorothea, who hated their appearance, was at her most welcoming and it hurt her all the more as Jamie clung tightly around his mother's neck as if never to let go of her again. That was not to be and after three hectic days filled with the Garrisons and other reunions, he was left bereft and in tears as the evil, hated captain took his mother away again.

They had been gone only a matter of days when Dr Amos Drew dried his hands with a fine white linen towel and looked up at the chubby face poking around his door.

'Show the young gentleman in now, please, Mrs Bellow,' he directed and Mrs Bellow, even weightier above but still light-footed below, went to fetch their new patient.

A few moments later the well-dressed young man was shown in but there was nothing to indicate that he might be an unwitting bearer of unwanted revelations. Amos Drew could tell at once that, despite the clothes, the young man was hardly a gentleman. To his eye, the squarish face had a common and not a well-bred look to it while his side-whiskers still struggled for mature recognition. There was also a lack of sophistication, if not confidence, in his bearing. Nevertheless, Amos Drew gave him his same, well-practised smile.

'Mr Trupp, I think you said,' he greeted.

'Yes, Doctor,' the young man replied, pleased to have been accepted and not turned away, and pleased too to hear the famous doctor speak his name. As someone on the way up he had chosen Amos Drew because of the doctor's fashionable reputation, even if it was going to cost him a lot more money. It would be another feather in his cap to be able to tell people that the same Dr Drew who attended to many Boston notables was his doctor too.

'And what is the problem, Mr Trupp?' Amos Drew asked.

'It's a rash on my arm, Doctor,' young Trupp told him and without further bidding removed his coat, undid his sleeve and rolled it up high to show his complaint. Amos Drew examined it. He rather liked the young man's skin. It was fine and warm to touch.

'How long have you had it?' he enquired.

'I guess a few months now,' Trupp answered.

A fly buzzed against the windowpane.

'Well, we'll see what we can do,' Dr Drew said, already thinking that, without voicing such a prediction, a few good coatings of gentian violet might clear it up.

'I guess it wouldn't have anything to do with what I do?' young

Trupp queried, deliberately giving lead to human curiosity about himself.

'And what *do* you do?' Amos Drew felt obliged to ask as he went about preparing a solution. Young Trupp was only too eager to talk about his success.

'In winter I have the ice cut up in all the ponds around Boston under contract for supplying Mr Tudor's ice-exporting business. In summer I'm laying on water into houses. Tanks, steam pumps, pipes, everything. I employ a lot of men now.'

'How interesting,' Amos Drew said dully, disappointing the young man with his apparent lack of enthusiasm.

'I got my start from somebody you know, Doctor,' Trupp said, trying another tack.

'Oh?' the doctor questioned. 'And who was that?'

'Miss Jackson,' Trupp replied.

Amos Drew did not particularly want to hear about Dorothea Jackson. He had been very relieved when he had seen her off to New York with the McBains and much disconcerted at her return. The only good thing about that was seeing the child. Although he had been kept up to date with the boy's progress he had found the changes amazing. And he was such a pretty boy. Too pretty for his comfort.

'Had it not been for her,' Trupp went on for lack of response, 'I might have been just nothing today.'

'And how was that?' Dr Drew asked as he stirred the crystals.

'She gave me a lot of money to carry water for her house,' the young man explained. 'I was only a kid.'

'I don't remember Miss Jackson's pond ever being dry,' Amos Drew said.

'Oh, it wasn't,' the young man said, keen to explain further, 'but she wanted it from the other side of town. Better for her roses, she said, but I don't reckon she minds me telling you the secret now. Kept me going six months, she did, and I saw the possibilities in it and saved nearly everything she gave me. Reinvested in the water business as you might say. Now look at me.'

Amos Drew looked at him, his curiosity at last aroused. What the young man was telling him was not only strange but made little sense.

'What kind of water was this?' he asked.

'The pond where the shot tower used to be before they pulled it down,' young Trupp told him.

Drew remembered the pond only too well. So strong had become the superstition surrounding it that a group of hysterical women had taken it on themselves a few years before to fill it in to make sure their children could never drink from it. For others, the incident had been of passing amusement and quickly forgotten.

'When exactly was this?' he enquired of the young man, but he was still not prepared for the answer.

'I remember that well enough,' young Trupp replied happily, 'because it was from the time Mrs McBain was confined until her poor little boy was born. Not poor any more though, is he?'

Amos Drew felt his skin creep all over his body. Mrs McBain's confinement had been all through the fall and winter months and no one watered rose bushes at that time. Not even with magic potions. As he brushed the fluid on the young man's arm, staining the rashed flesh purple, he did not hear him go on with his self-adulation and aspirations. Unthinkable and totally unacceptable thoughts were piercing his mind like arrows, and all of them frightened him.

After he had got rid of the young man who insisted on making immediate payment, he stood at a basin, washing his hands over and over again with his scented soap. Until then there had been no real foundation for his vague suspicions about Miss Jackson other than his own fear of being found out. Now, that had changed. It was inconceivable that she could have had anything to do with Mrs McBain almost dying in childbirth and the sickly, brain-damaged child born to her by using some unknown poison. That would have been attempted murder. Yet he felt that foundation heaving under the soles of his boots like a gigantic block of solid granite and a bead of cold sweat trickled down his temple.

'I'll be going out a little more than usual over the next two weeks,' he told his housekeeper that evening without explaining why. And in all the time he could spare in that two weeks he made calls on every public institution where insane women were held. It did not surprise him that he himself was met with some suspicion. It was only recently that another Dorothea, Dorothea Dix, had had her declaration on the cruel and inhumane treatment of the insane recorded in the State Legislature and keepers were on their guard. But they did remember Miss Dorothea Jackson, although she had long since stopped visiting them. To his questioning he discovered that in every instance the pattern was the same. The selection of a woman isolated for her own safety. The request to be left alone. The destruction of her gifts. All his instincts told him to turn away. If that pattern had any hidden meaning to it, he did not want to find out what it was. Yet, like some witness mesmerised into unwanted fascination by the mangled flesh and bone of a gory accident, he continued to investigate, eventually arriving at the asylum where he was met by the keeper in the huge and formidable shape of Miss Blossom. No longer was the stout stick stuck through her belt for all to see. And she was clearly very nervous.

'I do the very best I can here, Dr Drew, sir,' she wasted no time in telling him defensively.

'I've absolutely no doubt of that, Miss Blossom,' Amos Drew replied.

'It's all right for them to criticise, Dr Drew,' Miss Blossom ran on as if she had not heard him. 'What right have they when they don't know what it's like?'

'Miss Blossom . . .' Amos Drew tried to interrupt.

'What am I going to do if I lose my job here?' Miss Blossom pushed on. 'What am I going to do? I've put my whole life into this place and I've saved nothing from what I get. I have no husband to turn to – no one. I live here, it's my home. I don't have anywhere else. What do they think I'm going to do?'

'Miss Blossom . . .' Amos Drew tried again.

'I'll be reduced to poverty if I lose my job,' she continued. 'What else could I do? What other work is there for women? God knows I've done my best. Do they think I've been beating women for the sake of it? God knows I've done my best. Oh God, oh God.'

And to Amos Drew's amazement and embarrassment this Amazon of a woman who could have thrown most men over her shoulder with ease began to cry.

'There, there, Miss Blossom,' Amos Drew tried to comfort, at the same time turning his head away so as not to see her. 'I think maybe you're mistaking my purpose here. It's got nothing to do with the things Miss Dorothea Dix has said. I've never even met the woman. And if anyone has criticised you or tried to lay blame on you for the way you run this institution I'll personally seek a retraction from them. I've seen for myself how well you do here. You have the most difficult job in the world and no sane man would envy you for it.'

That did comfort Miss Blossom considerably although it was hard to tell since the tears of self-pity that she wiped away with the back of her large hand would not stop as easily as they began.

'I came to ask you, in the strictest confidence, of course, if you can remember anything about the visits paid by Miss Dorothea Jackson.'

At the mention of that, with his head still turned away, he did not see the look of fright that came into Miss Blossom's wet eyes.

'If there's anything you can tell me, I can assure you that it will be kept between ourselves and won't go outside these walls. Neither will it go against you in any way whatsoever.'

Miss Blossom did not reply. Amos Drew waited a few moments. He was being given his final escape and sought to take it. He glanced at the keeper, then turned to go.

'I'm sorry if I've upset you, Miss Blossom. Perhaps some other time.'

'That wasn't my fault either, Dr Drew,' Miss Blossom blurted after him and he stopped, trapped again.

'What wasn't your fault?' he asked quietly, his back turned to her.

'I saw her,' he heard Miss Blossom go on, 'saw what she did.'

Amos Drew started to turn around to face her, wishing he had never come here, wishing he had never asked, but there was no stopping her. She was only too eager to redirect the blaming of cruelty away from herself, even if she had been beating lunatic women for years in the frustration of trying to keep order.

'I went down the corridor to get something and saw her with Lucy May. One of my quietest. I never touched her in my life. All the other inmates did that to her. Miss Jackson didn't know I was there but I saw her through the space between the hinges.'

Amos Drew clasped his hands together, holding them tightly, feeling a mounting sense of horror although he had, as yet, been told nothing.

' "You recite me the Constitution," she kept telling Lucy May who knows nothin'. "You recite me the Constitution an' you can have this pretty Chinese fan," an' I could see Lucy May all the time tryin' to reach for it. She went on and on about it, askin' over and over until she had Lucy May cryin' for it. Then she broke the thing over her knee and tore up all the printed silk of it, Lucy May trying to pick up the pieces.'

Although Miss Blossom had not finished, Amos Drew felt his stomach turn.

' "You're a very, very bad woman, Lucy May," she went on at her,' Miss Blossom ended, 'and Lucy May started screaming. When I went in, Miss Jackson says to me like she done every time before, "Don't strike her, don't strike her, she didn't mean to do it".'

Amos Drew stood staring at the huge figure of a woman. What he had not wanted to hear was ringing and burning in his ears. He could find nothing to say.

'People like that should never have been let in here, but that wasn't my fault, was it?' he heard Miss Blossom say further after a pause. 'It wasn't me asked her to come here. I never touched nobody in my life except if it was needed.'

134

When Amos Drew left, Miss Blossom felt somewhat consoled at having got it out, especially since it was Dr Drew himself who had recommended that Miss Jackson be admitted there as a credited visitor. The doctor sat in his carriage, his head spinning. He had no more idea than Dorothea herself why she felt so compelled to punish such helpless, incarcerated women for nothing. And not aware of her other secrets, he knew nothing of her deep, subconscious desire to replace the child she had killed. All he could see was a madwoman, a torturer of the damned walking the earth in the guise of a kindly and charitable lady. The responsibility of being the only one outside an asylum who knew it almost overwhelmed him. He told himself he had been incredibly stupid. If only he had shut his eyes he could have pushed everything aside as coincidence. He was a doctor, not a law-enforcer. But the possibility of Mrs McBain having been deliberately poisoned was no longer just an outrageous conjecture. It burned in his brain.

'I have something important to do,' he told his housekeeper on reaching home, 'and I don't want to be disturbed.' And he retired to his study to sit down and open his inkwell with the intention of writing to a friend in authority. Nothing came. Every resolution he made to himself to expose Miss Dorothea Jackson came into his head with the weight of lead only to float out again like wood. A dozen or more times over days he sat down to put pen to paper but never a word went down. Too many things got in the way. What could he say? What would he be letting himself in for if he said anything at all? People were bound to want to know why he had not detected poisoning if he made any such suggestion. He could make himself look an incompetent fool. And how could he explain to Captain McBain that his son might be in grave danger in the care of his wife's aunt? It would all be an awful scandal with himself at the centre of it. He began to tell himself that he was being much too hasty, that it might not be as bad as it first seemed. Was there not every possibility that Miss Jackson had recovered from her terrible madness? That she had not made any visits to institutions in Boston since her return from New York was evidence of it. And what possible danger could the boy be in? He was growing up handsomely beyond all expectations for everyone to see and Drew himself had taken a good deal of credit for it. After only ten days of crawling through his dark tunnel, Amos Drew came back into the light of escape, having convinced himself that by far his best course was to do nothing.

Not too distant in a classroom of the Landon Classical Academy, James McBain junior sat at his own desk amongst the sons of well-known Bostonian fathers, trying to pay attention. Mr Allburn, a tall, thin man in long, dusty coat-tails, was writing the conjugation of a Latin verb on the blackboard, pronouncing at the same time. Jamie's mind drifted away, past the bas-relief of Jesus on the wall, past the statue of Socrates, and out the window towards far and vague horizons. There were other things he was being taught.

'You mustn't be thinking of your mother all the time,' Aunt Dorothea had told him more than once in sympathetic and understanding tones. 'It isn't good for you. Pining for something they can't have only makes people ill, and you don't want to be ill, do you?'

'It's a great pity your father took your mother away,' she told him another time, 'and that she chose to go. The captain's a very strong-minded man and sometimes I fear he'll never let her go now she's proved her worth to him at sea. You poor child. But never mind. God always has His reasons and you always have me, you know, and I love you more than anyone.'

'You mustn't pay too much attention to anything Mrs Garrison tells you,' she had warned him one day. 'I know she's a good friend of your mother's and she probably means well but I wouldn't put any trust in her. It's not as if she's our own flesh and blood.'

The indoctrination of Latin, Greek, English and Aunt Dorothea was gradual, almost timeless.

'McBain!' Mr Allburn said, frightening him.

'Yes, sir.' Jamie started.

'If your father showed as much inattentiveness to the running of his ship as you're showing to me,' Allburn told him, 'he would never get across the ocean.'

The other boys tittered. Jamie lowered his head, and Allburn accepted it as shame. He was wrong. Jamie's mind was far too choked with a mixture of confusion and burning anger to give it room.

Chapter Thirteen

Two years after Jamie had been taken away from New York, South Street on the East River had become more crowded than ever. Atlantic packets had reached a massive 1000 tons. Along the waterfront a forest of masts soared ever higher towards the sky. Beneath the huge bowsprits overhanging the street itself, boys jostled for space as they herded sheep, pigs and cows for delivery to ships' barnyards, guiding them between horses and carts, barrows, boxes, barrels, bales, grocery victuallers, seamen, longshoremen, men in tall hats and a vendor of pies.

Four storeys up in the counting house of Kimball and Jay, Mr Kimball lit up a large Havana as he got down to details with Mr Jay.

'We must consider it carefully,' he said.

'Not get too carried away,' Mr Jay returned.

For some time they had been making a review of their situation and had already come to a decision as to where to invest in the future for the best profits. Others were already making fortunes.

'We mustn't appear too keen,' Mr Kimball said, 'not let him think he's the only one.'

'Not offer him a cigar even,' Mr Jay suggested.

'All the same, I think we should be prepared to go to fifteen per cent,' Mr Kimball said.

'I'm sure he wouldn't settle for any less,' Mr Jay agreed.

'But,' Mr Kimball cautioned, 'if we offer him fifteen you can be sure he'll want to raise us. So if we offer him ten and let him lift us to fifteen we'll all be happy.'

'That is fair,' Mr Jay replied, although Mrs Jay had loudly and strongly advised him that, if he was to succeed, he was going to have to stretch himself. The little lady knew as well as he did that it was not going to be easy to get Captain James McBain back for their new project.

'Past friendship should account for something, too,' Mr Kimball pointed out.

'It should do,' Mr Jay concurred but felt a little doubtful about it. James had become a name. On Merriman and Rudd's big new packet he had broken another record, this time for the easterly run between New York and London, making it in the incredible time of only twelve and a half days. Several women's journals had written articles on his navigator wife and the New York *Weekly Museum* which covered the social scene had reported that she could charm winds out of Aeolus's cavern like no one else while her husband took every last bit of advantage of them.

'All stupid, goddamned pretentious nonsense,' Eastlake had tried to tell everyone in reply to that. 'It's luck and not a damn thing else. McBain's no better than any other packet master.'

In response to Kimball and Jay's hand-delivered letter, James, who had just arrived back in port, duly put in an appearance. They had said only that they wanted to put a proposition to him without saying what and James, intrigued, had been unable to resist that.

'James, James,' Kimball and Jay said, both rising from their desk, 'sit down, sit down, sit down.'

'A cigar, James,' Mr Kimball said, offering him the box.

James smiled. It could not have been clearer to him that whatever it was they had up their sleeve, they very much wanted him to be part of it. He was at an advantage from the start and knew it.

'Good to see you again, gentlemen,' he said in sincerity and both seem delighted by that.

'Good passage back over?' Mr Jay ventured.

'Very good, thank you,' James replied.

'How are things then, James?' Mr Kimball enquired.

'Couldn't be better, Mr Kimball,' James told him.

'Good,' Mr Kimball said, unable to wait any longer, 'then we'll come straight to the point. We're going to have a new ship built, James.'

'For the tea trade,' Mr Jay explained.

'Canton, Amoy, Foochow, wherever is best,' Kimball added.

James might have sat bold upright with interest at that if he had had less control of himself. For many days on his trip back he had sat talking with a ship designer returning from a visit to England. The man had fascinated him by discussing his theories on hydro-dynamics and the speed of ships' hulls. He had produced drawings of a vessel as big as an Atlantic packet but as sharp as a little Baltimore clipper. James had been very excited by that. The only question was, who might risk having such a vessel built? It was a radical concept that might not work.

'Why are you telling *me* what you intend doing?' James asked as casually as he was able.

'We're looking ahead, of course,' Mr Kimball admitted.

'Planning forward,' Mr Jay put in.

'But we want the right master for her,' Kimball went on, 'and have drawn up a short list.'

'Well, shortish,' Mr Jay contributed.

'And I'm on it, is that it?' James said, showing little interest.

'Yes, you are, James,' Kimball assured him. 'Yes you are.'

'At the top, in the middle, or at the bottom?' James smiled, putting them on the spot, and he watched Mr Kimball and Mr Jay glance a little anxiously at each other for the answer.

'As far as primage is concerned,' Kimball said, finding it first, 'at the top, James, at the top. Indeed, with you, we'd be prepared to go as high as ten per cent.'

No one could ever have told that James's heart was running fast under his waistcoat at the possibilities that might be opening for him. He pulled at the heavy gold chain to bring out his watch to look at the time, as if to suggest he was running late for something more important.

'Is that all, then, gentlemen?' he said as if prepared to go.

'Twelve, James, and that's it,' Kimball offered.

'We can't do better than that,' Mr Jay added in support.

'Do you realise,' James said after a pause, 'that if you built a ship big enough and fast enough, carrying tea from China you could pay for the cost of her building in one single round voyage?'

Both Kimball and Jay looked at him in feigned surprise as if they didn't.

'Could we?' Kimball gasped.

'Could we really?' Mr Jay repeated.

James felt like bursting out laughing at their performance but the moment was not appropriate.

'Fifteen then, James,' Kimball upped with a wave of his cigar.

'For old times' sake, James,' Mr Jay half pleaded.

James looked from one to the other as they waited. 'I think you might be better off with Captain Eastlake,' he advised.

Fist clenched on desk, Kimball tried not to thump it. 'What in the hell do you want, James?' he demanded to know. 'The shirts off our backs?'

'Only the buttons,' James told them, 'and I'm sure you'd have no trouble getting new ones sewn on. If I considered this at all I'd want a ship design of my own choosing and be given shares in her.'

'*What*?' Kimball and Jay exclaimed aghast and in unison.

'I thank you for thinking of me, I appreciate it,' James said politely, risking all as he reached for his tall hat to rise, 'but the truth is I'm very settled the way I am. Captain Eastlake will still make you money. I hear he's signed the pledge again.'

'Goddamnit!' Kimball shouted at him. 'Sit back down there and let's discuss this sensibly!'

'Reasonably,' Mr Jay requested.

It was no lie for James to say he was settled. Having been able to keep Amy he had taken a much greater interest in his son and, whenever time made it possible, dashed up to Boston with his wife between sailings. If these visits were invariably rushed with so many people to see, it was an arrangement that, nevertheless, had worked. Amy saw her son while James, as dutiful father, not only provided for all the boy's material needs but assessed and guided his education.

Amy, clothes packed ready for a quick dash up to Boston, waited aboard for James to return. She was not particularly curious as to why Kimball and Jay wanted to see him. There was always someone wanting to see him – merchants, shipowners, newspaper reporters, societies and all kinds of people. Social invitations to attend functions were regularly extended.

It had taken only a few Atlantic crossings for Amy's English challenger to disappear completely into the London gloom, but it was not because she felt any threat of another emerging that she continued at sea. Strong and powerful a man as James was, it had come as a blinding light to her just how much he needed her with him. It had nothing to do with her mastery in the art of navigation either, it was simply for his stability and happiness. She had been profoundly shaken when she came to realise that this seemingly self-sufficient man who could face a hurricane without as much as flinching lived in a real and constant fear of losing her again. Yet that and her love for him was still not all of it. She got a tremendous satisfaction from her job. It gave her purpose, made her more than wife and mother. It provided her with a separate identity in a world where very few women ever got such an opportunity. While others struggled upstairs, lamp in one hand, fat baby in the other, Amy McBain would be going nimbly down a companionway to bend over her charts.

'Am I being selfish?' she had questioned Sophia on a previous visit to Boston, feeling guilty about leaving Jamie yet again.

'Don't be so silly, Amy, of course you're not,' Sophia had reassured her. 'My God, you couldn't have done more for him than you have. Everyone still talks about it. And although your aunt is inclined to cosset him a bit and I don't see as much of him as I'd like, he's growing into the most charming young man. You should all be proud of each other in the McBain family. Clever father, clever mother, and clever son.'

140

It was what Amy needed to hear and she was quite unaware of what she was letting herself in for. Neither was she told that it was not only Jamie who pined for days after each hurried departure but the dog Bosun, too. And she had no idea just how relieved Aunt Dorothea was to see the back of her. Only Captain the cat whose days were numbered and who seemed determined to sleep the rest of them out in peace remained unaffected.

James returned to her as she waited on the wharf in New York and she could tell immediately by the way his eyes were lit up that something had happened.

'You know that ship Nat Miller the designer showed us the drawings of on the way back?' he grinned. 'The one you said looked back to front for an ocean-going vessel?'

'What about it?' Amy asked.

'I think she's going to be built.'

'What?' Amy explained in surprise. 'Who for?'

'Kimball and Jay,' James told her, 'but keep it under your hat for now, they don't know it yet and they're nervous enough as it is. And you, Amy, you can start thinking about what you reckon might be the quickest route for taking her to China.'

Amy stared at him in astonishment but that was nothing compared to Mr Kimball and Mr Jay who, after conceding to James's wishes in order to get him back, saw what was happening. When they looked on the actual shape of their new ship rising from the yard at the bottom of Corlears Street they nearly fainted. They were conservative businessmen chasing dollars, not innovators or experimentalists. They began to worry to death as what they had decided to call the *Cirrus* grew higher.

'Are you sure, are you positively sure?' both Kimball and Jay asked Nat Miller almost every day.

Every time James and Amy returned from another passage back from London, they had hardly put a foot ashore when they found themselves confronted by the anxious faces of Mr Kimball and Mr Jay.

'We want your assurances on this, James,' they demanded.

'I've given you all I can, gentlemen,' responded James who had put all his trust in Nat Miller. 'It's a matter of hydrodynamics.'

A lot of good that was. They knew perfectly well he knew no more about hydrodynamics than they did, which was almost nothing.

'You come and have another look,' they commanded, practically dragging their hostage to the yard again, a worried Amy at their heels. Every day Mr Kimball and Mr Jay lived on the edge of a cliff with their dilemma, undecided as whether to jump into the deep blue sea or pull back with their loss until they had reached the point of no return and it had become too late. But if Nat Miller and James McBain had any confidence in the new ship being built, no one else had. Knowledgeable men who had spent their entire lives on the seas around the world looked on in disbelief at such madness.

'With that flat bottom and those sharp bows she'll go into the first big ocean swell she meets like an arrow,' they said, 'and keep right on going. Right to the bottom.'

Mrs Jay woke from a nightmare about it all and blew like a loudhailer right into Mr Jay's shattered ear, 'Why did you let him do it to you, you stupid man!'

Captain Eastlake who had immediately left Kimball and Jay in a rage over their arrangement to give McBain their new ship and who, despite his reputation for unreliability, had managed to get command of an Atlantic packet, gloated.

'It serves them right,' he told everyone. 'If no one could see McBain's failings before they sure as hell can now and going along with a ship being built the wrong way round proves it.'

The matter became a topic in Boston, too.

'My poor Amelia, my poor Amelia,' Aunt Dorothea grieved prematurely to some visiting charitable ladies, knowing that Jamie could overhear. 'What has he done to her?' And each night Jamie knelt by his bed praying that his mother might be saved but giving his father not a mention. And, as it got closer to the time, the subject even arose during a morning break at the Landon Classical Academy.

'Is it true this ship *Cirrus* your father's going to captain is going to sink?' boys demanded to know from Jamie, wanting the outcome settled.

'Captains think they know everything but they don't,' Jamie answered them. 'They don't know Latin and Greek to start with, do they?'

'Aeneas did,' a smart boy told him and three others pinned him against a wall, intent on a definitive resolution.

'Sure she's going to sink,' Jamie told them but not because he was afraid of being hit, and he hated fighting.

'How do you know?'

'I'll show you, I'll show you,' Jamie said and as they took their hands off him, he took a coin from his pocket. 'Heads she sinks and tails she floats,' then spun it in the air and slapped it down on his hand as it landed. Luck was with him. 'There, heads, see, she sinks.' They might have been satisfied by that had he not added, 'Except my mother might save her.'

142

He himself was only saved by the intervention of the elder of the Garrison boys who sometimes tired of having to see to it, on the instruction of his own mother, that Jamie McBain did not get injured in the rough and tumble of school. Although Jamie had become as fit as any other boy his age, he was still seen as someone who needed extra protection because of his earlier years.

For Mr Kimball and Mr Jay back in New York there was yet more horror to come. Nat Miller had decided to change the rig plan he had first shown them in favour of another he had come up with. When the masts were stepped, not only did they look far too slender, but they were raked back with the impertinence of a pirate. It was as if Miller himself had finally come to doubt the survival of his creation and by making the masts lean back was making a desperate effort to get her to hold her head up even before she ever caught sight of a wave.

James and Amy returned to New York from London to find Mr Kimball and Mr Jay going frantic and almost chewing their top hats as riggers set about weaving an endless web of shrouds and stays that was needed to support these spars. As James stayed there doing his best to appease and comfort the distraught Kimball and Jay, Amy escaped temporarily by making a dash to Washington. She had recently heard of a Lieutenant Matthew Maury of the US Navy there who was researching winds and currents around the world. Invalided ashore with a lame leg, Maury had been put into a room at the Depot of Charts and Instruments, a man forgotten. There, he found himself surrounded by old ships' logbooks. For want of something else to do he started reading them and, to his surprise, found patterns of weather and sea conditions starting to emerge and had begun to collate them for what he saw as valuable information.

'Madam,' he said in even more surprise as the extremely pretty woman was ushered in to see him.

'I'm navigator to my husband, Captain James McBain, sir,' Amy began by telling him,' and we're soon to set sail for China – that's if we get that far since everyone thinks we'll not get a day beyond Sandy Hook on the ship which is of new design.'

The lieutenant had heard of McBain's successes and although Amy had come in like a fresh, warm breeze out of the cold, he did not appear much interested at first. He had become an embittered man, not because of the pain his leg gave him or for having been cast ashore out of the way. He had initially been very enthusiastic over his self-appointed task but his enthusiasm had waned. The Navy showed no interest. No encouragement had been given to him. Sea-serving officers dismissed what he had already discovered.

They were not having any gammy-legged landbound junior of limited experience telling them about the sea. It had become clear to Maury that he was alone and that he never would be given either recognition or promotion. A week before he had decided to abandon his work and had just been sitting there in depression.

'I'm sorry, Mrs McBain,' he said, 'but I can't help you with anything on design.'

'Not on design,' said Amy, 'on the things you know. For years I've been asking questions about winds and currents and no one's been able to tell me. But recently I met this man who said you'd been working on it and that you were probably the only one in the world who might be able to help me.'

Maury sparked up a bit with that. The beautiful young woman was somewhat more than just a warm breeze. After an hour he found himself being lifted by her enthusiasm for his subject. Her faith in him was touching and he began openly to confide his past findings.

'The Gulf Stream's higher in the middle than it is at the sides?' Amy exclaimed in wide-eyed astonishment.

'Yes,' Maury confirmed, 'and because of it there are ways of telling where you are on it so as to take advantage of the strongest current.'

'Tell me, tell me!' Amy cried like an excited girl and after the lieutenant explained it, he rose and limped to a shelf to take down a bundle of charts that had been overmarked with many lines, arrows, wind forces and scribblings of his own. He spread them on the desk and pored over them with his fervent pupil. Not in all the time he had been in that cluttered room had anyone shown appreciation for all his hard labours and here was this vivacious young woman navigator who obviously knew what she was talking about almost falling over herself with it all, hanging on his every fresh revelation with amazement. It was like a tonic coursing through his tired and defeated veins, giving him new life.

'You must publish all these things, sir,' Amy told him eagerly.

'Maybe one day I will do,' the lieutenant smiled out of his clean-shaven, pleasant face, 'but there are still a lot of gaps in my information as you can see.'

'Never mind the gaps, sir,' Amy insisted, 'you must, you must!'

If it was to be just another long winter's day for everyone else in the Depot of Charts and Instruments, it was to be all too short for Amy and the lieutenant. Together, as snow fell over the rest of Washington, they travelled the weather patterns of the Atlantic, went around Cape Horn, across the Pacific, to the Java and South China Seas, and reached down the Indian Ocean on the Mozambique current, stimulating each other further as they went.

144

'It's incredible!' Amy told him. 'You'll be famous!'

By the end, so refreshed was Lieutenant Matthew Maury that he could hardly wait to resume his work. And Amy returned to New York with pages and pages of notes, her head whirling with all the new knowledge. James was pleased and relieved to see her back but he looked weary and a little dispirited.

'If my ears look red and swollen,' he told her, 'it's because Mr Kimball has been hammering the left with misgivings and Mr Jay bashing the right with anxieties.'

'This will cheer you up,' Amy said, giving him her notes which he immediately read. He was as astounded as she had been. In them was everything from the best way of attacking clearly defined doldrums to fresh information on the uncharted reefs of the South China Sea.

'How could he have found out all this sitting at a desk?' he wanted to know, a little scepticism showing.

'He looked,' Amy told him, 'and still is looking. Through thousands of old logbooks.'

'Do you trust him?' James asked.

'Do you trust me?' Amy rejoined.

James knew full well the value of what he held in his hand, but the question of whether the *Cirrus* would plunge to the bottom or keep her bows up still hung over the East River like the sword of Damocles.

It was the first launching of their lives Mr Kimball and Mr Jay tried to keep a quiet affair but although it was not advertised, the crowd stretched halfway up Corlears Street, the hot corn vendors doing a roaring trade. New Yorkers enjoyed being critics.

'Crossbreed if I ever seed one,' said one old salt, 'father a cotton packet, mother a yacht. Damn me if her spars ain't headed for the deck already. Don't know what Captain Jim was thinkin' of. She's for the seabed all right.'

It did not stop the *Cirrus* being launched, and the critics eventually drifted away to the warmer climes of the bars along the waterfront to continue with their comments there. All that remained was to find out if they were right and Kimball and Jay could not afford to wait. Although the middle of winter was the wrong time of the year to set out for China, James was forced to sail.

After they cleared the Floating Light off Sandy Hook and headed down the Atlantic on Amy's course, James took the helm himself for six-hour watches, sleeping only two between. It was essential for him to get to know the ship. In what was only a good breeze he piled on the canvas and he hardly needed to be told by the constant putting down of the log to check her speed that she was fast. But each time the bows plunged into what were only moderate waves, it was to bring on board seas that came rushing down the deck. Nat Miller had told him to expect that but it meant that seamen had to be careful not to be swept off their feet all the time.

'We're in for a gale,' Amy forecast, two and a half days out.

'The glass is steady,' James pointed out.

'I know,' Amy replied, 'but the cat's getting restless.'

There was no arguing with her over such matters. The behaviour of cows, birds and porpoises was also part of her calculations as was the attitude of a new moon. And she and the cat were right. Within a few hours the sky began to turn harsh and gaudy with torn cloud formations and the glass began to fall.

'Well, now we're going to find out,' James said to his wife, referring to how the *Cirrus* might take it. But it was dark before the gale struck. James fought with the helm himself to try to nurse his new ship at an angle over the waves but with every one a fresh tumbling of sea smashed down on the foredeck and came roaring aft like a cataract. Amy was bracing herself in the saloon over a chart when it happened. She heard the loud, quick succession of cracking reports that might have been gunfire, but she knew what it was. The snapping of rope under unbearable tension. Within seconds the topgallant masts of the *Cirrus* were crashing to the decks in a tangle of splintering wood, rigging and canvas as men dived for cover. Grabbing a hurricane lantern she rushed out in fear for James but it was almost impossible to see anything. Spray lashed at her face.

'All hands, all hands!' she could hear the mate's voice yelling over the wind then, with relief, James's. 'Get it cleared, damn you! Get it cleared!'

There was no time to assess the situation and no telling whether anyone had been killed. Knee-deep in rushing water, seamen hacked with axes and knives in the darkness. Four men were brought aft, soaked in a solution of diluted blood. It was no time either for Amy to think of feeling squeamish. Back inside the saloon, she attended to their wounds. They were not as bad as they looked. One had a broken arm that she put in splints and bandaged but the other three were suffering only from cuts and half stunned from blows to the head. James, looking as if he had just been pulled from the sea, put in a brief appearance.

'Any of them dead?' he wanted to know.

'No,' Amy assured him, 'they'll be all right.'

'Good,' James said and disappeared again.

'Do you want me to give you a course for the nearest port?' Amy called after him, but she might have known the answer. The idea was far too embarrassing to contemplate.

'No,' he called back to her. 'When we get sorted out we'll carry on under jury rig until we can make our own repairs!'

Amy could not blame him for that but she feared for all of them. It was a fear that was to be justified. In the way it so often happens at sea, disaster called in reinforcements to help finish the job it had started. In the battle to clear the tangle that was still going on, no one noticed the gale undo the end of the gaff line, urging it to snake down and lash out towards the head of the man James had put to the helm. The first he knew was the feeling of being horsewhipped across the eyes. Automatically putting a hand up to the blinding pain and trying to duck away from it at the same time, he lost his grip. Suddenly the wheel was wrenched from him, spinning so fast that it threatened to snap like dried twigs the fingers of anyone who tried to touch it. Before he could retrieve the spokes, the *Cirrus* slewed beam-on into a giant trough and a thundering mountain of sea lifted her and started to send her over. Amy and the men she had attended to were hurled across the saloon like rag dolls, sea coming rushing in the door to flood over their bodies. Amy had never thought about her own death, not even when she had been so desperately ill after the birth of Jamie. But then there had been something to fight against. Now there was nothing. Now the sea was in command, not herself. Yet, as she faced the inevitability of it and it was there before her, all fear left her and she felt strangely calm, just waiting. The trivia of life was all that was left to observe and it did not seem at all the height of silliness to wonder, during these seconds, when the lamp would go out.

Chapter Fourteen

The early summer sun that shone along the busy East River did nothing to warm body or soul for Mr Kimball and Mr Jay in their counting house. Ever since the *Cirrus* had sailed there had been an air of loss and impending doom around their desk. And the months of waiting in agonised suspense for an announcement of one kind or another had taken their toll. Mr Kimball's round, ample waistcoat sagged for want of filling and it had already been taken in at the back once, while Mr Jay's thin, whiskered cheeks had become positively hollow. Not a morning went by without long silences passing between them. They had heard not a whisper of their ship and it was far from easy not knowing over such a long period if they were ruined. The insurers in London, because of the controversy surrounding the building of it, had only agreed to cover half of what she had cost.

'It's June now,' Mr Kimball said, as much to himself.

'June,' Mr Jay echoed.

'Another month, maybe two, and we should know,' uttered Mr Kimball.

'Two,' returned Mr Jay, giving himself more time.

Although neither could have been accused of being mercenary, it was not the bodies of Captain James McBain, his wife and his crew floating on the sea that were constantly to the forefront of their minds. Rather a vision of their lost asset lying at the bottom. Certainly they had been able to keep themselves afloat by trading in flour and grain but there was little comfort and no fortune in it. For Mr Jay it was a little worse. Each time he took his wife for a drive in their carriage, Mrs Jay did little else but loudly point out to him the carriages of the wealthy, sensible merchants.

'If Mr Morse had constructed his ingenious telegraph wire to China instead of Baltimore,' Mr Kimball fantasised in vain and forlorn hope, 'we might at least know if she ever got there.'

Up in Boston, it was not money that James McBain junior thought about. Every night he knelt to pray hard for his mother's life, aware of the paradox in that so doing he was asking for his father's, too. He could find no way around that except to detest ships, the sea and everything to do with it, and it was not because of anything Aunt Dorothea told him that he had refused to put a foot aboard Mr Garrison's fine yacht on invitation. He hated his father for robbing him of his mother and more than once gave Aunt Dorothea a curious, sad sense of joy by shedding a tear into her welcoming bosom.

'There, there, poor child,' Dorothea comforted, 'it's little but cruelty they've shown you but you must forget all that. The Lord giveth and taketh away and although He's given me you, I don't think He'll ever take you away again. I'll always be here when you need me.' And she held her child against her. Her child and no one else's. And to him, the only one in her entire life, she gave genuine love, patient for the day when it might be genuinely returned.

Sophia Garrison, too, worried about the fate of her friend and made Hinton call at Topliffe's News Room almost every day to get the latest report on shipping movements.

'What if a ship comes from this Canton place and they say they didn't see them there?' she questioned. 'What do we do then?'

'There will be nothing we can do,' Hinton replied, 'and we can't assume anything either. For a hundred different reasons they might have been forced to go somewhere else, to some other Chinese port. For all we know they might have been blown far off course and ended in India or Australia or somewhere.'

Sophia looked at him tight-lipped. It was always difficult for Hinton to get her to see practical matters and this was no exception.

'There's no need to try and humour me, Hinton,' she said. 'I want the truth.'

'I'm giving you the truth.'

'Amy would never be blown off course. Never. And no one could be blown to Australia. It's more likely they were attacked by pirates in this Sunda Straits place people talk about, wherever it is, isn't it?'

'You think James would have sailed fifteen thousand miles to the other side of the world and then let himself be caught unawares by pirates?' Hinton pointed out.

'How do you know he sailed fifteen thousand miles?' Sophia demanded to know with perfect illogicality. Hinton did not like these kind of conversations with his wife. They made him feel frustrated.

'You mustn't make me angry, Sophia,' he told her. 'You know you don't like me when I'm angry.'

'I never said I didn't like you when you're angry,' Sophia replied. 'I said I didn't like you when you're impossible.'

'Then I won't be impossible,' Hinton agreed, escaping for his waiting carriage to go and attend to business affairs of his own. He had as much affection and respect for the McBains as anyone but he simply could not go on day after day speculating as to whether or not they might still be alive. And it would have been much too upsetting for Sophia to tell her of the decision he had already made. That if it was all eventually for the worst and their bones were lying on the seabed, God rest their souls, he would provide for the boy's financial welfare if necessary. He did not know the extent of the captain's estate but as James was a risk taker and might have made bad investments with his earnings there was no telling. Hinton had no more idea than anyone else that it would not be months before he could resolve these issues. At that moment, news of the fate of the *Cirrus* was approaching New York, only a day and a half out from Sandy Hook.

It was after midnight when the lookouts on both Navesink Highlands and in at the New York Pilot Station sighted the white flare calling for a pilot. At the pilot station, where two pilots were playing cards for a lot of money, the man hurried down from the roof with his information.

'Why couldn't the son-of-a-bitch lay off till daylight?' complained the one who was losing, but the winner wasted no time in taking action and soon the two-masted pilot boat was raising sail and heading out into a strong night breeze. There was no moon and clouds were scudding across above but as the pilot boat quickly closed on the ship, heeled over under full sail, even in the dark there was no mistaking her. There was nothing else like her.

'Jesus, it's the *Cirrus*,' the pilot gasped.

The pilot boat manoeuvred skilfully alongside the hull and the pilot leapt for the rope ladder and clambered up. Captain James McBain was standing behind the helmsman, ready to greet him, and even without a light he could see that the captain was grinning almost from ear to ear. Beside him stood his wife, all dressed up complete with hat firmly pinned to her bundled hair, looking for all the world like some lady arriving on the railroad from Newhaven except that without having to take a grip this lady was standing on a heeling deck as steady as a rock. There was no need to ask if they had actually got to China either. Despite the wind blowing it away, the whole ship was permeated with the scent of tea.

'Congratulations,' he said, shaking both James and Amy warmly by the hand. 'By God, congratulations.'

'I take it no other ship's recently in from China?' James asked him. 'No.'

'Thought not,' James smiled. 'Others left before us but although we had to beat against south-west monsoons all the way down the South China Sea, I'd hoped to show them all my heels. So take her easy. You're standing on the fastest and most beautiful ship in the world. There will never be another built like her.'

The dumbfounded pilot found that easy to believe. The *Cirrus* had made it to China and back a whole month quicker than any ship had done before and he was still to learn the rest of it.

'Dismasted too?' the pilot uttered, in even more astonishment at the record being broken so decisively with such setbacks.

'That was a night I'll not forget,' Amy said. 'I thought we were capsizing right over.' But she did not mention how readily she had accepted the oncoming of death.

'She righted again but with a list because of our ballast shifting,' James explained, 'but we got her trimmed again. It took four days to make full repairs,' and he glanced up at the full masts with some pride, 'and that's them, still holding.'

The grizzled, side-whiskered pilot was not an unimaginative man. He did not have to be told the details. As an experienced seaman he could visualise it all, feel their fears and their pain, see the chaos. The huge ship on her side, half the tangle tossed to the sea. The men working up to their waists like horses to recover it, the ones in the hold bending their frantic backs to move the ballast over as quickly as possible. The furious pumping of shipped water. Under jury rig, going on, the carpenter with a team sawing, chipping, shaving and splicing in new spar sections around the clock, the blacksmith with his little forge and big anvil on the rolling deck hammering red-hot iron into supporting bands. The bosun and his own team splicing rope and stitching heavy canvas until their fingers were raw and bleeding. The hands hauling as inch by inch the repaired masts were raised back into position, secured and well stayed. Then McBain piling on the canvas once more, undisputed master of his new bride and familiar with her ways.

'She'll be all right, I've got the hang of her now,' was the way he had put it to Amy at the time.

'Did you lose crew?' the pilot enquired.

'Not one,' James returned. 'It's something I try to avoid. Can't stand feeding able bodies to the fish.'

The pilot felt highly honoured at bringing this ship in. And in no time, the news schooner was trying to keep up alongside, eagerly calling through a loudhailer for the amazing story of the *Cirrus*'s performance, but James refused to spill wind and was slow to accommodate them. He was not giving away a single minute of his passage time.

152

In darkness, both Mr Kimball and Mr Jay were woken by messengers banging on their doors. In their separate homes they could scarcely believe it.

'My God, my God, we're in the money!' Kimball shouted as he struggled out of his nightshirt to get into his clothes.

'It's a fortune!' Mr Jay proclaimed as he struggled out of his, and for the first time in two hundred days, little Mrs Jay, sitting up in bed with her night bonnet fallen right down to her eyes, was silent.

Nathaniel Miller, too, was happy to be raised from his sleep, his reputation assured.

What Amy did not mention to anyone was the marvel of finding a gap in the doldrums where Lieutenant Matthew Maury had said to expect it. In only three days they had been through it, but she did not intend breaking what she saw as the lieutenant's confidences. Already she had composed a letter of gratitude to him and had laboriously copied out every page of her logbook to send him in case it should be of any further help to him.

As the sun slipped up out of the sea, people were flocking to the East River to have a look. There, the *Cirrus* rode at anchor, all sails furled neatly on the yards of her impudently raked masts, black paint stripped here and there from along her hull. Small craft were already surrounding her, many of them carrying newsmen from every newspaper and journal there was. Along the wharves, captains of other ships were blowing their congratulations on their long, trumpet-like foghorns.

'Now that's what I call a ship,' said the same old salt who had forecast she would dive straight to the bottom. 'Big as she is, if she can go at a clip like that she got every right to be called a clipper and Baltimore be damned.'

James was not going to disappoint his audience. He had his own boat lowered, his seamen dressed in their pumps, white trousers, checked shirts, navy pea jackets, silk scarves, and black, shiny hats, each of which was adorned with a full fathom of flowing black silk ribbon. As he and Amy were rowed smartly ashore by the best-dressed men in America and the cheers rose in a wave from the waterfront, he got to his feet in the middle of the boat and stayed there, raising his tall hat in acknowledgement to both the crowds and to New York in general, enjoying every minute of it, then pulling Amy up to stand beside him and holding her there. It was as well that Captain Eastlake, across the other side of the Atlantic, was not there to see such a sight at first hand or he might have exploded and rushed off to break the pledge again in frustration at McBain's undeserved luck.

Although, on urging, Amy waved herself and was delighted to be back after a round trip of thirty thousand miles, and so pleased for James, too, a tinge of warning at such public adoration rose unwillingly from somewhere at the back of her mind. A vague sense of danger lurked behind it all, as obscure as some hidden, unknown reef but real enough for all that. There was little time to think about it.

Waiting to the forefront of the spectators on South Street to pump James's hand and throw their arms around his wife in turn, Mr Kimball and Mr Jay had the air of conquering heroes. They had already done their sums. With a full cargo of the freshest tea ever to come from China into the West, the profits they would make from it, all in that one single voyage, would pay for the cost of the *Cirrus* twice over. If there was any touch of regret it was in the enormous sum of money they were going to have to pay James for the share he had insisted on. But it was not the time to let it get them down.

'God knows whatever made us doubt his judgement and ability,' Mr Kimball said.

'I think a little bit of apology may be due,' Mr Jay suggested.

Due to a combination of semaphore and Mr Morse's wonderful invention which had also been taken up in Boston, it was only hours later that a messenger boy ran from Topliffe's to Hinton Garrison's elegant banking house with the news. Hinton read it quickly with surprise and pleasure and immediately redirected the boy to his home.

'I knew they were all right!' squealed Sophia. 'I knew it!' and, dropping everything, made a dash to the school.

'Mrs Garrison is waiting in the hall to see you, McBain,' the chalk-dusted Mr Allburn called out over the whole class, and Jamie looked up from his books, puzzled. Mrs Garrison had never before interrupted him at school. 'It's about your father, I believe,' Allburn added, then impatiently, 'well, come on, come on.'

Jamie rose with difficulty from his books and slowly made his way down through the class, every pair of eyes stuck to him like limpets. The question that had almost been forgotten by them had suddenly arisen again and they were curious to know the answer that obviously awaited. Jamie's head and stomach were in a turmoil and he thought he might be sick. If there was news, why had Mrs Garrison come to tell him and not Aunt Dorothea? Was it because Aunt Dorothea had been unable to face him with it? For a moment, such was his dread, he felt like turning to run away from it all, not wanting to know anything. Yet his unwilling legs went on at snail pace. But the moment he reached the hall and set eyes on the smiling face of Sophia, he knew at once that all was well. Sophia almost

154

rushed to him, but resisted the temptation to throw her arms around him. He was beginning to be so grown up and she thought it might only have embarrassed him.

'Your father's broken the record to China and back by a whole month, Jamie,' Sophia told him breathlessly. 'They got into New York early this morning. Mr Garrison just heard and I knew you'd want to know straight away.'

Jamie could have wept with relief to learn that his mother was safe but he had other, conflicting emotions to deal with at the same time. Her captor and keeper was there, too, as if standing in front of her, keeping her apart, looming larger, more powerful and more famous than ever, and he had not a single weapon with which to fight back at him. More than ever people would expect him to shine out of the shadow of the captain's glory and he would have to suffer the pain of it in silence. But for Sophia, who knew nothing of his deep resentment, he smiled.

'It's very kind of you to come and tell me, Mrs Garrison,' he said, 'and I know my mother will appreciate it, too. It's the most wonderful news.'

Sophia could have kissed him for his youthful handsomeness and gracious manners but she could not do that either.

When Jamie returned to his classroom, he began to make his way quietly back to his desk in the surrounding silence and curiosity, but Mr Allburn stopped him.

'Well, McBain?' he asked. 'Do you have nothing to tell us?'

'No, sir,' Jamie replied and went on to sit down, every boy there ready to kill him for making them wait. Had they been students of human behaviour and had known his father, they might have just noticed that their classmate's conduct bore certain similarities to Captain James McBain.

Aunt Dorothea had to hide her fury at Sophia Garrison taking it upon herself to inform her child instead of telling her first and letting her do it in her own way and she determined to keep Mrs Garrison more distanced from Jamie than ever.

'Who can blame her for taking all the pleasure of telling the poor child?' was the charitable way she put it to her ladies of charity, allowing them to infer for themselves that Sophia was one who only snatched at the good and that had the news been different Mrs Garrison would have left if to poor Miss Jackson to toll the bells of death to the boy.

The *New York Herald* of the same day eulogised. 'It is doubtful,' they ran in part, 'if the outstanding performance of the uniquely designed *Cirrus* in the masterly hands of Captain James McBain will be bettered in our lifetime.'

155

Whether that might be true or not made no difference to Mr Kimball and Mr Jay. So carried away were they that within twenty-four hours of having sprung from their beds they were ordering the keel of another ship to be laid and announcing that Captain McBain would be her master.

'You can't say that before we've come to terms,' James tried to tell them amidst the bedlam of their counting house where tea buyers loudly competed with each other and sparmakers, rope-makers, lumber merchants and all kinds of people were clamouring for business.

'Later, later, James,' Mr Kimball pleaded.

'Patience!' Mr Jay called impatiently.

'The same arrangement or there's no deal,' James said.

Amy, who felt desperate to get up to Boston and Jamie, was swept up amidst more confusion. If there were a number of men who saw her as a threat to their male superiority with her navigation activities and who would have liked to throw buckets of filth over her pretty head and sent her scurrying back to her kitchen, she found herself besieged by women, some simply for rubbing social shoulders, others campaigners eager for her to endorse their causes on everything from total Temperance to more practical ladies' fashions, from anti-slavery to women's education. Considering that, after such a long voyage, she was about as disorientated as a sea nymph suddenly thrown ashore and put in the fish market, Solomon might have been proud of her.

'I don't condone regular drunkenness and believe in the rights of every human being,' she answered a swarm of them. 'At the same time I don't know if a sober woman physician in trousers with her hair cut off is necessarily the cure for all our nation's ills. For myself I only sail with my husband so I can be by his side as his wife.'

Flummoxed by such statements, the campaigners were unsure as to whether to make her their heroine or not. In Washington, however, there was one left in no doubt. On receipt of the news of the *Cirrus* success the discarded Lieutenant Matthew Maury felt the greatest satisfaction, silently thanked Mrs Amy McBain for her faith in him and put his nose and pen to his project more enthusiastically than ever.

Being the right time of the year, only two days after James and Amy's arrival, the ships that normally sailed on the China run for the fresh tea clippings were already weighing their anchors.

'We have to turn right around and go with them, James,' Mr Kimball pointed out.

'The quickest possible repairs and off,' Mr Jay added.

156

James knew every bit as much as they did the enormous financial advantage in sailing as quickly as possible, but he had Amy to think of. Such was his fear of losing her that he was not prepared to risk her discontent if she were not given enough time to spend with their son.

'How long can you give me?' he asked.

'The yard assures us they can have new masts stepped and rigged in a matter of days,' Kimball said, waving a giant Havana. 'Five days to be precise.'

'Maybe even four,' Mr Jay suggested more hopefully.

James did not blink an eye as he glanced calmly from one smiling face to the other. He could not explain to them and they were also forgetting something.

'A month,' he said sternly in his captain's tone, taking their smiles away, 'a month or we find her a new master.'

It was that 'we' which stuck into them like a marlin spike. Sometimes they were inclined to ignore the fact that James was part owner of their vessel. Mr Kimball argued hotly, looking horrified and becoming angrier by the minute, while Mr Jay interjected with expressions of disbelief. But yet again James stood by his guns and waited until Mr Kimball thumped his desk in desperation. He could never figure out how two such astute businessmen had such a blind spot for his bargaining technique, but it was to work again.

'Three weeks and Mrs McBain is put on the pay sheet,' he declared in what to them by that time seemed like surrender and they eagerly shook hands on it. It was not until after James had left that they saw it as a defeat.

'Goddamnit, why do we let him do it to us?' Mr Kimball moaned.

'I don't know,' Mr Jay replied, but without saying it, both knew perfectly well. They had already made a small fortune out of Captain James McBain and, with any luck, stood to make another one. It was just the humiliation that hurt.

It was to be three days after getting into New York before Amy was able to clear away for Boston, and James, in brand-new dark suit and tall hat, was by her side. But if she was a little disappointed at only having a clear fortnight with Jamie, it was compensated by Kimball and Jay recognising her worth by putting her on wages. That was very flattering. It would be the first money she had earned in all her twenty-nine years of life and gave her a standing and sense of independence that very few women in America enjoyed.

'You sure you didn't press them for it?' she questioned James.

'Why in the hell would I want to do that?' he rejoined. 'You have all the money you need and more. I suppose they wanted to make a gesture to you and when they suggested it I felt sure you wouldn't want me to turn it down.'

'Quite right, and I must write them a letter of thanks,' Amy returned, any little suspicion she might have had dissolved.

'I guess they'd appreciate that,' said James, pleased to have got away with it.

Soon after, Amy was to stand staring at her son. It seemed to her that the boy she had left only six months before was no longer there but had been replaced by a much taller youth. At first she did not quite know whether to kiss him and hug him or simply shake his hand. Then her arms were around him, tears squeezing from her eyes. But his words were different, too.

'You mustn't tell me how I've grown, Mother,' he said to her, 'everyone says that. But it's a natural process I believe and hardly worth the comment.'

Amy hardly knew what to make of him. On the one hand she felt he was so pleased to see her that he was close to tears himself. On the other he seemed remote, so removed from her.

'Have you been well?' she asked him, still holding him, conscious of his young hands on her back, so tentative, shy and inhibited.

'Yes, I've been very well, thank you. Hardly a day of sickness. It's yourself who's been in all the danger.'

'Why and I've been perfectly safe all the time,' Amy assured him. It was so much like the rather nervous renewal of acquaintance as it had once been in the earlier years with James each time he returned from the sea that it pained her. But she was wrong in thinking it was the same, if the other way round, and that all they needed was a little time to readjust to each other. Nor was time to be on her side. The Garrisons insisted on holding a large dinner for them on their very first evening and it was to be only the beginning of a whirlwind of engagements.

'I want to know everything about China,' Sophia said eagerly and impatiently to her, 'absolutely everything, Amy.'

'I'm afraid there isn't much I can tell you, Sophia,' Amy told her, disappointing half a dozen other pairs of ears anxiously listening in. 'We anchored at a place called Whampoa Reach where there's a tall, stone Chinese tower, but it's miles down from Canton and they don't let foreign women go there in any case. I only know what it's like from James and he'll be able to tell you much better than I can.'

'But you're not foreign, Amy!' protested Sophia before James could open his mouth. 'You're American!'

'In China, Sophia,' Hinton interjected swiftly to save his wife any further embarrassment, 'everyone who is not Chinese is foreign.'

'Yes, of course, how silly of me,' Sophia confessed without a blush and was much more pleased when James allowed Amy to go on to describe the fleet of great painted tea-deckers coming downstream to tie up alongside and load them, the non-stop, beehive activity of so many Chinese labourers sweating through day and by torchlight at night, their skill so practised that not a finger could be pushed between the tea chests and when finished the top layer was so perfectly flat it might have been part of the deck itself. But so as not to offend the sensibilities of Sophia and the other ladies present, and not put them off drinking their favourite beverage, she made no mention of how the Chinese charge hands cruelly laid whips across the backs of their men if they showed any signs of slowing. Not even James had been allowed to interfere with that. Nor did she tell of the anxious moments as they ran the gauntlet of almost naked Chinese pirates through the Sunda Strait, the *Cirrus* in any case being too fast for their junks and able to outrun them.

'Mr Samuel Cunard's steam packet service doesn't worry you then, Captain?' a gentleman asked James.

'Not in the slightest, sir,' James replied. 'I don't consider steamships real ships at all. A vessel like the *Cirrus* can show any of them her heels, and without having to be half laden with coal either. In the end, these ventures will prove to be unprofitable.'

It was hardly the right thing to say amongst people who were so proud of Mr Cunard having made Boston his American terminus that they had given him wharfing facilities free, but because it was Captain James McBain giving his honest opinion he was forgiven for it.

The following day it was a lunch reception and in the evening another dinner. Amongst the guests was Dr Amos Drew who felt ill at ease having to converse with James and Amy, knowing what he knew. It was another there who was to make an impact on James, the strong, whiskered and bearded face of Henry Longfellow, the famous poet and professor at Harvard. Although the professor showed a keen interest in sailing ships and had a good knowledge of them, he was everything that James was not and James was very much aware of it. If Amy had avidly read most of what Longfellow had so far written and talked with some excitement to Mrs Longfellow about it, he himself had not scanned a line. That did not disturb him. He was master of his own craft and let others be masters of theirs. Indeed, the two men greatly enjoyed the pleasure of each other's company, perhaps because they recognised the romanticism in each other's soul. It was not any inadequacy in himself that James began to think of but that in his son. So

159

impressed was he by Longfellow's literary knowledge and understanding of mankind, he felt that if James McBain junior could reach such heights of scholarship and learning as this man he might be proud of him. As a result, he declared on the following day, since the boy had still not come to a decision regarding his future, that Jamie would go to Harvard when he was ready and become a man of letters.

'My, how time has flown,' Aunt Dorothea said in concealed relief when the two weeks were up, but there was to be no relief for Jamie. On the same day the *Cirrus* sailed from New York bound for China again, he found the aged Captain the cat dead in the garden. And he dug a hole and buried him there, and while old Bosun pined between his paws within the cottage, Jamie knelt on the turf in the sun and wept bitterly against all the injustice in the world.

Chapter Fifteen

Under the shadows of the green elms, sixteen-year-old Jamie McBain walked out of Harvard Yard with grim and determined steps, but no one saw him go. That he turned towards Cambridge was only from habit of natural gravitation. It might as well have been any other road. It made no difference. Although he had been a student at the college for a year he carried nothing but the clothes in which he was dressed and the few dollars in his pocket. If he had one rational thought it was the knowledge that he would never return there. The rest was a turmoil of confusion at the centre of which was an overpowering desperation to know who he was and what he was supposed to be. He had told no one what he intended doing and, indeed, did not know himself. Going was all that seemed to matter. If any of his friends had been asked when this disturbance in him had begun they might have dated it to around the time two months previously when his old dog Bosun could no longer walk and Dr Amos Drew had kindly offered to take the animal away and destroy it for him.

'Thank you, sir,' Jamie had told him, 'but it's my dog and it's my duty,' and he had borrowed a gun and, choked with guilt and heartbreak, shot his friend between its almost blind, rheumy eyes. But his fellow students would have been wrong to assume that this was the time. How were they to know how far back in his life the accumulation of events had been gradually building to bring him to this?

Jamie had been quite happy at Harvard to start with. There was the novelty of it, the apparent freedom he had never had before. The staff had found him a capable and responsible young man, even if they did know that he sometimes held secret drinking parties in his rooms and it was rumoured he had once smuggled in a whore to add spice to the occasion. Although both were frowned on, such lapses were only to be expected amongst exuberant youths trying to find their feet. His fellow students had found him pleasant and likeable, especially as he was so generous with loans and hand-outs from the bank account his famous and wealthy father, generally known to the public as 'Hurricane Jim', had set up for him. And if they were quick to notice he was inclined to slope off when a good, serious fight was offering, no one had sought to accuse him of cowardice. Even in laughter and normal rough and tumble they were careful with him. There was something about him that inhibited a direct challenge of fists, something unknown.

It was only when the novelty wore off that Jamie became more and more aware that the captain had followed him into Harvard and that James McBain junior himself was no one and nothing.

'Look what your father's done now,' students would say to him as they thrust yet another newspaper at him which gave a glowing account of the captain's latest achievement. Three times Captain James McBain had reduced the time to China and back and twice to Rio. As 'King of the Sea' and 'King of the Clippers', as they sometimes termed him, no one could touch him.

Jamie walked right through Cambridge and on towards Boston, for no other reason than the road was under his feet and there was nothing to stop him, and his eyes were unseeing.

Reaching the outskirts of Boston by evening, going home to the cottage and telling Aunt Dorothea what he had done did not as much as enter his head. It was not only Harvard he was running from blindly in his desperation to find his identity but from everyone and everything that had ever concerned him. Aunt Dorothea stifled rather than encouraged his meagre attempts at independence. It had been two years ago when he first felt that her unceasing affection was suffocating him. Then, ship's fever had been raging in Boston and she had anxiously kept him imprisoned in the cottage for the entire summer with no one allowed to come near him in case they were carrying the deadly infection.

'I'll be disconsolate, Jamie, disconsolate,' she said with a wringing of her thin hands when he went off to college and she made him promise to come home to her every weekend. She had filled him with guilt at being unable to be to her what she wanted him to be. Once he had even plucked up enough courage to try to discuss her attitude to him with Dr Drew in the hope of finding some comfort or advice, but it had only seemed to embarrass the doctor, who refused to be drawn.

Jamie never knew why he eventually gravitated to the waterfront. It was without thinking. And there, down Purchase Street and many others he walked into a torchlit and lamplit pandemonium. Half of New England it seemed had crammed themselves into the area in search of transport to California and the recently discovered goldfield there. Amongst the rolling, brawny seamen, some with their pockets already burning with the wages from a long voyage were bakers, butchers, clerks and people from all walks of life, all fevering to buy a passage to the great wealth awaiting them. Some were even already armed with picks and shovels over their shoulders. Old ships put out of commission and ready for the graveyard were hurriedly being put back into repair to accommodate them. No greater contrast to the learned peace of the Harvard campus might have been imagined and Jamie felt that here, until he decided what to do next, he could safely stop for a while. Intent on losing himself further he pushed his way into a rum mill where the air was so thick with tobacco smoke charged with the heavy smell of urine it stung his eyes.

'Rum, please,' he said, showing his money.

'Please is it now? An' ye can please yer bloody self.' The harassed barman's Irish voice came back at him as if the politeness had been an insult. But Jamie got his drink, quaffed it down and ordered another to help drown his confusion and misery. A small man with a squint in one eye edged to his side.

'Where you from?' he asked.

'Nowhere,' Jamie replied.

'Get a bunk for California then, did ya?'

'No.'

'Ah, I's thought not,' said the man. 'Ya can tell from the faces of them that got them and them that ain't. I'm a kinda agent tryin' to help folks. I might be able to get ya on a fine stout vessel sailin' in two days. At a price, mind, at a price. Ain't easy. Ain't easy at all.'

Even with two stiff rums in him, Jamie was not fooled by the trickster for a minute. At the same time, suddenly the idea of escaping all the way across to the other side of the American continent seemed a way out. He had money in his bank account. He could go there on the following day and withdraw it. No one would yet know what he had done. It would take time for everyone to realise he had gone. And if he could not ship out immediately he could hide until a vessel was ready for him.

'The only problem is I hate ships and I hate the sea,' he told the squinting eyes. 'I'd rather go overland.'

That threw the man into some confusion. He had made no provision for offering fares on non-existent wagon trains to those who sought to cross the entire continent. 'But that ain't no good,' he said. 'It would take ya years to get overland. An' if the Injuns didn't get yer, all the best fortunes would be dug up by the time ya got there.'

'In that case,' Jamie replied, 'I reckon I better get myself a gun

163

and start walking now,' and he left the bar to head for another one, leaving the disappointed 'kinda agent' scratching his head at having picked on such a lunatic. 'Where ya come from?' he asked, edging up to another man who looked as if his luck was out.

Jamie had, of course, heard of the finding of gold in California but had given no thought either to that or to Britain's recent repeal of the Navigation Act, opening up the Eastern sea routes to non-British ships for the first time, which meant that American vessels could bring cargoes from the East into Britain. But the result of both was to create a mad scramble by American merchants to build new and even faster ships.

Several bars later, Jamie found himself staggering down over the cobbles of the narrow Broad Street, giving very serious but very fuzzy thought to California. If only he could get advice on how to go about getting overland, that was his solution. Music blared out of a dance hall. A whore hung an arm around his unsteady neck. 'A dollar with them on, two dollars with them off,' she whispered in his ear, and feeling thoroughly befuddled he took her into Miss Culpeper's Bar for a drink.

'Where you from?' the bewigged and powdered Miss Culpeper asked him as he held on to the counter for balance. Jamie focused on the smiling lady with the rose-coloured bow lips. Since everyone asked him this it was obviously a very important question requiring a very serious answer. He concentrated and vaguely waved an arm in the air. 'Up there,' he said, 'up Salem way.'

Miss Culpeper measured him up. Whatever else he was, the young man looked healthy and fit. Just the ticket.

'What's your name?' she enquired, leaning over closer to him in the friendliest manner. Jamie found himself focusing deep down into the soft valley of her large breasts and imagining for a moment he could even see the pink rosettes of her nipples.

'Hills,' he said.

'Friends and family with you, Mr Hills?'

'I have no family,' Jamie slurred.

Rarely did Miss Culpeper go to such trouble with her victims but the young man was different from the usual type. Even full of grog he gave the impression of being lost in the wood. But business was business and there was no place for sentimentality. She gave him a drink and Jamie struggled to get the coins out of his pocket.

'No charge,' Miss Culpeper smiled, 'this one's on me.'

Jamie thanked her and drank. A few moments later the world began to turn. The last he remembered was not the figure of Miss

Culpeper but a brief image of a man with big, wide teeth with a gap in them grinning into his face.

He did not know how much later it was when his body fell to what felt like solid wood. He turned and opened his eyes to see a man standing over him. There was the sound of something heavy squeaking over his head and distant voices. The air was foul. His head was splitting in pain, and he thought he might vomit at any moment. For a few seconds he reasoned that he must have died and gone to hell. He became aware of wooden bunks on either side and two other tortured souls trying to struggle to their feet.

'Get up,' the man ordered, giving him a kick in the ribs, and he did his best to rise to the Devil's command. His suit was torn and dirty. The boots had gone from his feet.

'Where is this?' he demanded to know, even the sound of his own voice threatening to crack his skull open.

'Jesus save us, we's aboard a ship,' he heard one of the other lost souls mutter.

'And consider yourselves lucky for it,' the man told them, 'for we're bound for California and half the world's payin' a lot of money to try and git there. You's is going' for nothin'. Git up there on deck, Mr Tyrrel wants to talk to you and Mr Tyrrel ain't a man to be kept waitin'.'

Jamie and the two other, much older wrecks, helped by pushes from behind, made their way to the shaft of daylight of the hatch, went up a short ladder and were taken aft to the mainmast. They quickly became aware that the squeaking sound came from the turning capstan, that the anchor was being weighed and that the ship was about to sail.

Mr Tyrrel, a man with a face like a red moon, complete with craters, stood with lash in hand so that, from the start, there might be no misunderstandings. Jamie could hardly believe it was happening to him. It was like a living nightmare.

'Name?' Tyrrel wanted to know from one of the others first and Jamie had to think quickly before his turn came. Despite everything, the last name in the world he wanted to speak was that of James McBain and be rescued because of his father. He glanced towards the shore. They were almost out in the middle of the river. It was much too far for him to consider making a dive for it and swimming. In his condition he would probably have gone down like a stone if they did not catch him first.

'John Marsh, sir,' he replied when the question came, showing the only defiance he could by using the name of a famous hell-raising student of Harvard's past who had become a legend for his rioting, drinking, burning, breaking windows and throwing a bucket of ink over a professor's head.

On the quarterdeck which he never left, the middle-aged, grizzle-cheeked Captain Beriah Gurley was taking them in from a distance, at the same time keeping a close eye on all the other activity involved in setting sail. The young man did not appear to him to be the right material to splice into a seaman.

'Any of you sailed before?' Tyrrel asked his three new crew members and they shook their heads in suffering. 'Right,' he went on, 'as from today you're sailors. And as from today, each of you owes the captain three months' wages since that's what it cost him from his purse to have you carried to your berths. Proper clothes you can buy from the slop chest and another month's wages will be debited to you for them. The captain and myself will have no disobedience, no buntline reefing and no talking back or it's belayin'-pin soup, marlin-spike hash or this here in my hand drawing blood from you backs. You understand?'

Jamie could not at first understand how in the hell he came to owe the captain three months' wages. He did not know of the new species called Crimps who had been suddenly spawned because of the problem of finding full crews, or indeed that he has been an early victim of a 'Miss Culpeper Special'. Three months of a sailor's wages was the price agreed for delivery of a body – any body so long as it was male and still breathing. But with his legs barely holding him up, his sickening stomach and his throbbing brain, he was still not in a condition to piece together all that had happened to him. Yet through the desperation of his plight, he thought he saw a glimmer of hope.

'Listen, sir,' he got in, 'if it's a matter of me owing the captain money, I can pay him back. I've got money ashore.'

He had hardly finished saying it when he saw the backhanded swipe and felt the tongues of the lash strike painfully across his face. 'So we got ourselves a smartass, have we?' Tyrrel glared at him and Jamie said no more. 'At four bells of the afternoon watch,' he went on, 'the three of you will jump lively back on deck here and be shown the ropes. Until then, get your miserable, goddamned souls back to the fo'c'sle and get yourselves shipshape for work.'

Jamie staggered back for'ard with the other two. Never in his worst moments or wildest imaginings had he ever thought his life could come to this. There were no curses or oaths strong enough to hurl against himself for his blind stupidity. Trying to escape he had run right into the worst of all possible worlds. It was *worse* than hell. It was a case of either throwing himself over the side to drown

166

or enduring it. Not being of suicidal tendency he had no alternative but to go into further debt for his seaman's knife, his sea clothes, dungarees and watchcoat.

Tyrrel did not know that the rather fiery-eyed young John Marsh had no need to learn the ropes. After the first few days of utter misery, something strange began to happen in the mind of Jamie. Information he did not know he had began to seep out from some lost burial ground of his memory, everything his mother had fed into it when he was a child without his conscious awareness of it. He discovered he automatically knew every bit of spar, every brace, sheet and halyard that there was, every block and more. Knew their purpose. Forced aloft he was surprised that he was not frightened hanging on so high above deck and sea, and although he was at first under the supervision of an able-bodied seaman, he found he knew exactly what to do without the telling. That he did not want or care for all this knowledge made no difference. It came pouring into his consciousness and he could neither stop it nor get rid of it.

In the fo'c'sle he was given no quarter amongst the rough, squabbling seamen and with no one else to look after him he had no alternative but to defend himself with his fists and earned a certain amount of respect by his determination not to be put down.

It was ten days after clearing the Boston Light and heading south into the North Easterly Trades when it happened. James McBain junior alias John Marsh had been put to holystoning and was on his bare knees, his fingers and palms rawed to bleeding, when he found Captain Beriah Gurley standing over him. Gurley had been watching the young man closely since he had come aboard and knew full well he had something very special here.

'Which ship were you on, Marsh?' he asked him.

'I've never been to sea before sir,' Jamie replied without stopping, but Gurley did not believe him. Had he known his real name was James McBain he might have looked for similarities. And seen them. But he did not. He also considered every man had the right to hide his past if he wanted to at sea as long as he did his job well.

'Take the helm,' he said gruffly, and Jamie stopped and looked up at him.

'Sir?'

'I said take the helm, damn you,' Gurley repeated. Jamie rose to his feet and the captain nodded him towards the wheel and followed him. 'Hand over to Marsh,' he ordered the man steering.

'Course sou'-sou'-east by south.'

Jamie was aware he was being put to a test but for what purpose he was not at all sure since Gurley was a man to show only the worst of his feelings and keep the best well hidden under his hat.

'Sou'-sou'-east by south,' Jamie echoed without even knowing he had said it and gripped the spokes as he was ordered. Never in his life had he grasped so much as the tiller of a jolly boat, never mind the wheel of a ship. Nor, in his defiance at being a prisoner, was he sure whether or not to deliberately make a total mess of it, make no effort and allow the vessel to take what head she wanted. He was existing day by day only to get to California, where he was determined to escape and never sight as much as an oar for the remainder of however many years God chose to give him.

'As she goes, Marsh,' Gurley growled from behind him.

If it was a tentative and reluctant start, uncertainty did not last long. Something even more strange began to happen to John Marsh. He could feel her in his raw hands, feel her hull alive under him, feel the power of the wind in the sail pushing her through and over the sunlit waves. Within him, some sense of being he had never experienced rose in him and enveloped him like a cloak that shielded him from his miseries.

I'll be goddamned, Gurley said to himself. For a full hour he had stood behind Marsh watching him, noting the young man's feel for the helm, easing her over waves when it was needed, every now and then glancing up as Gurley did himself to ensure that all sails were filling to their fullest. He was left in absolutely no doubt that Marsh was not only a thoroughly experienced seaman but an intelligent one too.

Jamie had no idea he had been there for as long as an hour but it was not until the moon-faced Tyrrel came aft and looked at him in surprise that he became aware once again of anything but the ship itself. And he was reminded that he had still not got back at the mate for striking him across the head with his lash for nothing and raising weals on his cheek. With a renewed confidence in himself, he looked for some fault that Tyrrel might be caught up on. All the background talk that had gone meaninglessly into the ears over the years, about rigging and dismastings and all the rest, had not been wasted either. And there, oh, my God yes, there. He had found it.

'Can I say something, sir?' he requested without turning.

'What is it?' Gurley asked.

'There are two fore topmast backstay shrouds on the starboard side need tightening, sir.'

Gurley looked at him briefly in astonishment and then directly for'ard along the starboard side and was suddenly roaring at Tyrrel. 'You need a goddamned boy to tell you your job, Mister!'

And with extra red on his face, Tyrrel was hurrying for'ard roaring his own orders. Jamie felt pleased with himself at that but dared not show it and Beriah Gurley said not a word to him about it, but he was nevertheless not quite finished with young John Marsh.

'Mr Tyrrel!' he shouted when the job was done and Tyrrel came hurrying aft again to stand before him. 'Mr Tyrrel,' he instructed, 'you will take Marsh out of the fo'c'sle and put him in better accommodation.'

Such was the unexpectedness of this bonus that Jamie nearly let go of the wheel, but some instinct told him he would only have angered Captain Beriah Gurley if he expressed his thanks. In any case the stern-faced master immediately turned away to head for his cabin. Tyrrel glowered at the upstart who had put him in trouble but decided it might be in his own interest to give him a wider berth in future.

At half past four in the afternoon, one bell struck for the beginning of the first dog watch and Marsh was relieved from the helm. But it was not so much relief he felt, rather that for the first time ever he had achieved some status for himself without any encouragement, or pushing. It felt very satisfying and it was a feeling which was to grow.

'You been to Navigation School, Marsh?' Gurley asked him several days later.

'No, sir,' Jamie replied.

'Pity,' the captain said, but still highly suspicious of Marsh's background without wanting to make any enquiries into it, he had a chart fetched and held it before him. Suddenly charts, too, came flooding into Jamie's head. He knew all about charts. He had been raised with them. Before he could even remember he had been sat on them, had been held over them, had been sick on them, wetted on them and later had scribbled on them. They had always been there as part of his life.

'Where do you think we are, Marsh?' Gurley wanted to know from him.

'I don't know, sir,' Jamie admitted, which was the truth.

'Make a guess,' the captain demanded.

Jamie looked at it. He had seen this old chart many times before. It was as familiar as the back of his hand. He stuck a finger vaguely at an area with no idea whatsoever as to whether he might be right or wrong. Stony-faced, the captain rolled up the chart and without as much as uttering a grunt, walked away. There was not the slightest doubt in his mind that young Marsh had been to Navigation School and had somehow been keeping track of where they were. That pleased him. He felt that if illness happened to lay him low, young Marsh would be able to keep his ship on course since Tyrrel was about as much use at navigating as a dead hog at a Jewish funeral.

Soon afterwards they were into the doldrums, the airless heat below insufferable, the unshaded deck fire to the feet, the sails above hanging limply from their yards. Nerves frayed in the fo'c'sle and two knifings brought Tyrrel into his own with Gurley's sentence of the lash. But here Jamie learned to take advantage of every capful of wind that sometimes came slowly streaking like shimmering fingers across the glass-like sea to help them on. It was to be a week before there was a steady breeze again and, without actually sighting it, they were clearing Cape São Roque, the most easterly point of Brazil that stuck out into the Atlantic.

Captain Beriah Gurley noted the change taking place in Marsh as they swept on down past Rio. The young man became much more authoritative with the seamen put under his control on his watches. 'You show me goddamn fair,' he was heard to say to them in determined tone, 'and it's fair I'll show you back,' and, somewhat surprisingly, as they were all hard-bitten men, they showed him fair. Furthermore, when disputes arose between them, it was to young Marsh they went to act as intermediary. His past was a mystery even to the carpenter and bosun who became his friends. It was the one thing he did not want to talk about. One minute he gave them the impression he was a college man, the next that he had been sea-born and had barely put a foot ashore since.

That James McBain junior might have inherited the qualities of both James McBain and Amy Hall did not so much as enter John Marsh's head as he went reaching down in fresh westerlies into the colder latitudes and no one was more surprised than he to realise that the sea had already seeped into his blood and that all the years of Greek and Latin had been wilfully scattered forever in his wake.

The dreaded Cape Horn lay ahead. 'You're holding course well, Marsh,' the captain said, giving him his first word of praise. 'You ever been round Cape Stiff before?'

'No, sir,' Jamie replied but Gurley did not believe that either. In preparation he ordered all canvas to be reduced to nothing but jibs, small staysails and reefed spanker. The rigging became alive with men eager to get the job done and return to the deck. Soon the ship looked almost bare-poled without a stitch on her yards. Wind and sea started to rise alarmingly, but it was not until the sails were hardened up to take her to windward that the full force of them became apparent. The wind screamed and the seas were charging mountains with great white crests driving freezing, flying spume before them. The heeled vessel rose and plunged and shuddered as if to split her timbers. Oncoming peaks of sea rose high above the bowsprit to smash down on the decks and come thundering aft as if to sweep anything in their path to destruction. Sodden, freezing seamen took hold of whatever they could find, some silently praying that the masts and planks would hold up to the incredible battering. It was just after a gigantic wave towered high above the bows then came crashing down as if intent on consuming the entire vessel in its bowels that an anxious Gurley, up to his knees in water, caught sight of Marsh hauling himself up the inclined deck to weather. It was the more unexpected because Marsh was supposed to be off-watch and could have been in shelter. Then, in surprise, he saw the young man start to climb up the rigging of the main, his watchcoat looking as if to blow right off him. There was no need for anyone to risk their life going aloft. From what he could see between his eyes being filled with sea, nothing had broken. No one had been ordered.

'What in the hell is he doing, Mister?' Gurley shouted to Tyrrel against the roar as he pointed. It was the wrong moment for Tyrrel to turn his head to look up. As he did so he was too late to duck the lash of spray that stung and drowned his face with such force he thought it was going to take his head off. Holding on, he had to wait to answer.

'I don't know, sir,' he replied when he was able but unlike Beriah Gurley he did not have enough wit to ponder on whether the mysterious Marsh might be about to deliberately end his life. They watched him go right up to the bare yard of the main topgallant and, when they were able to look again, on up to the royal.

'*Get down, goddamn you!*' the captain yelled but his words had hardly gone a yard when they were thrown right back in his face.

It was up there, clinging on with all his strength, the rising and falling and whipping mast threatening every moment to hurl him like a stone from a sling to the howling jaws below, that Jamie looked to the north. He could just make out the distant grey cliffs of Cape Horn and it somehow confirmed to him the sudden revelation that had struck him like a bolt of lightning and had him springing from his cabin to go aloft. High above this wild, tossing fury where God and Devil met to fight for the souls of the drowned, he felt no fear, felt no cold on his flesh or in his bones. If it was impossible, it was still true. The answer he had so long despaired of ever finding and the search for which had sent him fleeing from Harvard was here before him. It was beneath him and all around him. No longer was there any thought of escaping when they eventually came to anchor at San Francisco. He had already escaped. This was his element. Where he belonged. The weapon with which to fight back was in his hands. Oh, God, how could he ever have been so blind as not to have known it? It was through the sea and only through the sea that he could ever cut the knees of Captain James McBain and bring him down. And under the dark scudding clouds he felt exalted.

Chapter Sixteen

The messenger boy who came down the road and turned in at the cottage gate did not so much smell the summer flowers, rather the scent of money. Women always tipped him better than men and the letter he carried was addressed to Miss Dorothea Jackson. Then he smelt something else, the sweet, mouth-watering air of fresh baking. There was every chance he might get a couple of cookies, too. Reaching the porch, he put on his best hangdog hungry look and knocked on the door which was open. From inside he could hear the voices of several women chattering.

'His raising and gentlemanly manners do you the greatest credit, Miss Jackson,' a charitable lady said, genteelly lifting a cup of very special China tea to her thin lips. It was what Miss Dorothea Jackson wanted to hear. Indeed, why she kept inviting them. Her whole life had come to revolve around her child, and she was never done boasting about his fine qualities and scholastic achievements. Never done, either, fishing for praise for him which naturally reflected on herself.

The messenger boy knocked louder.

'I think someone's at the door, Miss Jackson,' one of the ladies told her and Dorothea went to find the hungry-looking child there, holding his thumb-marked envelope.

'A message for Miss Jackson, ma'am,' he said, 'and I been told I was to get a reply.'

'I'm Miss Jackson,' Dorothea said, taking it from him to stick a bony finger into the flap to rip it open. The boy, thinking only of his tip and his cookies, watched her read it. He saw the thin hands tremble and the face above them turn pale. Then she was suddenly glaring at him and he could almost feel her eyes physically striking at him.

'What mischief is this?' she demanded.

'It's a m-m-m-message, ma'am,' he stuttered.

'It's mischief, that's what it is,' Dorothea told him again, 'pure and utter mischief. Now begone with you!'

In apprehension and bewilderment the boy began to back away

down off the porch on to the path, but stopped there for a moment. 'I was to get a reply, ma'am,' he tried to tell the old lady.

'Be off with you or it's my stick you'll get!' Dorothea cried and the boy ran, tips and cookies fallen to the bottom of his priorities. Attracted by the commotion the ladies came tentatively to the door in curiosity.

'Is everything all right, Miss Jackson?' asked one with concern.

'Yes, of course, of course,' Dorothea answered, 'it's just some mischief,' but they could tell from the look of her that it was far from all right. Most certainly not. Dorothea Jackson hardly knew where she was. On the one hand she was shocked, on the other convinced that there was nothing to be shocked about since it had to be an evil lie, and no one better than herself knew all about those.

'Dear Miss Jackson,' the letter read:

It appears that your ward and our student, James McBain, has not been present at college for three days, an absence foolishly concealed from us by his friends until this morning. As his possessions and spare clothing are still in his room we are left to conclude that he has gone home to you where he has given some plausible explanation for his departure. On enquiry it seems that he neither sought permission for his leave nor notified anyone of his intent and we therefore expect him to give reason for this remissful conduct to us in writing. Meanwhile, we would be most obliged to have you confirm by messenger return that he is indeed safely in your hands.

(Signed) Mr J S Maynes

Dorothea mentioned nothing of this to her visiting ladies and although she ushered them all back inside, such was the disturbance in Miss Jackson that the happy chattering of the tea party was killed stone dead to be replaced by anxious glances amongst her guests, and soon after they were all making their excuses for leaving. Indeed, they were all dying to discuss among themselves what might have happened. It was very unlike Miss Jackson to become embroiled in anything untoward.

Only an hour later, Dr Amos Drew heard his bell ring and a short while after his housekeeper knocked lightly on his study door and poked her chubby face in.

'It's Miss Jackson, Doctor,' she told him.

'Miss Jackson?' he said unhappily. God, how he hated having to examine Miss Jackson. It was so embarrassing for him he could hardly bear to look at her.

'She says it's urgent,' the housekeeper added.

'Show her in, please,' Amos Drew instructed politely, and a moment later Dorothea was striding through his study door. 'Ah, Miss Jackson,' he greeted with his practised smile before he noticed the almost demented look on her face.

'I've been the victim of a very serious mischief, Doctor,' she announced without waiting.

'Sit down, sit down, please, Miss Jackson,' he said with the smile gone from his face, but Dorothea remained standing.

'I want you to help me do something about it and at once,' she said and it sprang immediately to Dr Drew's mind that someone else had discovered Miss Jackson's secrets and let them out. And that worried him to death in case his own name had been dragged in and his silence would be exposed. Dorothea handed him the letter and it was almost with relief that he read it. 'It's a lie, isn't it?' he heard Miss Jackson say.

'You know it is?' he questioned.

'Of course I know it is. Jamie would never go anywhere without telling me. He would never leave me like that. Never.'

'Where is he then?'

'Where is he? Where is he? He'll be at college, of course.'

Amos Drew gazed at her worriedly then glanced at the letter again. It had been written in fine copperplate hand on Harvard notepaper and did not at all give the impression of a trick, but he did not realise at first what he was dealing with.

'But if you are certain he's safe in college and know this to be untrue, Miss Jackson, what exactly do you want me to do? I have simply no idea who could have forged such a letter, or why.'

'I want you to take me to Harvard, Doctor, and see for yourself that he's there,' Dorothea declared, 'Now, Doctor Drew.'

Amos Drew stared at her, stunned. To see for *himself*? It was no business of his to see for himself, anxious as he might have been for the boy if he had, in fact, disappeared, since it was becoming clearer to him that Miss Jackson was in some doubt about it. So odd was her behaviour that, despite the fact she was a strong Temperance campaigner, his nostrils surreptitiously sniffed the air for the smell of drink. If it was there it escaped him.

'What did you reply to this . . . this mischief, Miss Jackson?'

'I replied nothing. You expect me to reply to an evil thing like that? I want you to take me there and I'll *show* you what an evil this is.'

'Miss Jackson,' he tried to protest, 'I can't just . . .'

'You mean after everything I've done for this town, and done for you, there's no one I can turn to?'

Amos Drew could not remember Miss Jackson ever having done anything for him, unless she meant refraining from publicly accusing him of his supressed attraction to boys. At the same time he was beginning to see that her disturbance was on the verge of being manic.

'We must be very careful before we start throwing stones, Miss Jackson,' he warned, hoping that it might have some meaning for her. It did not, but he got the strong impression that she might get close to violence if he did not humour her.

'Miss Jackson,' he said patiently, 'it would be long after dark before we could get to Harvard. They would all be retired.'

'What has that got to do with it?' Dorothea demanded, her ageing eyes blazing.

Amos Drew became aware that no matter what he said, Miss Jackson in such a condition might be prepared to try to bring hell down on his head if he did not do what she wanted. Knowing what he did of her, he considered her capable of anything. That she go hire a carriage for herself instead of getting him to take her in his he did not dare suggest under the circumstances. But he told himself that it was to clear the matter up for the sake of Captain and Mrs McBain that he went.

'He would never leave me, that I know,' Dorothea kept repeating in the doctor's carriage as his driver whipped the horses along the road.

'I'm sure, I'm sure, Miss Jackson,' Amos Drew had to say over and over again.

Amos Drew had been more than half right about the college being asleep when they got there. Only a few lights shone from windows and the porter took a long time in coming to the imperative ringing of his bell.

'I apologise for the hour,' the doctor told him, 'but I must see a Mr Maynes on a matter of urgency.'

Eventually, he and Miss Jackson were led to Mr Maynes's day room where a lamp was lit for them and they sat and waited. But Dorothea no longer spoke and although still looking manic, now stayed tight-lipped.

Joshua Samuel Maynes, a tall, fiddle-faced man with a weak chin, hurriedly dressed before attending to them. Although he guessed what it was about, he was annoyed at being raised from his bed. It was not the proper time to resolve the matter of James McBain's negligence and he was rather surprised when he entered his room to see that the student he was determined to make pay for all his trouble was not there. He glanced at Miss Jackson whom he

176

had met before but the lady was looking straight ahead of her and gave no sign of recognition. Amos Drew introduced himself and produced the letter.

'I'm sorry about all this, sir,' he said, 'but I must ask you if this message is from yourself.'

Maynes glanced from the doctor to Dorothea and back again, wondering if they might both be mad. Who in the hell else could it have been from? But he caught the meaning.

'I take it, then, ma'am,' he said, 'that your ward is not indeed with you?'

For Amos Drew, that cleared the matter up immediately. Not for Miss Jackson. 'He is not my ward, sir, but my child,' she almost spat out straight ahead of her without giving either of them a glance, 'and he is here in your care. You will present him, sir, and now.'

Both Maynes and Amos Drew stared at her for a moment but it was only the doctor who was beginning to understand and he found enlightenment unwelcome.

'Miss Jackson is naturally most anxious,' he apologised quietly to Maynes. 'Is there anyone I can question on Miss Jackson's behalf? I've been a friend of the family for many years.'

Young men, some with the sleep still falling from their eyes, were brought, but Dorothea sat stiff-backed and stiff-lipped throughout, not giving a glance to any of them, not asking a single question, not so much as opening her mouth.

'He spoke to me often about going to Chicago, sir,' the elder of the Garrison boys volunteered.

'Why Chicago?' Amos Drew wanted to know from him.

'He said, sir,' young Garrison replied with a little embarrassment, 'that it was about as far away from the ocean as he could think of, even if it was on the shores of Lake Michigan. Everyone knows he has a great dislike of the sea, sir.'

Dr Drew did not and if Dorothea Jackson knew she was not saying.

'He hasn't been himself for a while, sir,' another youth admitted, 'but he wouldn't tell us what the matter was.'

When the interrogations were spent, Mr Maynes offered a few words more calculated to distance both himself and the college from any responsibility for the missing student than to express his sorrow. It was not the first time a young man had suddenly been lured away from Harvard by some romantic dream hovering over distant horizons.

'I have little doubt, ma'am, that you'll hear from him soon,' he added as Amos Drew led Miss Jackson back to his carriage but he might as well have been talking to her black hat. For the doctor it was to be an even more troubled journey. Several times on the way back towards Boston through the night he made efforts to reassure the stony-silent Dorothea.

'There's bound to be some simple explanation we'll probably come to laugh at when we know it, Miss Jackson,' he said. 'I'm sure all will be well.' But such were the emanations of aggression coming from her that, tired as he was, he was afraid to close his eyes even for a moment. It was with the greatest relief that he finally arrived at the cottage to drop her off.

'You'll find there's nothing to worry about,' he said as a farewell, 'nothing at all.' But Dorothea made no reply as she went into her cottage and slammed the door behind her. Amos Drew felt sure that she would calm herself and that Jamie would soon reappear, but he was wrong on both counts.

It was just on daylight when Sophia and Hinton Garrison were woken by a maidservant tapping on their bedroom door.

'What is it?' Hinton asked, raising his head from his pillow, and as the door came ajar he could see the nervous figure of Sophia's maid only partly dressed.

'I'm sorry, sir,' she said, 'but Miss Jackson's at the door wanting to see you. In fact she's inside the door in the hall. She's a bit upset. She pushed her way in and would have no patience with me, sir.'

Hinton and Sophia sat up in bed in surprise.

'Good heavens, whatever is it?' a worried Sophia asked but she had hardly finished her question when Dorothea came bursting through their bedroom door, waving a stick, all guns of paranoia blazing.

'You bitch!' she yelled at the shocked Sophia. 'You've taken Jamie and hidden him! Well, don't think you're going to get away with it! I'll find where you've put him and will be taking you to court on it!' And, with that, she raged back out, smashing a vase and almost knocking the frightened maidservant off her feet. Had he not been so surprised Hinton would have sprung from his bed to fend off the uninvited intruder. As it was, he and Sophia were left gaping at each other in astonishment. There was not even time for Sophia to become hysterical.

'What was she talking about?' Hinton managed to get out at last but Sophia had no more idea than he had.

'She must have gone mad,' was the only explanation Sophia could find to make then, realising what she had said, did become a little hysterical. 'You must get Dr Drew, Hinton. Get Dr Drew. Get Dr Drew!'

178

From a bleary-eyed Amos Drew, Hinton soon got the whole story, throwing Sophia into even more distress.

'You must find him, Hinton,' she demanded of her husband. 'Find him!'

The practical Hinton was quick to discover that Jamie's bank account which contained a considerable sum of money had not had a withdrawal in some time. For Sophia, that could not have been more ominous.

'Oh, my God, he's dead!' she cried, throwing her hands to her mouth in horror, and it took the best part of an hour for Hinton to settle her. But for two months, as Hinton did everything he could to try to find out what had happened to Jamie McBain, she agonised every day for Amy.

In her innocence, Amy had every reason to be happy as James lowered his telescope, turned to smile at her and said, 'Congratulations, Mrs McBain, you've done it again. Sandy Hook dead on target and another record,' and he would have kissed her and hugged her and swung her around for joy had it not been for the mate and some of the crew looking on. Then it was the news schooner and the pilot, both showing the greatest respect for 'Hurricane Jim' and his wife as information was exchanged. McBain had become more than 'King of the Sea'. He was part owner of three different clippers with Kimball and Jay, owned real estate on Wall Street and in Boston.

'You'll find the East River bedlam,' James and Amy were told. 'With this gold strike in California it seems like half of Europe's here clamouring for transport to San Francisco.'

But then it was Mr Kimball making very hard work of it as he struggled up the rope ladder, the nimbler Mr Jay behind him. It was unusual for them to board before the ship had come to anchor and both James and Amy could tell straight away by the expression on their faces that something was wrong. And then it came, Mr Kimball, charged with the duty by letter from Hinton Garrison, for once doing all the talking. He told them as gently as he knew how that their son had mysteriously disappeared and that Mrs McBain's aunt, suffering ill health, had been put into a home for a rest. Little did they know that Miss Jackson, screaming foul language and making meaningless accusations, had had to be dragged there by two powerful keepers.

James did not have to look at Amy to know the blood was draining from her face. And Amy was hardly aware of James taking her hand in his to give her some comfort and support. But it was not for

179

nothing she had sailed through tempests in awesome seas that did their uttermost to claw men to their graves and while fearing for her own life had had to tend terrible injuries on impossibly heaving decks. If her heart had sunk to the pit of her stomach she stayed steady on her feet.

'Thank you for letting us know, Mr Kimball,' she said.

Amy did not hear the cheering of the usual crowd as she and James were rowed ashore. And, for once, James did not raise his tall black hat. And his real feelings he could not show either. Inwardly he had begun to fume in rage for the son he had never come to understand inflicting yet more pain on his wife. He had thought that to be all over and for the first time in a long while a sense of insecurity rose in him again. Two years before she had talked of going ashore so that she could give Jamie a little time in what was left of his youth. He had made no argument against it and had said nothing, but he did not have to. Amy knew and had stayed. And he did not have to be told what she was thinking now.

'If anyone's to blame, it's me,' he told her as they shipped for Boston, not only believing it but hoping it might help to relieve her. 'But he never raised anything but anger in me. I could never find any meeting point with him. He was always a stranger to me. He stood off and wouldn't be thrown a line. I guess I should have made more effort in the time given me. Forgive me, I'm sorry.'

Despite her world falling apart, Amy was still thinking clearly enough to see that as rather ironic. It was too late for it. She could not have told the number of times she had tried to bring father and son together. What had always seemed incredible to her was that they were so much alike yet found it impossible to see the similarity in each other.

The crowd of friends who stood on the chilly Boston wharf, the Garrisons and Amos Drew amongst them, looked like a gathering of mourners waiting patiently for the arrival of the coffin. All were there to extend their sympathies and tell of the individual efforts they had made. Amy did not feel she could face them all at once but, with no alternative, yet again stayed steady. Sophia was already shedding tears and was the first to receive Amy's arms while a long-faced Amos Drew hurried to intercept James, offer his soft, limp hand and, most reluctantly, discharge the duty forced on him.

'Captain,' he said quietly and confidentially. 'I'm very sorry to have to tell you this but only two days ago Mrs McBain's aunt ran away and so far has not been found.'

'Ran away?' James exclaimed overloudly, bringing Amy hurrying to them in the belief that it was information she should know. 'What do you mean, ran away?'

'I was just explaining to your husband, Mrs McBain,' Amos Drew said in some embarrassment, 'that your aunt's ill health is not so much to do with her physical condition – indeed she appears to be most healthy in that respect. Rather is it . . . ah, a stress of the mind. I did ask for every precaution to be taken but despite that she . . . appears to have tricked her keepers and decided to go elsewhere.'

Amy never knew how she managed to withstand this fresh blow, but she did. Surrounded by so many people there was little else she could do. But it was perhaps as well she did not know that she was the cause of her aunt escaping. Dorothea had cunningly planned her disappearance the moment she was told that her Amelia and the captain would soon be coming to see her and wouldn't that be nice. Nice? Merciful God! Were they not two of the conspirators in the kidnap? They were probably coming to kill her to silence her. They were all conspirators, every one of them. That became crystal clear when she found so many Bostonians hesitant to sign her petition which she had intended presenting to the State Legislature, calling for just retribution on the perpetrators and for the return of her child. Even her so-called charitable ladies for whom she had done so much had turned out to be conspirators. Bitches to a Bloomer, every single one.

James and Amy thanked all their friends for their thoughtfulness and concern but it was not until Amy was being ushered into the Garrisons' carriage that she stopped and turned to the gathering. It was more than simply her usual impulse, rather an overwhelming compulsion to tell them what she herself had come to know, as sure of it now as there was a God in heaven, as sure as the world was round.

'I know what many of you are thinking,' she said, 'and I don't blame you for it, but I can assure you that wherever he is, Jamie is not dead. If he were, I would know it.'

There were some nervous little smiles at that but later, when Hinton had James alone, he said, 'James, it's hard for me to say this but I know you'd want me to be frank. I fear the worst.'

'You heard what Amy said,' James replied, surprising him.

Hinton had taken Amy's pronouncement as purely the wishful thinking of a stricken mother but, father as he was, James was another matter.

'You believe it, too?' he frowned.

'Hinton,' James assured him, 'I've been with Amy a long time now and she's never steered me a wrong course yet. My main worry now is for how long I'm going to be beached. Amy will never leave here until we find out where he's gone and I can't risk not staying with her and going back to sea without her. I need her with me, Hinton. I need her companionship. She's the only one I have. Being stuck here when there's so much to be done is going to be the hell of it. Not once in his life have I raised a hand to him and maybe I should have done. This time when I find him I'm going to bloody keelhaul him for putting her through yet more. That I swear. I never claimed to understand him but I always did my duty by him. And more. I've seen more worthy men given twenty lashes for less. Not even a note to her. Nothing.'

With the scramble to get to California and new factories opening which paid good wages, it was only with the offer of a lot of money that James was able to find half a dozen good men willing to spread out throughout New England and beyond in search of two people – James McBain junior and Miss Dorothea Jackson. And since it had become common knowledge amongst his friends that Jamie detested everything to do with the sea, ships and waterfronts were not even a consideration in the hunt.

'You'll report back to me here at weekly intervals in any way you can,' James told his assorted bunch of amateur detectives, 'and you'll keep a true and honest account of expenses with proper receipts or they'll not be paid.'

Hinton found James's faith in Amy's belief touching but he was not so sure about Sophia's sudden conversion. Like most converts she was an instant zealot.

'I never of course doubted for a moment he was still alive,' she almost glowed as she readied for bed on the very first night of the McBains' arrival, 'and I'm just pleased Amy herself was able to confirm it. There's every reason to be hopeful, Hinton. He could reappear any day.'

'Yes, my dear,' Hinton replied patiently as he pulled off his boots, keeping his opinions to himself to please her, aware too that Amy might need such an optimistic disciple. 'Every reason. Any day.'

Indeed Amy was to find Sophia's support a comfort for which she was very grateful. But it was for hardly more than a day that she allowed herself the indulgence of inactive distress. She then set about playing her own part, going over the ground Hinton had already covered by questioning everyone who had ever had any contact with Jamie, with Aunt Dorothea not forgotten either.

'Previous to this,' she enquired of Dr Drew, 'did you ever see any

182

strange behaviour in my aunt that might have given warning?' Amos Drew might have blushed scarlet at that had he not expected the question eventually. Prepared, he kept himself under control and, clasping his hands together, he raised his head slightly for a moment as if in thought, then lowered it again to look her straight in the eye. 'No, no. Nothing I was aware of, Mrs McBain,' he answered.

Amy was left to conclude that it was because of Jamie that her aunt's mind had been turned and she blamed herself for that, too. She should never have given her the responsibility for him. It had clearly been too much for her. It seemed to Amy that *nothing* she had done had been right. But as time passed without result, she began to have yet another pressure put on her. By James himself. Although he had not once uttered a word of complaint, it started to become clear to her that it was he who was suffering the more by the waiting. And she knew it was not pretence or any attempt at moral blackmail on his part. He was just changing. Letter after letter came from Kimball and Jay urging him to return to New York but he ignored them. Invitations to speak to societies began to be turned down. Day after day she watched him just sitting there, assuring her when he was asked that he was all right. Removed for so long from the sea when so much maritime activity as never before was going on, when America was surging ahead of the rest of the world with faster and faster ships, he looked as if he was turning into an old man before her eyes. It was as if his restless soul had stopped struggling and become still, as if a barnacle had been prised from a hull, taken indoors and put before the fire to shrivel up and die. It was unbearable agony for her.

'James, you must go,' she almost wept.

'I'll go when you're ready, Amy,' he said, and there was nothing she could do.

The first snow fell over Boston before salvation came. James, who had been opening any mail addressed to Aunt Dorothea in case it should reveal anything, recognised the handwriting immediately. It bore the postmark of San Francisco and he tore it open. There was no sender's address on it. 'Dear Aunt Dorothea,' it read:

No doubt I've caused you considerable anxiety by now and for that I'm extremely sorry. My only excuse is that my departure was rather more hurried than I had originally anticipated and this is the first real opportunity I've had of making good my remissful conduct as our Mr Maynes of Harvard might have put it – he was very fond of remiss, Mr Maynes, and no doubt he remisses me very much.

Please, you mustn't worry. I'm perfectly safe and happy. Indeed, I've never been happier. For the first time in my life I can see things clearly, know exactly what I'm doing and know the purpose of my future. But if you have any regard for me I ask you to accept that I do not want to be found, so if anyone is looking for me, please have them stopped. That is my sincerest wish and I trust you will let my mother know this, too, when you see her. Where she is as I write I'm not sure but presume it to be somewhere in the Indian Ocean. You will give her my love.

Once again, I ask that no one be concerned for me.

Trusting this finds you well.

Love, Jamie.

For a wide-eyed Amy, the knowledge that he was safe and happy was a burst of summer sun. 'Why didn't we think of California?' she said. 'It was so obvious. It's where half the world is headed!'

For James, what he quickly saw as his release was like a large injection of brine. 'We can go there if you like,' he said. 'Who knows, you might even run into him.'

That was something Amy was unable to resist and with James promising to keep his little army of land crabs crawling ever west in search of Aunt Dorothea, he wasted little time in having Kimball and Jay organise a cargo for his latest clipper to take to San Francisco, pleasing Mr Kimball and Mr Jay very much.

'But what am I to do with your wife's aunt if these people find her?' Amos Drew asked the captain, hoping it might sound like strong reluctance on his part to have any more to do with missing persons, but if he thought he was going to get Miss Dorothea Jackson out of what was left of his whitening hair so easily he was mistaken. The revived James was having no objections put in his way, by Amos Drew or anyone else. 'You will have her brought back and do what you can for her, Doctor,' he instructed with an authority that Amos Drew found impossible to combat. 'I must trust your professional judgement on that. And I've arranged with Mr Garrison to pay your fees and any expenses you incur.'

Shortly after, Amos Drew washed his hands with his perfumed soap and dried them with pure white linen, but it did not help.

'Good luck and God bless!' called a much happier Sophia, waving a handkerchief on the icy Boston wharf as James and Amy's passenger barque slipped her mooring. Beside her, Hinton, only a very recent convert and pleased to be one, raised his arm aloft in salute and soon the McBains were gone.

184

Had he not been Hurricane Jim, James would have found it a lot more difficult to find a full crew. As it was, among them was an Italian who spoke hardly a word of English, two Norwegians and a Dutchman. But only ten days later, under low, dark skies over New York, his hold laden with everything from flour to factory cotton, from preserves to playing cards, he weighed anchor.

On shore, a beaming Mr Kimball in a large woollen coat with a luxurious astrakhan collar, large cigar in hand, stood watching, Mr Jay in more conservative dress beside him.

'Fortune smiled on us again,' Kimball noted. 'I thought James might not want to go to California. All going well, I think we're about to make another pile.'

'May Cape Horn be kind to us,' Mr Jay returned, almost as a prayer.

But only John Marsh knew that James McBain junior was no longer in California. Indeed, during the short time his ship had been anchored off San Francisco in the waters already being termed the Golden Gate, he had not put a foot ashore.

Chapter Seventeen

When Jamie had arrived at San Francisco, he felt he could actually smell the excitement that was coming from the land. It was as pungent as woodsmoke. And he was quickly to learn more about the power of gold fever than Miss Culpeper had taught him. Hardly had they furled sail and dropped their hook when three of the crew were suddenly throwing themselves over the side and swimming for their lives and their fortunes towards the shore, Captain Beriah Gurley hurling curses after them to no good effect.

'The boats, damn you, Mister, lower the boats!' he yelled at Tyrrel in the hope of catching them. That was going to take time. The boats were still securely lashed in position. Jamie took quick note of that delay, resolving that when it came to his own purposes in future he would see to it that, at all times, the boats would be ready for lowering before they had even spilled wind. But it was by no means the only confusion. Not far away, coming towards them was a fleet of small boats engaged in what could only be described as a miniature sea battle. Each was rowed frantically by men who, almost overnight, had become merchants, wholesalers, and agents, and had quickly discovered that there were ways of making a fortune other than trusting to Lady Luck with a pick and shovel. Even a four-month-old penny newspaper from back East was fetching a whole dollar, a mark-up of one thousand per cent, so the competition to get to a cargo first and buy before the captain knew what the latest prices were was, to put it mildly, fierce. As they closed on the ship and her treasure, they did all in their power to eliminate each other. In fascination, Jamie saw several boats turned turtle, their owners spluttering and screaming vengeance as they surfaced. On one boat, the oarsman produced a gun and shot a hole in his nearest enemy's waterline. On another a man sprang up and with a great, herculean swing, did all but decapitate one of the opposition with the blade of his oar. On deck, Captain Gurley, who had disappeared only for a moment, reappeared brandishing his own gun.

'The next man who tries to leave this ship without my permission,' he roared at the crew, 'gets shot between the shoulder blades!'

'Lower away! Lower away!' Tyrrel shouted but by that time it was too late to put the boat in the water. Already, directly underneath it, stopping it from being put down, were three fighting merchants trying to tie up to the hull. It was not surprising that the first three seamen to jump ship to head for the goldfields got away.

'Don't let these men aboard your ship, Captain!' shouted the first merchant who managed to reach the deck. 'They're thieves and robbers and would have your eyes out while you're not looking! My only purpose is to do straight and honest business and I'll take whatever you have! Is it a deal, sir?' But with that, another having grabbed his coat-tails, he went backwards over the side to land cursing in the ship's boat still dangling halfway down the hull. It took Gurley some time to restore order to his vessel but Jamie did not at first realise that it was all going to be to his advantage and would push his plans forward faster than he might have imagined.

When the business was done, every item on the cargo manifest bought at prices Gurley could hardly believe, the arrangements made for unloading, it was natural that he should send the moonfaced Tyrrel to have the merchants' banks confirm payment while he himself kept armed guard over his crew. He should have known better. If Tyrrel was strong of hand, he was weak aloft. Hardly had he put a foot ashore in the thronging, mushrooming town when he was stricken by the fever. The promise of gold rose from the earth. It floated in the air and in the clouds. It radiated from the sun. And he, too, took the opportunity of deserting to head for his fortune. When Gurley discovered it, such was his rage it was surprising no innocent seaman was shot for it. As it was, corn could have been roasted over the fire of his curses. But none of it was going to bring Tyrrel back and he feared for how he stood. It called for desperate measures and he shouted for the only man left aboard he felt he could trust.

'Yes, sir,' Jamie said, standing a little nervously before the captain's gun which was pointing at him.

'Marsh,' Beriah Gurley told him, 'you have two alternatives. Either you try to leave my ship, in which case I swear to Almighty God I'll come after you and blow your head off, or you stay as mate for the return voyage and a bonus of two hundred dollars when we get back. Which is it to be, Marsh?'

At first, Jamie was stunned. Although he looked older, he was aware that he was still only sixteen. Since rounding Cape Horn he had thought it might be at least a year before he would get such an opportunity and was prepared to wait for it. Gurley was not so patient.

'I asked you a goddamn question, Marsh!' he said.

'I have no intention of jumping and leaving you, Captain,' Jamie replied happily. 'And I thank you for your generosity.'

'All right, Mr Marsh,' Beriah Gurley instructed him. 'See to it this vessel and her crew are kept in good order. I can keep alert for at least another twenty-four hours but when one of us bunks, the other will be on armed watch covering bowsprit to stern, Mister.'

To Mr Marsh, it did not seem so simple. It was going to take two days to lighter off the cargo and it was not just a matter of gold fever. The men had been at sea a long time and he felt he was not at all ready to handle a mutiny. They had become surly and dourly threatening as it was at not being allowed ashore.

It was the middle of the night when Beriah Gurley was woken from his first rest by the commotion and still fully clad he sprang from his bunk, grabbed his own gun and ran out on deck which was lit up by many lamps. He stopped and looked on in disbelief. Two men were fiddling jigs on violins. Men were dancing with women, stopping as often as they could at the barrel of drink where John Marsh was dispensing it with magnanimity. Already some of the crew were half drunk while others were staggering off to shadowy spots on the deck or to the fo'c'sle with their girls who were squealing merriment.

'What in the hell is going on, Mister?' Gurley demanded of his new mate.

'Just a bit of recreation, sir,' Jamie replied.

'How the hell did they get here?' the captain asked, pointing in astonishment to what were obviously a bunch of whores.

'Well, sir,' Jamie explained, 'since the men couldn't go ashore I saw no harm in bringing a bit of the shore to them.'

Gurley stared at Jamie again, not quite sure what he had in this young man. 'I gave no permission for such a thing, Mister!' he shouted above all the noise.

'I didn't want to wake you for it, Captain,' Jamie excused himself, 'but you can see they're getting drunker all the time and the drunker they get the less they'll be able to swim. And since the ladies here come very expensive, I'm sure the crew will all be in debt to you by morning, sir.'

Beriah Gurley's eyeballs almost fell out at that. 'You mean I'm paying for this?' he gasped in shock.

'Not paying, Captain, just advancing,' Jamie pointed out.

Whatever else he was, Gurley was not stupid. The clever young man's reasoning made perfect sense, but he was damned if he was going to let him know it.

'You have the tongue of a lawyer and the morals of a hog, Mr Marsh!' he said, spat to a scupper in disgust, swung around and strode back to his cabin. Jamie thought that a bit rich coming from a captain who had no compunction in using Crimps. They were there in San Francisco too, much aided by an infamous lady with the name of Miss Piggot who, by means of a wooden lever, dispatched many an unfortunate drunk through a trapdoor into their hands, a subtlety Miss Culpeper might have admired. It was part of every waterfront scene that John Marsh was going to make a close study of for his future purposes.

In the meantime, that night gave him the chance to write his letter to Aunt Dorothea and on learning that the mail was much quicker going through the Panama Isthmus and on by small steamer, he had one of the girls take it for posting ashore.

It was only with great effort and every precaution being taken that as few as two more seamen managed to slip away but Beriah Gurley, red-eyed from lack of sleep, was not going to wait for the Crimps to deliver replacements on this occasion. He was far too anxious to get away before he had no crew left at all and was prepared to risk his ship for it.

'Weigh anchor, Mr Marsh,' he ordered Jamie while the last barrels of flour were still coming out of the hold and Jamie was taken by surprise.

'But what about the victualling, ballast and clearance, sir?' he questioned.

'I said weigh anchor, Mister!' Gurley blasted at him.

The hatches were still open, the boat still upright on the side deck, the discharging barely completed as they sailed from the Golden Gate. Gurley ordered every piece of spare equipment there was into the bottom of the hold, including the boats, but as far as ballast was concerned it was a spit in the ocean and as soon as they got into even moderate seas she was rolling like a cork. Sometimes she was almost right on her beam and by spilling wind at appropriate moments, Mr Marsh and his depleted crew fought day and night to keep her upright, if for no other reason than to save their own lives. Mr Marsh, reduced to a diet of 'salt horse', unleavened bread and biscuits like the rest of them, learned a lot by it. And from that unstable world and without any encouragement or tuition whatsoever from the captain he learned to take accurate readings on the sextant and went to work on his own on the maze of figures in the Almanac.

After forty hectic days of it, Jamie was looking worriedly at the darkening clouds when he heard the voice behind him.

'You fear for my ship, do you, Mr Marsh?' Captain Gurley asked him.

'Not fear, Captain,' Jamie replied without turning, 'but I'd say if we're going to try and get back round Cape Horn like this we'll never make it.'

'You don't have to tell me, Mister,' Gurley said, 'so pick a port on the chart we can put into and take us there.'

Puzzled, Jamie turned to look at him. It was in some terror he noticed that the captain's eyes were like watering embers and that, despite the breeze, he was sweating without effort. Gurley was going down with sickness and expected him to take over and see them safe. All on his own. Had there been a road to run down at that moment of realisation, Jamie might have run. But there was no such road. All around them, north, south, east and west was the Pacific. The vessel heeled dangerously to a creaking of timbers and the cracking of backwinding sail. He was not ready for total responsibility. If he knew what navigation was about, he had only just begun to practise it. The idea of being entirely alone with no one else in the world to confirm or deny his capabilities shook him to the depths. For two whole hours he stood behind the helmsman in silence, praying that by morning the captain would recover. But the captain did not oblige him. By morning, Gurley was not only still in his bunk but delirious with fever. Sheer desperation and necessity drove James McBain junior to be master, mate, navigator and nurse all rolled into one. He had the ship scrubbed from stem to stern with vinegar until it was almost pickled. He lived on his nerves rather than salt horse, only able to snatch sleep for an hour at a stretch. There was no time to appreciate that his crew, in a much-changed mood, were giving him their full support.

It was ten days before Captain Beriah Gurley came back into the world of the living, the fever passed, and he was aware that his ship was not moving.

'Where are we?' he mumbled and Jamie, relieved, was quickly at his side.

'In Valparaiso, Captain.'

Hitting Valparaiso on the Chilean coast so accurately had given Jamie an enormous sense of satisfaction, especially as he had brought the unballasted ship through some heavy squalls without damage and no one else had taken sick, but it was as well he did not expect the old man, now gaunt of face, to praise him for it.

'Spanish harlots you have all over my decks now, is it, Mr Marsh?'

'No, sir,' Jamie replied. 'We're anchored in quarantine and a doctor has already looked at you. He'll be coming back this afternoon. But we've been allowed to take on some fresh food.'

'Speak Spanish, do you, Mister?'

'No, Captain.'

'Thought there was something wrong with you,' Gurley grumbled and closed his eyes again, very grateful for what John Marsh had done.

It was in Valparaiso that Jamie started to pick up Spanish and he did not find it difficult. Then with Gurley recovered, ballast and some mixed cargo was taken on before heading south again. And this time Jamie was thrilled by the speed the ship made over the huge seas around Cape Horn as they ran before the wind only partly canvassed.

Up into the Alantic, John Marsh took it on himself to start experimenting with the tuning of the rig and getting more speed out of the sail. Gurley had been turned in only an hour when he was tumbled over the lee board of his bunk on to his cabin sole with a thud and hurried on deck, at first unable to believe his eyes. It was blowing near to a westerly gale but every bit of canvas was aloft, the vessel heeled over so much the main-course sail yard to starboard was almost touching the water. Two men were fighting with the wheel to keep her head from forcing itself to windward. His ship was surging on a reach such as he had never seen, like a mad dog racing over hills, foaming at the mouth and about to crack its ribs and burst its stays. Fear and awe were showing on the faces of the watch. 'Sweet Jesus Christ,' he exhaled before finding full voice. 'What in the hell do you think you're doing?' he roared at his young mate in fury.

'Making good time, sir!'

'Who the hell do you think you are? Hurricane Jim? Get those royals and topgallants in before we're dismasted! Now, Mister!'

Disappointed, Jamie shouted his orders for men to jump to the sheets and sent others scurrying aloft to do Gurley's bidding, but the captain might have lost his grip and been swept to the scuppers had he known it was not only the son of Hurricane Jim he was shouting at but that the young man was sharpening his sword for the sole purpose of cutting his father down. And there were to be other echoes of Hurricane Jim that even Jamie himself was not aware of.

'I suggest, sir,' he said to Gurley at the first reasonable opportunity, 'that if you have no trust in me, we put into Rio where you might be able to find a mate you have more faith in.'

That put Captain Beriah Gurley in a quandary. He knew what he had in John Marsh. There was no doubt in his mind that, given a few years, Marsh would get his own ship. Clear, too, that it was a driver he wanted to become and not just another master. But he could not bring himself to say any of it.

'You realise that giving the master of a vessel an ultimatum is tantamount to mutiny, Mr Marsh.'

'I didn't mean it to be an ultimatum, Captain, but if that's the way you want to take it then lock me up and choose my replacement from the crew if you can find one willing.'

'Damn you to hell!' Gurley exploded and struggled to calm himself. He did not want to lose either Marsh's talents or his goodwill. He needed the mate more than the mate needed him. 'Don't think I don't know what you want,' he went on. 'You want me to give you your head with my ship, don't you? Well, I'm not giving it to you, Mr Marsh,' but as Jamie opened his mouth to speak, Gurley quickly raised a commanding hand to shut him up. 'But . . .' and he paused for a moment before continuing. 'But,' he repeated emphatically, 'if you were to ask me for half of it, that I might consent to giving you,' and once more he stopped Jamie from getting in with 'And!' before adding, 'You can keep your damned thanks in your teeth, because if you so much as snap a halyard or crack a yard I'll deduct it from what I owe you, and if you lose a man to the deck or to the sea I'll deduct the lot. Is it an agreement, Mr Marsh?'

'It's an agreement, sir.'

Thus was Jamie allowed to push the vessel harder than Gurley would have done but not as hard as he would have liked. It was a lot better than nothing and by having the log put down almost constantly he was able to study the effect on speed with sail trim, angles of heel and the way in which the ship was helmed over the seas. These were things Beriah Gurley had taken many, many years to learn and already this young man was catching up on him. He looked on in wonderment but without comment while Jamie did all he could to ensure nothing got broken and no man went over, often going aloft himself to supervise.

It was many days later off Cape São Roque when the lookout aloft called the sighting of a ship far inshore and Gurley fetched his telescope. Since you could sail ten thousand miles without ever seeing another vessel, a sighting was always an event. On a heading north, the captain had stood well out at sea for rounding Brazil's easternmost point but had fallen into a hole and become almost becalmed, much to John Marsh's annoyance as he fought to take advantage of every puff of air. Gurley raised the glass to his eye and picked up what was obviously a clipper, amazed to see that she was so close in she might well have been on the rocks. It was a very dangerous place to be and tradition had it there were also strong, adverse currents there that could have a ship sailing astern. But the clipper was neither becalmed, aground, or being pushed back. Instead, heading south under a full suit of canvas right up to her skysails and with every staysail set, she was heeled over and reaching at speed in a fresh breeze which might have been specifically conjured up by the god Aeolus himself for her passing. But although the house flag could not be made out, there was no doubt whatsoever in Beriah Gurley's mind as he lowered his telescope and turned to his mate.

'There's only one man I know who'd sell his soul to the devil like that for wind, Mr Marsh,' he said, 'and you have to admire him. It has to be McBain. Hurricane Jim and no other.' And hardly had he spoken the name when, to his surprise, his mate was seizing the telescope from his hand without so much as a thank you and thrusting it to his own eye. Oddly, it had not occurred to Jamie that, despite his request to Aunt Dorothea that no search should be made for him, his mother, on receiving the information of his where-abouts, might head for California in the hope of finding him. But he sensed that was what was happening. And somewhere under those distant white sails there she was. For her he felt pangs of guilt and remorse. She was so, so near, so, so far away. On the one hand he felt desperate to let her know he was there, on the other aware that, no matter what, he would have to keep himself and his secret well hidden until he was ready. But that did not stop the pain of knowing how she must be feeling. He had imposed a heavy burden on her and she would have to endure it until his plan had matured. He was sorry about that but there was no helping it. To mail any more letters might only result in sending her on other wild-goose chases. In the mean-time there were still so many things he had to do, so much more to learn before he struck.

Skimming along the distant shore like a bird, the clipper moved further and further south. Several times Gurley had moved away and returned to find his mate still there with his telescope glued firmly to his eye. Jamie did not know how long he had stood there.

'You intend neglecting your duties for the rest of the day, Mr Marsh?' Gurley growled at him at last, returning him to the deck of his own ship, although with the sails hanging there was little to do.

'I'm sorry, sir,' Jamie replied, handing him back his telescope.

Gurley nodded towards the disappearing clipper. 'That who you want to be like, is it?'

'No, sir,' Jamie answered.

'Then that's one disappointment in life God's saved you from,' Gurley told him and walked away.

Jamie could hardly have told the old man that he was determined not only to be as good as Captain James McBain with a ship but better. He had to be. And he had no time to waste about it either.

'All right, stand by to get the lady off her backside!' he shouted at the watch as he saw a ripple coming across the water, and shortly after had her under way again, sheets and braces hauled and eased as he took advantage of every breath of wind he could get as if every extra sea mile gained was more important to him than his life.

Three hundred and two days and 30,000 miles after Jamie McBain had fallen to a Miss Culpeper Special, the mate John Marsh, now turned seventeen, pushed his ship up through Nantucket Sound, the buds on the trees ashore beginning to burst into leaf. As four hundred days to San Francisco and back was considered a respectable time for such a vessel, Captain Beriah Gurley was mighty pleased. But, as usual, it was not his way to show it.

'The luck of fair winds, Mr Marsh,' was the best he could bring himself to say and Jamie had to smile at that. It was not just the winds and the old man knew it well enough.

'You're welcome to stay on as my mate, Mr Marsh,' was as near as he got to telling Jamie he appreciated him while he paid him two hundred dollars in wages which included Tyrrel's money and the other two hundred he had promised in San Francisco. He liked Marsh. And despite the fact that Gurley was the man who had taken him from a Crimp as just another unconscious body in debt to him, Jamie liked him in return and was grateful to him.

'Thank you, Captain, but as much as I'd like to I can't,' he told him.

'Thought not,' the captain said gruffly and handed him a sealed letter addressed 'To Whom It May Concern' which was a reference. And so, as was often the case with men who had sailed long voyages together, they shook hands, wished each other luck and parted.

Dressed and rolling like a seaman, kit slung over his shoulder, Jamie kept a sharp eye open as he made his way along Boston's Central Wharf. He could not risk hanging around for fear of being recognised. And with four hundred dollars in his pocket there was no need to risk going near his bank account either. He immediately shipped out for New York to get himself on to a good clipper from there and learn best how to make her go.

The voyage of Captain James McBain to California was an entirely

195

different matter. Between his driving and Amy's navigation his clipper shattered the previous record for the run by making it there around a storm-battered Cape Horn and up to San Francisco in one hundred and three days. And if he was disappointed for Amy's sake that no trace of their son could be found and that he, too, suffered a loss of crew to gold fever, there was to be an overwhelming compensation. More astute in business than Beriah Gurley, James held an auction to sell his 75,000-dollar cargo which fetched a quarter of a million. It was a profit that paid for the building of the clipper three times over!

When report of their new riches reached Kimball and Jay via Panama, New Orleans and Mr Morse's telegraph wire, their faces beamed brighter than the Floating Light on a moonless night.

'We'll have the keel of a new clipper laid for him,' Kimball suggested. 'And right now.'

'We can do nothing less,' Mr Jay smiled.

'She'll be the biggest and best there could ever be,' Kimball declared with a wave of his huge cigar.

'Masts two hundred feet high,' Mr Jay envisaged.

'We'll call her *Wings of America*,' Kimball announced.

'Excellent, excellent,' Mr Jay enthused.

Smashing the record again for the return passage, James and Amy eventually sailed back into New York to a riotous welcome, but there was only one thing that occupied Amy's mind and that was her missing Jamie.

'It is doubtful,' reported the *New York Herald* euphorically on Hurricane Jim's latest exploit, 'if the man will ever be born who will surpass him. The world can only wait to see what more incredible feats he achieves with *Wings of America*, a clipper vessel of 1,200 tons already started building, the likes of which may never be seen again in our lifetime.'

There was some exaggeration in that for although the air along the East River was alive with flying sawdust in the race to build other clippers less impressive, another along the lines of *Wings of America* was rising from the stocks in East Boston on order from a New Yorker. She was to be called the *Flying Star*. That did not worry James in the slightest when he heard about it, and worried him even less when he discovered she was to be captained by East-lake. Several times the pledge-taking master had been on the verge of being sacked from transatlantic packets for being shot in the neck and legless in front of passengers and had only saved his career in the end by marrying a lady ten years his senior who was as vociferous as she was unattractive but was the daughter of a wealthy merchant ship owner. It was only Amy who worried, and not about ships.

'There's still no news of either of them,' she told James forlornly as she returned from yet another visit to the Post Office.

'They'll turn up, I know it,' James comforted and it was in a letter from Hinton Garrison two days later that Hinton informed him of a Scotsman called Allan Pinkerton who had set up a private detective agency operating out of Chicago, suggesting that he might be usefully employed in the search. James immediately wrote to Mr Pinkerton with all the details of James McBain junior and Aunt Dorothea, raising some fresh hope in Amy that Mr Pinkerton might find them.

Both would have been astonished had they been able to see, and known why, at that very moment, their son as Second Mate John Marsh was driving another clipper for all it was worth down across the Atlantic towards the Cape of Good Hope bound for China. Little did either of them know that of all the people in the world this was the man Captain James McBain would come to fear.

Chapter Eighteen

Sophia's face was stricken as she looked at her husband. The information was not only confusing to her but shocking.

'It can't be her,' she insisted. 'She would never dress like that to start with. Never. And she didn't have a sister. Amy would have said. The woman must be mad to say such a dreadful thing.'

'Sophia,' Hinton reminded her, 'it's a madwoman we're talking about. And there are similarities.'

'It's not her, I'm sure of it,' Sophia declared and set about finding something to do to try to take her mind off it.

Hinton who was looking after the matter while James and Amy were back at sea, *Wings of America* still building, studied the message from Pinkerton's National Detective Agency again. Whoever this woman was who refused to give her name, she had to be checked out. He headed for Dr Drew's.

Secure in the belief that it was going to be another happy summer day, Amos Drew had Hinton admitted to his study, gave what was almost a genuine smile, and held out a limp hand which had been freshly washed under a faucet from the new public water supply.

'Ah, Mr Garrison, sit down, sit down, sir. Not too much of a troublesome ailment I hope?'

'I'm not yet sure but I'd say it looks like it,' Hinton replied and soon the summer was draining from Amos Drew's face, gradually becoming laden with doom as he listened to the tale of the lady in Chicago attired in fashionable, bright green dress, purple bonnet, red lace gloves and orange boots, found attacking young couples in the streets with a stick, accusing them of having stolen her children and demanding them back. When confronted by the man from Pinkerton's she boasted that she had murdered her sister and would murder him too if he did not leave her alone.

Amos, who had hopefully thought to be rid of Miss Dorothea Jackson for good after such a long interval, felt his stomach turn. From out of the dim, distant past of his boyhood came the memory of being told of the tragic drowning of the younger Jackson child. It had not meant much to him then and had soon been forgotten.

199

Now, on top of all his other discoveries, it became bathed in a sinister, bloody glow. There was no question in his mind that this Chicago woman was none other than Dorothea Jackson. But to have dragged up that drowning or anything else might have led to him being closely questioned on all he knew and why he had concealed it.

'Do you know if she has a sister, or did have?' he heard Garrison enquire.

'Not to my knowledge,' he lied, and knowing what was coming next, did all he could to resist it. 'I can't go all the way to Chicago to make an identification, Mr Garrison, if that's why you've come,' he got in quickly. 'I just couldn't afford the time and I have my patients. I'm very sorry.'

'So am I, Doctor,' Hinton said, both disappointed and displeased. 'Surely you could get another doctor *locum tenens* in the meantime?'

'Oh, that's not so easy, Mr Garrison. Not easy at all. In fact I'd say it's impossible at the moment. Besides, I'm sure this woman is not Miss Jackson. It doesn't sound at all like her. What little information there is I'd say is pure coincidence. The condition of mind bringing on such behaviour is not unique.'

'Dr,' Hinton persisted firmly, 'we still must know for sure. And if it does turn out to be Miss Jackson the best must be done for her.'

'I realise that, but at the moment Chicago is impossible for me, sir.'

Hinton felt angered by Drew's lack of co-operation and aimed to let him know it.

'I thought it was the arrangement Captain McBain made with you and that you agreed to, Doctor. Are you going back on that now? Myself, I hardly know the woman and I can't ask Mrs Garrison to go. It would be much too distressing for her. There *is* only yourself.'

Amos Drew had been slow to wake up and suddenly realising what he might be letting himself in for was struck with dread. But it was not the wrath of the famous captain that had flashed into his head, nor any condemnation by the Garrisons. What came to him like a bolt of lightning was that if Dorothea Jackson had deteriorated to the extent of openly confessing to child murder, which was very possibly the truth, what else was she saying? He had to hear it for himself. For his own safety he had to convince everyone that anything at all she said was no more than the demented ravings of a lunatic. As a doctor his word would be taken for that but he had to start on it now. If Hinton Garrison noticed he had quickly gone a little pale, he was not in the mood to express his concern.

'You're perfectly right, of course, Mr Garrison,' Drew came back, surprising Hinton by the sudden change of heart. 'Of course I must go to Chicago. It's no less than my duty and I'll prepare to go straight away.'

Recovered and relieved, Hinton hurried to the telegraph office and wired Pinkerton's to the effect that if the woman was not claimed by anyone else in the meantime she was to be held in some secure place for her own safety on the authority of Dr Drew of Boston who would reach Chicago as soon as possible.

Wishing for all his life he had become a lawyer instead, Amos Drew recruited Miss Blossom and another lady keeper who, if she was not up to Miss Blossom's proportions, was as strong as an ox, and set out armed with enough paraldehyde to subdue a herd of stampeding buffalo.

'You must not be surprised by anything she says,' he warned. 'Her mind has completely gone. She will probably make outrageous accusations against us but she is only to be pitied.'

'The lady will get nothing but understanding from me, Doctor,' Miss Blossom assured him in case some supporter of Dorothea Dix's continuing campaign for better treatment of the insane was in earshot.

After weary days of travel, Amos Drew arrived in Chicago and after settling in was led to a house where Miss Jackson had been locked up in the cellar. But if the doctor thought he was going to grab his patient and rush her back to Boston just like that he was mistaken. Word of someone coming who was responsible for the lady had quickly got around and the crowd of angry people on the sidewalk waving bits of paper at him barred his approach.

'Make way there!' Drew demanded.

'The hell we will!'

'You don't take this woman from here until we's paid!' they shouted at him, pushing at him and shoving him back.

'I'm a doctor,' Drew protested. 'And I'm not even sure who she is.'

'You can be the goddamn President, mister,' a shop-keeper bellowed at him on behalf of the mob of other shopkeepers, costumiers and hotel owners, 'but you ain't gonna find out until we's bin settled!'

Despite having Miss Blossom, who alone put two men to the ground, her colleague, and the man from Pinkerton's, a highly embarrassed Amos Drew had no choice but to retreat from Dorothea Jackson's creditors. Even with Mr Morse's wonderful invention it still took two days to get the money Hinton was holding

201

for James to pay them all off. Only then did Drew get into the house.

The cellar door was opened cautiously and a lamp held up. Below, Dorothea Jackson was perched on the makeshift bed looking like a bedraggled South American parrot. Miss Blossom was first to go down.

'Hullo, Miss Jackson,' she said. 'Remember me? Miss Blossom?'

Whether or not Dorothea did, she gave no particular sign of recognition. She rose, pulled herself to her full height and asked haughtily, 'What have you brought for me?'

'Comfort, Miss Jackson,' Miss Blossom replied. 'Comfort.'

'What's it made of?' Dorothea enquired.

It was a mistake for Amos Drew to think it was safe to go down. As soon as she caught sight of him at the foot of the steps, Dorothea flew at him with hand upraised to strike. 'You beast!' she screamed at him and Miss Blossom quickly pinned her.

'I told you,' a trembling Amos Drew said, 'I told you.'

Heavily dosed with the drug which had to be forced down her throat and with her two keepers constantly at her side, Amos Drew got the half-conscious and confused Dorothea Jackson back to New England where he had her admitted to a new, progressive, private home for the insane at Worcester with wide corridors and open spaces instead of chains and dungeons. There, to all the staff, the doctor forcibly made his point about her wild, outlandish, and often foul imaginings on all things and on all people. And Amos Drew breathed more easily. So did Hinton Garrison. 'Thank God for that,' he said. 'One down and one to go.' But he was mistaken if he thought Pinkerton was going to find the other so easily.

Some good time later the 'one to go' in the shape of the mate of a clipper, then fifteen thousand miles away, looked on in idle curiosity at the activity taking place on a British ship anchored near him in Whampoa Reach, several miles down from Canton. Although he was constantly on the lookout for anything that might help him in his odyssey to bring his father down, he did not know at first as he watched how much use this was to be to him.

A sampan had come alongside the British ship and tied up. Then, from it, a coffin was hauled up over the bulwarks on to the British vessel, a European in a black silk suit and black hat and not a Chinaman seemingly in charge of the casket. There was nothing odd about that, perhaps. Seamen died in port as well as at sea and, if they did, they were buried on land, even if it was Chinese territory. But then Jamie noticed something strange and his curiosity was no longer idle. The British Union flag was still fully hoisted on its signal halyard and not half lowered which was usual for the death of even the lowest hand aboard. Jamie's suspicion was further aroused as he watched the coffin being carried into the main cabin. It was not the place to be keeping a corpse, particularly in that heat. Hurriedly he fetched the telescope, took up a position on deck from where he could not be easily seen from the British vessel and focused it on the ports of the main cabin. He was lucky. If the light had been reflecting off the glass he would have seen nothing. As it was he could make out that the coffin had been placed on the cabin table although he could see only half of it. Its lid was removed. By moving from one port to the other he could see what appeared to be the captain and the mate in attendance, moving about and talking to the man in the black suit. Then a few minutes later he found himself staring with the one eye that was stuck to the glass. It was not a body that was being loaded into the casket but packages bound in sacking. Dozens of them. Jamie knew almost immediately that what he was witnessing was a smuggling operation. Neither did he have to guess what the packages were. He had already learned that despite the agreement Britain had made with China eight years before after two years of war over it, the English were still managing to get opium from India into China for great profits. But it was not that which concerned Jamie, it was this cousin of Miss Culpeper and Miss Piggot in the black silk suit he was interested in. Putting away his telescope he hurriedly sought out the bosun who was an old hand on the China run. The bosun smelt like a distillery.

'See that?' Jamie said to him, nodding towards the British vessel where the heavy coffin was being lowered back on to the sampan. The bosun glanced, removed his hat, crossed himself and said, 'God rest his soul.'

'I didn't know we had a European undertaker here,' Jamie said and the bosun turned back to him.

'Ain't exactly European, Mr Marsh. American. Name of Lymann Cobb. Seaman once. Got permission to set hisself up to bury all the Christians who dies here. Foreign devils, Fan Kwai, the Chinks might call us but they got an almighty respect for the dead. Specially ours. Gives 'em a wide berth.'

Lymann Cobb was exactly the kind of person Jamie was making a study of around the waterfronts of the world in case they could be of any use to him. And although most of them had come to him through hearsay, he already had quite a list. But for some reason, probably because he had heard no word against him, he wanted to make quite sure about this undertaker. At the first opportunity he had himself rowed upriver. He had already seen the exotic sights of Canton with its crowded scene of moored junks, Mandarin boats, exquisite flower boats, trading sampans darting about between them, the jammed, noisy hongs ashore and, further back, the line of three-storeyed buildings housing Western agents from Russia, France, the US, Britain and several other countries, all showing their flags. But it was only the Christian cemetery he was interested in now. Given directions he found it well clear of the city to the south. And there, in the British plot, he knew he need enquire no further on the character of Mr Lymann Cobb. The names on headstones of John Smiths and John Browns were all over the place, even a few John Does, all seamen, all 'Sadly Missed'. They were missed all right. Jamie was absolutely sure it was nothing more than ship's ballast that occupied their caskets with not a bone to show between the lot of them. He took out his notebook and, under the name of 'Miss Le Fevre – New Orleans/Crimps', entered 'Lymann Cobb – Canton/Op. Smug'. Pinkerton's back in the States who were searching for him might have been proud of their quarry's methods. And shocked by his motive.

Within a week, John Marsh's clipper, loaded with tea, sailed downstream, dismissed the Chinese pilot at Macao and headed out into the jade-green waters of the South China Sea with all its dangers of hidden reefs and lurking pirates. And since his captain was a driver he was allowed to push the ship as hard as he liked and do all the navigating as well, a skill he found had come like second nature to him and was now much aided by the second edition of Lieutenant Matthew Maury's *Winds and Currents and Sailing Directions*. As he stood on deck, legs apart, and shouted with authority for a hardening of starboard sheets to all sails, the duty watch jumping to his command as he insisted they put their backs into the hauling, he felt he was ready to make his move. All he needed was the right set of circumstances to come together. And the shifting patterns of profit and trade were conspiring to do just that for him.

Many thousands of miles away on a heading south-east by south as he made his way down the Pacific from another highly profitable voyage to California, Hurricane Jim stood on his quarterdeck to weather, shouting at his mate for adjustments, urging for greater speed. If he was not a perfectly happy man it was only because Amy had been disappointed once again at finding no trace of their son. He had even gone to the lengths of having leaflets distributed around the goldfields offering a substantial reward for information on the whereabouts of the young man called James McBain, learned in Latin and Greek. But they had resulted in attracting only hoaxers and tricksters trying to get the money for nothing. Little did the captain know that it was himself who was being hunted and that the hunter stalking him with such determination was his son.

Amy appeared on deck, sextant and deck watch in hand, the hem of her dress fluttering about her ankles as she made her way to the bulwark rail to brace herself against it for the shooting of the sun.

'Need a hand there, Mrs McBain?' James called to her.

'No, thank you,' Amy called back.

He had done all he could for her, given her all the love and attention of which he was capable, but although he knew she appreciated it and gave him her love in return, it was not quite the same. Part of her remained empty and he knew that only the reappearance of her son could fill the gap. Time, it seemed, did not heal everything as he had once believed. He had even willed himself to stop cursing his offspring for all the harm he had done to her in the hope that that might help. But the child, the boy, the youth, and somewhere now the young man, was always there between them.

'Amy,' he had tried to tell her in so many different ways, 'it's no good keeping on living in the past. It wasn't you he ran away from, it was me. It was me who made all the mistakes and even if I went down on my knees and wept for it, it would make no difference. What's been done's been done and I can't go back and undo it now. Unburden yourself, Amy, it's the only way.'

'Yes, I know,' Amy had always replied, but it being easier said than done kept right on looking back.

At the rail she raised the sextant, a few locks of her dark hair freeing themselves to stream in the warm wind. In her own right she had achieved more fame than most women would have dared to dream of. Two of the more liberal learned societies had condescended to mention her abilities in lectures on maritime affairs. Newspapers gave her space with respect and without ridicule as they did to some other notable women. She had been held up as a shining example of progressive womanhood by every women's organisation and every women's journal in America. But if any of it was intended to indicate her success as a wife as well as a navigator, the only effect on Amy herself was to deepen her feelings of failure as a mother. She believed that if she had fought to bring father and son together with the same tenacity she had applied in raising Jayjay from retarded child to normal youth it would all have been different. She was still deeply hurt that Jamie had left without a word of explanation to her. And there was Aunt Dorothea, since she was yet to learn that her aunt had been found. Now, on top of it all, she had

205

another growing concern. For James himself. Each time they weighed anchor he seemed that little more desperate to take his ships to the very extremes of their limits twenty-four hours a day, to make more and more speed, to do better and better. Each time they made port there was an added anxiety in him as he rushed to find out the passage times made by other ships across the world. She hardly needed to have it pointed out to her that there was a mounting fear in him of losing his lofty crown but she felt it was bound to happen sooner or later and the longer it went on the worse it would be for him. He was forty now, much older than any of his crew, even the grizzled cook whom they called 'Old Man Calibogus'. But although James laughed it off and denied it, she could see for herself that after he had spent a whole night on deck in a gale, sodden through as he kept driving his ship, there was often that bit of stiffness in his joints. Sometimes even a little pain he did his best to conceal. But it was not until the weather had turned cold and the albatross gliding astern heralded their approach to Cape Horn that she broached the subject.

The salt dish slid from the fiddles at one side of the table and back again, and they had to hold their plates down as they ate, but they were well used to that.

'Is there really any need to take up this new ship, James?' she asked. It was such a strange question that, at first, James was not sure if he understood.

'What do you mean?'

'I mean is it really necessary to go on any more? You've already done everything and no one can ever take that away from you. But isn't it time you enjoyed some of the rewards? You have more money than you know what to do with. If it wasn't for Hinton making investments for you it would be piled in a building a mile high. You could do anything you liked. Build ships yourself. Become a merchant.'

James who had stopped eating was staring at her as if unable to believe his ears. 'A shipbuilder? A merchant? What are you talking about? *Sailing* ships is all I'm good at. It's the only thing I know.'

'What utter nonsense. My God, how many times have I seen you running rings around merchants. You drive a harder bargain than any of them. Come to that, you needn't do anything at all if you don't want to. We have enough to live in the greatest comfort for more than the rest of our lives. You're rich, James, don't you ever think about that?'

'Of course I think about it,' he returned, which was the truth since he was always conscious of his poor beginnings, without

206

education and without boots to his feet. 'But are you seriously suggesting that just because we have money I go rot on the shore? Good God Almighty, Amy, I'm just at my peak. Look what's yet to come. With *Wings of America* we'll show our backside to every other ship so fast they won't even know which way we've gone. You read what the *New York Herald* said. She'll be the greatest the world has ever seen or likely to see ever again.'

'James!' Amy shouted at him in exasperation. 'Every goddamn ship you've ever had is the greatest the world has ever seen! To hell with the *New York Herald*!'

As it was very unlike Amy ever to swear, the intensity of it took James aback, so much so that he temporarily lost his grip on his plate which went flying down the table, jumped the fiddles at the edge and crashed to the cabin sole. Reprieves might have come in stranger ways but James welcomed this one. It gave him time to collect himself. First, a few moments of silence were accorded the departed meal of mutton stew, corn and potatoes as it slithered to leeward with little broken rafts of china towards the feet of a sofa, then it took several more minutes for the cabin boy to be called to clean it up.

James had a lot to consider. There was not the slightest doubt that Amy had meant what she said. Naturally it crossed his mind she might have been thinking that retiring ashore, with the ensuing publicity, might somehow result in Jamie returning. But that might be to misjudge her. He was very much aware that it had not been an easy life for her and she was simply tiring of it. As beautiful as she still was at almost thirty-six, she was not getting any younger. She deserved all the comforts he could give her. With every single voyage he made he was exposing her to dangers. There were many strong ships that went to sea under competent masters and never returned. And there would be no reward for her if that should happen. But to stand at the Battery in New York like some spectator as crowds cheered *Wings of America* as it set out under the hands of some other captain to try to overtake and destroy what it had taken him thirty years at sea to build up and leave him stranded as a has-been was unthinkable. Only if he broke records that could *never* be beaten would his brine-rimmed soul ever be at rest. Yet for Amy's sake he knew he had to listen. Apart from wanting to please her, he was every bit as much afraid of losing her as he had ever been. As much as losing his gilded crown.

After normality was restored and some trivial conversation followed, he decided to throw in and make his plea. 'Amy,' he said, surprising her, 'if it's what you really want it's what you'll get. It's your due and I've no intention of keeping it from you. But you must let me take the new ship first so we can show the world what we can do with her. Then I'll look around to see what might interest me. That I promise, Amy. Just one more year or less. Then we step ashore together and, no matter what else happens, we stay there.'

It was a measure of his total faith in *Wings of America* but Amy knew just how hard it must have been for him to agree to abdicate at all, and so quickly. Nor was he one ever to go back on his word and for a moment she was almost sorry she had pressed him into it like that. But as it was for his own sake she had done it, it made her a much happier woman.

For an hour in their bunk they held each other tightly. And despite the mounting waves and the howling wind shrieking through the rigging, to Amy the world seemed a much more hopeful place. A year was nothing. It would pass in no time and might bring all kinds of good things. Then, as Amy returned to her charts, James returned to the open deck, prepared for the worst of Cape Horn.

But Cape Horn would have seemed as nothing had they known that within the year they had agreed Captain James McBain would become engaged in the greatest battle of his life. With the entire Western world looking on.

Chapter Nineteen

Rain was falling steadily across the East River on a March day in 1851, but it did not stop the work. In the yard at the bottom of Seventh Street, *Wings of America* was almost finished, except for the most important thing of all. Steam engines clattered, puffed and hissed, winches turned and derricks swung as the massive bottom sections of her masts were raised vertically high above and then lowered, steadied with control ropes. On her deck, supervised by builder, designer and sparmaker, workers in dripping clothes stood with upturned faces and upstretched hands to take hold and guide them through, others far below waiting to set the heels to their sturdy steps on the keelson.

From the shelter of a shed, James, Amy, Mr Kimball and Mr Jay stood looking on at the already famous ship which had a constant stream of curious and admiring visitors. From head on, the uptilted concave bows receding to the keel looked as proud as a patroon and as sharp as a razor. From the stern she was as elegantly curved as a glass of champagne. To the mariner's eye, the long, gentle sheer of her fore and aft line was almost humanly seductive and James was itching to get his hands on her.

Even on such a day, the heavy gold ring with the large ruby on Mr Kimball's finger flashed its shining opulence as he gestured with his cigar.

'Up until now, James,' he declared, 'you've only astonished the world. And I mean no disrespect to Mrs McBain's own outstanding beauty when I say that with this graceful lady I think you might astonish God Almighty Himself.'

Mr Jay felt a little irritated at not being able to find anything to add to that, but Amy gave him the opportunity. She was not going to stand there and let Mr Kimball off scot-free.

'I would say the graceful lady, considering she's so large, is somewhat muscular too, Mr Kimball,' she came back at him.

'Exactly said, Mrs McBain,' Jay agreed hurriedly. 'Exactly said.'

James was amused by this little bit of parrying but felt obliged to put in a few words of his own. 'She's a big girl all right,' he commented, 'but wait until all her limbs are on and she's fully clad. My God, what a sight that's going to be. There will be no trifling with this one.'

At least Amy felt pleased that this was to be his last. After his final fling with her there would be no more and he would be safe from any downfall and humiliation. It was more than she could have said for her missing son about whom she knew nothing. More than she could say even for Aunt Dorothea who had already fallen. At first relieved to hear on reaching New York that her aunt had been found, the rush to Boston and Worcester had not only proved to be depressing but fruitless. Despite the comforting of the Garrisons and the warnings of Dr Drew as to what she might expect, she had not only hoped to talk to her aunt like she always had but to question her on where and why Jamie might have gone. But her aunt had had a bad week and was so heavily sedated that she was not even allowed to see her. For four days she had waited before James managed to coax her away from the smell of madness that permeated the home. And Amos Drew could make no predictions whatsoever as to Dorothea Jackson's future.

From the yard, the quartet retreated in Kimball's carriage back to the counting house where Amy was invited to sit in on the discussion around the desk. It did not take long.

'With almost every ship on the seaboard chasing Californian money,' Kimball told James, 'there's no guarantee these profits are going to last. But while it's still going on the fortune now to be made from getting fresh tea directly to England is being somewhat overlooked.'

'Indeed, severely neglected,' Mr Jay amplified.

'The British tongues are hanging out for it,' Kimball went on. 'Prices are going up all the time. London merchants are trying to charter every fast American ship they can lay their hands on for the next season's clippings. But it's first to make England with it who'll get the biggest prize.'

'Get the cream on the cookie,' Mr Jay interjected.

'With any luck, the cost of building *Wings* could be more than paid for in a voyage,' Kimball continued.

'All right, Canton it is,' James said and glanced questioningly at Amy in case she had any objections. As she was not allowed ashore there it was a longer voyage for her than it was for anyone. But Amy wanted to get it all over with.

'I'll check to see if Lieutenant Maury has gathered any further knowledge that might help,' she contributed.

'You see?' James smiled at Mr Kimball and Mr Jay. 'You need

have no qualms whatsoever about who'll be first from China to London. And by a very long way. Without any luck at all that's a guarantee. The prize is in your pocket.'

'The shares the same, James,' Kimball offered finally, or hoped to hell it was final as both he and Mr Jay held their breaths. It was only out of sheer devilment that James hesitated, making them wait as he studied their faces. Although very wealthy men they still stood like hound dogs with bared teeth over their pennies. James was almost an equal partner already in financial terms and without the burden of overheads.

'Agreed, gentlemen,' the captain said at last, bringing smiles of relief.

As there was no secret about these plans, Jamie alias John Marsh, who had recently turned eighteen and was shadowing the captain's every move, had picked up that information within twenty-four hours but it did not really surprise him. Other astute merchants, he had gone out of his way to learn, were thinking the same thing, among them the owner of *Flying Star* which was near to completion in East Boston. Keeping his head well down from being recognised, Jamie had looked both on it and on *Wings of America* and from what he could make out there was little difference between them. But although he felt the time had come, it was with some anxiety he sought out Captain Eastlake. What he did not know about the man already he had taken much trouble to find out and, smartly dressed, looking like a mature and experienced twenty-year-old, he eventually presented himself at Eastlake's home and gained admittance.

'Sir,' he said, introducing himself, 'my name's John Marsh and I'm very keen to serve under you on your new ship as first mate,' and he offered his two excellent references. Eastlake took them but studied the young man for a few moments. There seemed to be something familiar about this mate.

'Do I know you, Mr Marsh?' he asked.

'We've never met, sir,' Jamie replied, 'but I've been an admirer of yours for some good time.'

'Of mine?' Eastlake questioned in surprise. 'Why me?'

'Because, sir, drivers like yourself represent the real backbone of our mercantile marine. Others like McBain have relied solely on dancing with Lady Luck and little else and if you'll forgive me, sir, I must speak my mind. I don't consider Captain McBain in any way deserving of his reputation.'

'My God, Mr Marsh!' Eastlake exclaimed in eager accord. 'I've

211

been trying to tell people that very same thing for years! And you think they would listen? No, they would not!'

'And a man without a soul by all accounts,' Jamie threw in, but he was far from finished with his charming flattery. He had noted before that even the hardest of men were vulnerable to it. Moments later he was expressing his annoyance at all the attention being paid to *Wings of America* just because of McBain when Eastlake's own new vessel was clearly her equal. All in all, Hurricane Jim came in for quite a bit of putting down by Mr Marsh.

It was not only that, however, which attracted Eastlake more and more to this highly sensible mate. In truth he was a little nervous about the big clipper. Masts soaring two hundred feet into the sky were something to think about. There were to be extensions to the yards, too, which could be put out to carry even more canvas in the way of 'studding sails'. And he had not yet been to China himself. Moreover, the references claimed Marsh to be an outstanding navigator and good mates with such qualifications were getting harder and harder to find because of all the new ships being built.

'Canton, of course, is better than Amoy or Ningshien,' Jamie pointed out knowledgeably. 'Good anchorage and I'm familiar with the procedures there.'

John Marsh was not surprised when Mrs Eastlake swept into the room to join them. He had already been told that Eastlake was not allowed to make decisions without consulting her. As much as the captain disliked it, it was part of the price he had had to pay for the saving of his career.

'Ma'am, it's a great pleasure.' Jamie bowed on being introduced and would have kissed her hand like a Frenchman if he had not decided it might be overdoing it. He could sense Eastlake's acute embarrassment as she perused his references. Master aboard the captain might have been, here at home he might as well have been before the mast. Jamie could not have been more attentive as Mrs Eastlake then talked non-stop in forceful voice for a whole ten minutes on the merits and demerits of ships and men.

'It's rare to meet a lady so well informed and perceptive, ma'am,' he was able to say at last.

'It's only a great pity I'm unable to sail myself, Mr Marsh,' she declared, 'but unfortunately God did not see fit to give me the stomach for it.' And Jamie guessed that Eastlake must have been exceedingly grateful to God for His omniscience.

'Do you drink, Mr Marsh?' she demanded to know.

'No, ma'am,' he replied and would have denied taking water had she wanted him to, so important it was to him.

Shortly after, Mrs Eastlake led her mate out of the room, leaving Jamie alone, anxiously waiting with his fingers crossed. There were other options with other new ships he could have tried but none as good as this one. It was ideal for him. Although it seemed much longer, it was only minutes later when they returned.

'My husband has decided to give you the job, Mr Marsh,' the lady announced before the captain could open his mouth, 'and will expect you to do your duty by him at all times.'

'But you'll understand,' Eastlake managed to get in, 'that your wages on *Flying Star* will be not more than they would be for serving on any other East Indiaman.'

'Understood, sir, and you may rest assured, ma'am, it's my duty I will do. I thank you very much.'

The sword was in Jamie's hand and if he felt the weight of it he also felt the power. But there was still much to be done before he could carry it into battle. One task was to find a good second mate he could rely on and who was as eager to drive a vessel as hard as any man. Constantly looking over his shoulder and around corners for fear of being recognised, he combed the bars and lodging houses along the East River. And his perseverance with the addition of a bit of luck turned up Finis Barr. Barr was a young Scot recently arrived in New York who had been a foremast hand on ships sailing out of the Clyde and who had come to America to better himself. Six foot tall, broad-shouldered, dark-haired and dark-eyed, Finis was grateful for John Marsh putting a feather in his cap while Jamie was more than grateful for Finis. And he had no trouble at all in getting Eastlake to agree to signing the man on.

'His name sounds more like a goddamn obstruction to a harbour,' was the only objection the master made.

As the day of the launch of *Wings of America* approached there was mounting excitement in the counting house of Kimball and Jay, and there, too, names were mentioned.

'I'm told our old friend Eastlake's claiming he's got the best first mate in the fleet,' Kimball remarked, and James laughed at that.

'Fallen off the back of the wagon again, has he?'

Only Amy was a little concerned as she worried about the slightest little thing that might prove to be a thorn in the side of James's final ambition.

'What's his name?' she wanted to know.

'Marsh. I think that was it,' Kimball replied.

'It is,' Mr Jay confirmed.

'Never heard of him,' James said dismissively and turned the conversation back to the arrangements for the great day.

*　　*　　*

The huge gilded eagle of a figurehead under the bowsprit, wings back as if at any moment it would swoop up to the heavens, shone brilliantly in the sun and it seemed as if half of New York were there to see it. Amidst a sea of flags and streamers champagne flowed, prayers were said, the bands played, the speeches were made, the hammers rang along the keel and Hurricane Jim's last bride, his ultimate pride and joy, slid astern. On deck, James felt choked with emotion as she hit the river, throwing up great spumes of white water to the thrill of taking life, and the massive cheer resounded right across to Brooklyn. *Wings of America* was born.

There were two other launchings of new clippers along the East River within a week, but neither gripped the public imagination like *Wings*. This was the vessel that everyone knew, under the hands of Hurricane Jim, would show every other ship in the world her heels. Indeed in London there was envy and anger amongst members of the Establishment at all these goings-on and it was in tones of desperation that the London *Times* tried to wake up British ship-builders. It was outraged by the audacity and success of these brash Americans in the New World.

'We must run a race with our gigantic and unshackled rival!' it thundered. 'We must set our long-practised skill, our steady industry, and our dogged determination, against his youth, ingenuity and ardour. It is a father who runs a race with his son and we must not be beaten!'

But neither they nor Captain James McBain nor Amy nor anyone else were aware that the symbolism of that last sentence was about to turn into a frightening reality as John Marsh made his preparations.

As for news of the launch of the *Flying Star* up in East Boston soon afterwards, New Yorkers took a certain amount of pleasure in ignoring her. Indeed, so did Jamie since it would have been much too risky to have appeared anywhere near the East Boston yard. The Garrisons, Dr Drew, Professor Longfellow and many others who knew him were bound to be there. It was not until she lay at anchor ready for her top masts to be added that he slipped quietly aboard during the night.

Ten days later the *Flying Star* weighed anchor to head for New York but hardly had she cleared the Boston Light when big Finis came aft from the direction of the fo'c'sle carrying the lifeless form of a man over his shoulder. He dumped it unceremoniously on the deck at Jamie's feet where it landed face up, its button eyes staring up at him.

'Foreign body, Mr Marsh,' he said and Jamie could see

immediately that it was. Dressed in ragged clothes complete with hat, holed gloves and boots with the soles hanging off, it had never had any life. It was a cleverly made dummy stuffed with straw for which Eastlake the night before had paid a Crimp three whole months of a seaman's wages.

'I'll kill the son-of-a-bitch!' the captain raged. 'I'll kill him! Turn this vessel around, Mr Marsh!'

Anchored back in Boston, Jamie and Finis Barr waited impatiently while for two whole days Eastlake roared around the waterfront like a charging bull in search of his thieving Crimp.

'He's no' in a very great hurry to get to China, is he, Mr Marsh?' Barr commented dryly.

'No,' Jamie smiled, 'but don't worry. Our time will come.'

Barr thought that a rather strange thing to say. He sensed an element of threat in it but made no remark. You did not pry into another man's business.

Unsuccessful, Eastlake returned like a bear with a sore head, but there was to be another short delay when they reached Sandy Hook off New York during the hours of darkness. The tide was on the ebb and pilot or no pilot Eastlake was not going to risk the embarrassment of trying to push against the current and possibly getting into trouble with his new clipper, no matter what assurances his first mate gave him.

'Drop anchor, Mr Marsh,' he ordered, and for another six hours they waited, but as Jamie had been warned by men who had sailed with Eastlake before, that was nothing compared with what was to come.

In the East River, the *Flying Star*, handsome as she was, was regarded as just another new clipper. *Wings of America* was the real star. And it was within sight of her that Jamie sat down and wrote an anonymous letter to the editor of the *New York Herald* so that the world would know. Then he arranged for an acquaintance to mail it, but not until after the very last vessel in the China fleet had sailed.

It was a beautiful, early summer day with blue sky and fleecy white clouds when the fleet weighed anchor and headed out of New York harbour. All except *Wings of America*.

'It's too early,' James declared. 'Another two weeks is plenty of time. There's no point in having to wait in Canton when we can wait here.'

That was not so much a measure of his confidence as consideration for Amy who, not being allowed ashore in Canton and with nothing else to do, was likely to dwell too much on their missing son.

At sea, the rest of the fleet soon spread out on courses of their own until they were all out of sight of each other. And as the *Flying Star* pushed down across the Atlantic, Jamie did more than guide her in the direction where, according to Lieutenant Maury, the doldrums were narrowest at this time of year. As if to varying keys of different wind strengths, John Marsh was never done tuning and retuning the rigging like the strings of a violin, all the time watching the speed and learning what was best for the ship. But what neither Eastlake nor Finis Barr knew was that he was also sandbagging, not making the vessel go as fast as he knew he could drive her. That would have been a mistake. To make too good a time for the passage to Canton would only have alerted the enemy. Instead he made careful calculations to ensure that *Flying Star* would show up no better than the worst of the others. He need not have worried on that score. As he had been warned, Eastlake was about to help him in that area, and it began to happen when they hit their first day of calm.

'The captain's a very happy man today, Mr Marsh,' Finis Barr noted and Jamie was fascinated by all the signs. Eastlake's eyes were almost sparkling as he strode light-footed about, finding fault with nothing. All day he was overanimated, his every gesture that little bit exaggerated. It was as if he were expecting something wonderful to happen. It did. In the morning, Jamie was called to the captain's cabin. He found Eastlake seated there with an unopened bottle of liquor on the table before him, a whole case of it at his feet. He was like a cat tied down on hot bricks.

'Sit down, sit down, Mr Marsh,' he directed and Jamie sat. It was common knowledge that when Eastlake broke the pledge he never did so alone, and that if he was short of volunteers he resorted to conscription. Going to hell with company, it seemed, was much more reassuring than going alone.

'Pour yourself a drink,' he said.

'Thank you, sir,' Jamie replied, and making himself the first sinner broached the bottle and poured one. Hardly had he done so than Eastlake was eagerly grabbing at the bottle to do the same for himself.

'By God, she's a fine ship I have, isn't she?' he beamed, and quickly downed his first in one go. He grimaced, gave a few quick shakes of his head and a little shudder and was launched, topping up Jamie's guilty glass and urging him to help himself. He then started off on a string of reminiscences he clearly thought were funny and before the first bottle was three quarters of the way down it was John instead of Mr Marsh.

Jamie vaguely remembered hearing two bells of the First Dog Watch at five o'clock in the evening. Then he succumbed to oblivion, finished. But Eastlake had only just begun and lurched out on deck.

'Come and take Mr Marsh to his quarters!' he barked. 'He's not feeling well.'

Finis Barr had just managed to get the ship moving again in the lightest of breezes but it was too late, for it was now his turn to join the captain whether he liked it or not. To Finis's credit he somehow succeeded in lasting all night. But the ship, captainless and mateless, drifted about and might have been going around in circles or headed back towards New York for all anyone cared.

After Finis Barr, and with Jamie in hiding in a locker with his suffering, Eastlake worked his way down through the bosun, the bosun's mate, the foremast hand and anyone else while he ordered the carpenter to make a set of bowls and skittle pins in order to show off his expertise in a bowling alley. But the quarterdeck of a ship rolling in a swell from side to side like a pig in swill was not quite the best place to prove it, especially when the self-acclaimed champion's legs kept buckling under him and the bowls quickly disappeared down the scuppers.

For three whole days, Eastlake kept his spree going without once closing his eyes. Then for another two he lay on his bunk in his darkened cabin like a dead man. On the sixth day he rose.

Men tried to avert their eyes when he reappeared on deck but they were given no chance to avoid the matter. Eastlake ordered all hands to be assembled on the afterdeck. He waited until they were all there and settled. Then, without a word, he picked up a bucket of Atlantic Ocean he had had placed there and poured it over his head as if in some ceremony of renewal or self-baptism. After that, he picked up a lash as if to reinstate his authority, pulled himself to his full height and like a red-hot evangelist threatening them all with damnation let forth in full voice on the evils of drink. If Jamie had ever had any doubts about whether he had chosen the right ship and the right master, they were all now dispelled.

The letter opened at the *New York Herald* caused an immediate stir of excitement. But it was also puzzling. Who was this man who not only had the impudence to denigrate Hurricane Jim but was daring to challenge him to prove his supremacy? No one had ever dared to do such a thing before. McBain was paramount. Other captains often raced against each other on a run on the issue of challenges but never against McBain. That would only have resulted in making a fool of themselves. And why did the man want to remain anonymous? He could not stay so for long. Which captain of what ship was so eager to suffer the humiliation of having Hurricane Jim chop his head off and have it laughed at as it rolled bloodily down the streets at the feet of the public? As *Wings of America* had sailed two days before, McBain could not be questioned on the matter, and neither could anyone else. The only way of communicating with China was by ship and they had all gone. It could have been a hoax but then who was the intended victim? The *Herald* had nothing to lose by reporting information it had been given, no matter how outrageous it appeared. Whoever was doing this was very clever. Delivery of the letter had clearly been delayed so that Captain McBain himself would know nothing about it and that was what made the mystery all the more serious. The news was put aboard the very first packet bound for London where it would reach the London *Times* and eventually spread like fire.

In no time, all the seaports on the Eastern Seaboard of America and throughout Europe waited in anticipation, and rumours abounded. It was said that the stakes for the winner were to be as high as a hundred thousand dollars, but they were not to know that the prize was going to be far beyond the measure of money.

Chapter Twenty

Making his way through the teeming waterfront of Canton, Jamie cautiously avoided attracting any undue attention as he worked his way towards the premises of the Christian undertaker. If Chinese lookouts were keeping an eye on him, he knew it was only to ensure he did not try to go near the forbidden 'City of Rams' which lay behind the great warehouses and on which no foreign devil was ever allowed to gaze.

When *Flying Star* had eventually reached Macao and paused by the old Portugese factory there to get entry clearance, pick up the Chinese pilot and go on upstream past the forts to the anchorage at Whampoa Reach, it came as no surprise to Jamie to learn that his ship was the last of the American tea clipper fleet to reach there. Apart from his own delaying tactics, Eastlake had twice repeated his pledge-ripping performance on the long passage. No surprise either to be told that, despite being last to leave New York, *Wings of America* had been the first vessel in.

In an alley, he entered a door on which a bell tinkled and stood at a counter. Around him were two blank headstones, a vase of flowers, a large, plain wooden cross and a gaudily painted figure of Mary and Child on a plinth. After a moment, Lymann Cobb in silk suit appeared from the back through a beaded curtain. It was the first time Jamie had seen him close up. He was tall with a pronounced stoop to the shoulders of his thin frame, aged probably in his late thirties, and under the dark eyebrows that arched right across his brow without a break was a longish face.

'Can I help you, sir?' Cobb asked, but with little interest.

'I'd like to speak to you in private,' Jamie told him, and he could tell that the undertaker was immediately a little worried by that. Since no one else was there, it was private as it was.

'You can speak free here, sir,' Cobb said.

'In private, Mr Cobb,' Jamie repeated firmly. Cobb hesitated, trying not to look suspicious. Then he nodded for Jamie to come around the counter and follow him through the curtain. Behind, Jamie quickly took in the exotic Chinese furnishings, the jade figures, the ivory carvings and silver. Tied to a stake with a light chain was a small monkey who bared its teeth at his presence.

'Sit down,' Cobb offered and both of them sat at the black lacquered table inlaid with mother-of-pearl. Cobb waited for his visitor to state his business.

'My name's John Marsh,' Jamie opened, 'but if you're willing to forget it, I'll be more than willing to forget yours.'

Cobb, not yet having acquired full inscrutability, had trouble disguising his growing anxiety at that and made no reply. If only he had been warned that this Marsh was coming to see him, he might have been able to do something about it. As it was, he had been taken by surprise.

'You have a very good business here, Mr Cobb,' Jamie went on, 'and I'm sure you wouldn't want to see anything go wrong with it.'

'What in the hell are you talking about?'

'My cousins, Mr Cobb.'

'Cousins?'

'My sadly missed British cousins. Their names were Smith, Jones and Brown and surely you must have heard of them since you buried them all. What I was wondering was whether the Chinese authorities would give me permission to have their bodies disinterred so I can take their bones back to England.'

Lymann Cobb's mouth fell half open at that but he was not an idiot. He knew full well that he was staring blackmail full in the face. Had the features been those of a villain he could have dealt with it, like to like, but they were not. Instead he saw a suntanned, sea-weathered, clean-shaven face with cool, determined blue eyes looking out of it. He had a strange feeling he had seen it somewhere before but could not remember where or when. But it was worse, much worse, than any villain's could ever be. He was frightened. This Marsh, clearly a deck officer, was a young man on some kind of personal mission, the kind who was prepared to burn in hell for principle rather than alter his course, the most dangerous kind of creature there was.

'What is it you want, Mr Marsh?'

'What I want, Mr Cobb, is for a man to be put aside for a while but I'd also want a guarantee he'd come to no harm.'

Lymann Cobb tried not to gape at him. Jesus, he was talking about kidnapping and it had to be someone important.

'That's not my line,' he tried to protest.

'I know that, Mr Cobb,' Jamie returned, 'and I wouldn't expect you to risk your fortune and your liberty by doing it yourself, no more than I would. But I'm sure you must have lots of good Chinese friends who'd be able to help. In fact I guess it would suit us both very well if this man happened to be taken by pirates for ransom. You know of any clever pirates who can be trusted, Mr Cobb?'

'I know of no goddamn pirates,' Cobb hissed, still hoping he might somehow escape.

'What a pity,' James said, and rose to leave.

'Wait a minute, wait a minute! For Christ's sake wait a minute!' Cobb shouted.

And Jamie sat down again, ready to detail exactly what he wanted, even producing a roll of dollars so that Lymann Cobb, smuggler of Indian opium and undertaker to countless bags of consecrated pebbles, would not find himself out of pocket over his expenses. As Mr Marsh pointed out, 'Nothing could be fairer than that, Mr Cobb.'

Miles downstream, Amy stood at the port bulwarks of *Wings of America* swinging at anchor off the island there, watching all the visitors circling around. It had not only been the Russians, the Swedes, the French and all the other shipowners' agents who had left their counting houses in Canton to come down and gaze in wonderment and envy on the latest great American clippers but the Chinese too. There had been a constant stream of them. Mandarin boats, flower boats, junks and sampans of all kinds, some of them trying to sell everything from fruit to monkeys. But if Amy was watching, she was not seeing. Her mind was everywhere else: New England, New York, California, and indeed roaming over half of America wondering where her son might be, what he was doing, how he was, why he so resented her that he did not think she even deserved a note of reassurance. It made all the years of struggling with him and loving him seem so futile. 'It is giving, not receiving, that makes life worthwhile', poor Aunt Dorothea had told her so many times, but all the sayings and supposedly wise proverbs in the world could not salve the ache. Indeed, she had long since come to the conclusion that the men who devised them so glibly had never experienced the ailments for which they offered such cures. But now there was something else. Over the previous few days she had begun to suffer a growing sense of unease, almost a nagging fear, but could find no explanation for it. Everything around her was as it should have been and she only hoped she was not coming down with some sickness. She turned away from the many Chinese eyes who were as much fascinated by the American lady sailor as they were by her clipper and went into the cabin where James was rechecking his figures. He knew almost to the ounce how much tea he would be able to load, but tea being light there had to be the exact weight of ballast to go with it for perfect trim which in turn meant optimum speed. It had been very satisfying to cut ten days off his own record between New York and Macao in his beautiful new ship but what was all important now was to make a time to London which would stand forever. That and seeing Amy happy as a lady of leisure were the most important things in his life. His only dilemma was whether to announce his forthcoming retirement in London or wait until he got back home to New York. He was also very much aware of Amy's concern and for that reason alone was impatient to get back to sea where she would be kept busy again.

'It won't be long now,' he said, hoping it might give some little comfort, 'and who knows what news might be waiting for us in England.'

In the large open-sided drying sheds along the Canton shoreline, the fresh tea pickings were being prepared for packing into their chests, many of which were made with one curved side so they could fit against the curved inside of the hull and cut out any wasted space.

Two days later, the great tea-deckers with their lacquered sides and single tall masts, all carrying enormous loads of the tea chests, came downstream to tie up by the waiting ships and start loading, every Chinese master with a whip in his hand ready to lay it across the backs of any native workers who dragged their heels. The whole of Whampoa Reach became a hive of ceaseless activity, the waters crowded.

The junk that came alongside the *Flying Star* was hardly noticed among it all and the respectably dressed Chinaman who clambered aboard with a written message addressed to Captain Eastlake was only another figure among many.

'Damn,' Eastlake swore on reading it, 'can't they ever get anything right?'

The owner's agents wanted to see him as soon as possible to sort out an adjustment to the promissory note offered to the Chinese 'Hong' for payment of cargo, not at all an unusual occurrence but a nuisance. The wealthy Chinese merchants were well known for their trust and honesty but some much more so than others.

'Take over, Mr Marsh,' Eastlake ordered his first mate and even Jamie was a little surprised at the efficiency with which his own instructions were carried out. Eastlake fetched his satchel of papers and boarded the junk to be taken up to Canton. But only Jamie kept an eye on it as, among the many other boats jamming the sea roads, it made its way upstream. It was in horror that he eventually saw it turn around and start back down. His heart leapt to his mouth in case Eastlake had somehow woken up to what was happening. But then the junk headed for the western side of the island and kept on sailing downstream and away towards Macao and God knew where else. On top of the relief he could only pray that Eastlake would come to no harm but felt that Lymann Cobb would have taken the greatest trouble to ensure his safety, in the belief that he was finished if Eastlake so much as lost a finger. Then he felt almost overwhelmed by the excitement. There was only one small hurdle to go and the *Flying Star* was his.

Finis Barr climbed up a rope ladder out of the hold and over the edges of the hatch with a look of amazement on his face. 'My God, Mr Marsh,' he said, 'have you seen the way they pack them in? You couldn't stick a prayer between them.'

'Yes, I know,' Jamie replied and told him that the captain had had to go back up to Canton to sign some adjustments.

'Well, I hope he signs something else while he's at it, Mr Marsh. There's nothing I like better than a wee dram but the captain's gaed me the worst sore heads I've ever had in my life and that includes the time a spar split my skull open.'

In torchlight, the arrival of more tea-deckers and the loading work on all tea clippers went on through the night, and it was just after dawn when the owner's agents, Mason and Wintruffe, came alongside in a boat wearing tall hats and anxious expressions.

'I expected Captain Eastlake might be with you, sirs,' Jamie greeted them when they reached the deck.

'We want to speak to you alone, Mr Marsh,' said Wintruffe, the taller of the two, and Jamie led them to the main cabin.

'Before we say anything,' Wintruffe gloomily requested, 'we want you to swear to the Almighty that you won't repeat it. For Captain Eastlake's safety that is absolutely essential.'

'I swear,' Jamie said, looking suitably concerned.

With Mason, very serious of face but saying little, Wintruffe told how Eastlake had been kidnapped by pirates, an abominable act, and that the ruffians would let them know within two or three weeks what ransom they wanted for his safe return. In the meantime, if the news reached the Chinese authorities or anyone else before that, Captain Eastlake would have his throat cut. It was almost word for word what Jamie had told Lymann Cobb to say but it sounded so much worse on hearing it back from the solemn mouth of Mr Wintruffe.

'I can hardly believe it,' Jamie said.

'Neither can we,' Mason agreed. 'The devils have kidnapped before, of course, but not Americans, and never so blatantly right off a ship lying here at anchor on the Reach.'

'But there it is, Mr Marsh,' Wintruffe went on. 'Needless to say we'll be doing all in our power to get him back safe but it might take some time – even months – and this is an extremely valuable cargo you're loading. Tea of the very highest quality. You get our point? It can't be left here indefinitely to go mouldy and we don't keep spare captains in Canton. There's the possibility we might be able to get one from Shanghai but that would take far too long and he might know very little or nothing about a vessel like this. It's in the interest of the owner she must not be delayed a day more than necessary. You know what I'm saying, Mr Marsh? You'll have to assume responsibility as master and get her to London. You have no choice. How you explain Captain Eastlake's absence to your crew is up to you but we'd advise you not to say anything at all until you're weighing anchor. For pilotage and port clearance purposes we'll notify the port authorities you've been appointed as the *Flying Star*'s new captain.'

Jamie's hand was almost shaking when he was asked to sign the alterations to the ship's papers. His sword was sharper than the pen and he could feel its razor's edge, ready to be raised.

Shortly after, Mr Wintruffe and Mr Mason were gripping his hand in turn, wishing him Godspeed and fair weather, and were gone.

'Mr Barr!' Jamie called and led Finis Barr back inboard.

'What did they want?' Finis asked when they were alone, since he could tell something had happened.

'You're not to breathe a word of this until we sail, Finis,' Jamie told him. 'That's their strict instruction.'

'Cut ma throat and hope to die, Mr Marsh.'

'You don't have to go that far,' Jamie said, not wanting to hear the expression again, 'but Captain Eastlake has suffered a serious misfortune.'

'Sacked?'

'In a manner of speaking. I have to take over as master so now you become first mate.'

Finis Barr could not have been more delighted. America was all he had been told it would be. A land of quick fortune and no waiting to step into a dead man's shoes. Foremost hand to first mate on an American clipper all within less than a year.

'Then it's faster we'll make her go this time, Mr Marsh.'

Jamie felt tempted to unload himself and bare his soul to Finis Barr. It had been a very lonely existence since the day he had walked out of Harvard and set out on his course. There was no one he had been able to confide in. But although he trusted Barr implicitly, he decided it might not be wise. Not yet.

'Faster even than you think, Finis. We're about to challenge Hurricane Jim.'

Finis Barr's eyes might have popped out at that had they not been so well embedded and he could not find a word to say.

'What's more, I want him to know it. It could rattle him and give us an advantage. But I went a long way with Captain McBain once and I don't want him to know it's me. As he knows my writing I want you to pen the note. I'll tell you what to say.'

'Are you being quite serious, Mr Marsh?' Finis asked, finding voice.

'It's been the ambition of my life, Mr Barr.'

Jamie's ambition had been for so long inflamed that he had not once allowed himself to think of the possibility of failure and had made no provision for it. That was left for Finis Barr to worry about and worry he did. He liked Marsh and had the greatest respect for him but on openly insisting on taking on Hurricane Jim his friend was asking to be left with the wounds of defeat and blushes on his face for the rest of his life. It would not be Captain John Marsh everyone would remember but something more like 'Limpin' Jack'. But he did not say so.

Sweat glistened on ranks of Chinese bodies and the river reflected hundreds of paper lanterns as the second night of loading went on, chop boats and junks delivering the last of the victualling and fresh water supplies. Pigs squealed and chickens squawked as they were tossed into their barnyards. On *Wings of America* a seaman appeared up over the bulwarks with a note addressed to Captain James McBain, handed it to the first man within his reach and disappeared again before he could be questioned. James was standing on the quarterdeck when it was given to him and in order to read it without the interruptions of flickering shadows, took it into the cabin where Amy was going over her charts in careful pre-planning for the voyage. As soon as the last tea chest was in place the hatches would be battened down and all the tea ships would be scrambling to be off. She looked up as James read, saw the initial worried and rather angry expression turn into a smile.

'What is it?' she wanted to know.

'Nothing,' James replied, now appearing very amused. 'I thought it might happen one day. Our friend's finally lost his tops'ls.'

There was a time when he would have been driven to fury by such an insulting note. Might even have rammed a man's ship for it. Now, famous, successful and wealthy as well as emotionally secure, he could afford to be much more understanding of other men's envy and failures. Amy went to him, took the message from his hand and devoured it quickly with concern.

'What in heaven's name does it mean?' was her first reaction.

'What it means, my dear Amy,' he told her, 'is that he's got a bottle in each hand and is about to try and walk on water by falling over the side. But don't worry. I'm not going to lower myself to his stupid level by answering it. He wouldn't be in any condition to read it anyway. The best insult I can give him back is to show him our stern and be discharging in London while he's still in the middle of the Atlantic, which is the way it's going to be.' And with that he went quite happily back on deck. Amy looked at the note again. It was insulting all right. 'Sir,' it said:

'For too long you have deceived people into believing you are monarch of the sea, putting yourself above all other men when, if the truth be known, the only substance of your sovereignty is a lack of care for others cloaked in your own conceit. The captain should therefore know his luck has run out and his rule is almost ended. No longer will you command the salutations of the public which you have so craved above all else. You are now challenged on the time of your passage to London by my vessel and should know that the eyes of the world are on you, waiting to bear witness to your defeat.

> Captain,
> *Flying Star*

Amy could not laugh it off. The more she looked at it, the more deeply anxious she became. It did not seem at all to her like the outpourings of an angry drunk. It was too well composed. The words appeared to have been carefully chosen and were written in a strong, steady, copperplate hand, not scribbled. There was an undisguised bitterness to them, the sense of a perfectly serious and genuine threat with no hollow ring to it. And as much as she might have wished to deny it, there was even an element of truth. And what was meant by the suggestion that the world was already watching for the outcome when the world could not possibly have known? Why had Eastlake neglected to add his signature? It became so darkly sinister she felt a twisting of her stomach. It was as if the piece of paper she held in her hand was the cause of her fears over the previous few days, as if by some prescience of mind it was what she had been expecting. So disturbed did she become that rationality deserted her. Donning a dark cloak and putting on a seaman's hat, making sure no one noticed her, she slipped over the clear side of the busy ship and down a rope ladder into the smaller of the two boats. Untying it, intent solely on facing Eastlake, she grabbed two of the oars and began to row across the bustling river of the night in the direction of the *Flying Star*.

At the foremast, Finis Barr stroked the bell once as a five-minute warning to a change of watch and began to come aft. He was still feeling astonished by the contents of what Marsh had asked him to write. 'You sure he won't kill us?' he had queried nervously. 'No,' the new master assured him with a smile, 'but it should stir him and that will be a help.' Then he caught sight of the figure climbing over the side on to the deck and stopped. With all the torches and lanterns he could see almost at once it was a woman, and not a Chinese one. As there was only one white woman known to be on Whampoa Reach, the lady navigator on *Wings of America*, he fully expected her to be followed by her husband brandishing a pistol and howling for the master's blood.

'Mr Marsh, Mr Marsh!' he shouted as a warning. 'A boarding to port!' And he quickly stuck his head over the side to see how many of them might be coming to the attack, surprised to find that there was no one else and only the empty boat there.

From near the mizzen, Jamie came hurrying, but when he was still a good five yards from the boarded figure he stopped dead in his tracks. The two stood transfixed, staring at each other, mother and son face to face. Amy had no idea what exactly she had been going to do and now she had walked into what might as well have been a dream. For the first few seconds it was not Jamie at all, but someone else who was just as familiar. So unexpected and out of context was he here on a ship in Canton, her mind would not at first accept it. And, of course, he had matured into a man. It was as if she had suddenly run into someone she had known intimately all her life and just as suddenly forgotten his name.

Finis Barr stood looking from one to the other. If he could not see the lines being thrown to pull John Marsh and Mrs McBain together, he could feel them and could not understand. He watched the woman step tentatively towards the new captain as if unable to believe what she was actually seeing.

'Is it you?' he heard her ask in doubt. 'Is it really you?' And he could tell, he could see, he could feel that Marsh was unable to reply because he was choked with emotion. It was even more revealing when, to his amazement, Marsh held out his hand to her and she took it. Then, without either of them uttering a further word, the emotionally charged couple started towards his cabin, Marsh leading her.

'Jesus save us,' Finis exclaimed under his breath. This was an assignation if he had ever seen one. The two were reunited lovers or his name was not Barr. It was not the first time an older woman had bowled over a younger man and Mrs McBain was an exceptionally pretty woman. But the risk! Christ save us again. The letter to McBain started to make sense to him. The challenge was not so much about ships but about one man wanting to steal another man's wife. And the man was no less a person than Hurricane Jim!

But Finis Barr was a loyal man and the protection of his captain became his first priority. Trying not to think of his friend already bunking the lovely lady, he nevertheless visualised McBain arriving at any moment with a boatload of armed seamen, intent on nothing less than waging bloody war and rescuing his wife. Or maybe killing her instead. He collected up the new watch, ordered them to arm themselves with marlin spikes, knives and belaying pins and posted them right around the ship on lookout, instructing them that anyone except the Chinese still loading was to be repelled at all costs, no matter who they were. Then he took up his own stance facing in the direction of *Wings of America* and, with eyes searching every movement across the dark water reflecting a myriad lights, stayed there.

In the cabin, in the wake of disbelief and improbability, the shock and amazement still with her, Amy clung to Jamie in tears of overwhelming joy while Jamie, himself wet-eyed, held her. A whirlpool of questions began to spin dizzily in Amy's head but it was a while before passions would allow either of them to speak.

'What are you doing here?' Amy blurted out at last. 'How did you get here? – where have you been? – look at you – what have you been doing all this time? – why did you run away like that? – was it because of me? – why have you been hiding? – what are you doing on this ship? – why didn't you ever write to me?' And assuming, since she knew he hated everything to do with the sea, that he must somehow have been there against his will, threw in for comfort, 'And don't worry, Jamie, we'll get you off here and quick.' He looked so much like his father.

'Mother, wait a minute,' Jamie managed to get in and very briefly explained how he had been willingly at sea for more than two years and did not want to get off. But that was only the first thing to leave her speechless and also temper her rapture, particularly after two more tight, spontaneous embraces when a sliver of clarity crept into her wild confusion and she not only remembered why she had come but became aware that it was in the captain's cabin she was standing. There was something out of joint and she could sense it.

'Where is Captain Eastlake?' she asked.

'He's been temporarily indisposed and won't be making the voyage but for his own safety it's not to be known. You must promise not to mention it. Not to anyone.'

'Has this First Mate Marsh taken over as master, then?'

'Yes.'

'I must see him, Jamie.'

'You're seeing him, Mother. It's me.'

Amy could only gape at him at first.

'You're Marsh?'

'Yes, and the new master.'

Amy gaped yet again. Apart from all else, even if he did look older to most people, to Amy he was her child and only eighteen. To be captain of a clipper at that age seemed inconceivable. But as if that were not enough she was thrown into yet further turmoil as the full and frightening realisation of the situation began to strike and sink home.

'You?' she breathed aghast. 'You wrote that to your father?' and needed no answer. It might as well have been James standing there before her. My God, it was a Captain James McBain. Another one. So much younger and still with the arrogance of youth shining out of his eyes. 'In God's name, Jamie, what are you doing?'

'What I have to.'

'Why, for God's sake, why? *Why*?'

'Because if I don't I'll never be me, that's why. But if you can't understand that, please just try and accept it. For me, Mother, please.'

'You'll never do it, Jamie, never! You'll never beat your father!' And immediately wished she had not said it. Not that it made any difference. She knew that no matter what she did or said there was going to be no changing Jamie's mind.

'I want you to swear you'll not let him know it's me,' he asked of her. 'He must think it's Eastlake.'

For so long Amy had prayed for Jamie's return and now she had so unexpectedly found him, it was only to also find herself facing the greatest dilemma of her life. It was son against father, her child against her husband, and it was with desperation that she wanted to help both but could not help either. For a few mad moments she contemplated staying with Jamie as his navigator but instinct alone told her of the complications and chaos that would have resulted. She also knew she had to hurry if she was not to be missed. Not finding her in the main cabin, James would assume she had gone to rest and would not disturb her, but her time was limited.

Finis Barr was not in the slightest surprised to see that the lady looked shaken as John Marsh, holding her hand, eventually led her back out on to the deck but he still could not wait for her to get off and be gone. He turned his head away as the couple embraced again but with all the noise going on with the loading, he could not hear her words.

'Try to keep up across the China Sea if you can,' she said to Jamie with concerned urgency. 'I know every reef on the courses I'll be taking. But after the Sunda Strait only God can help you.'

Out of the corner of his eye, Finis saw Marsh help her over the side and back down into her boat. He breathed an enormous sigh of relief as he saw her row away to be quickly lost in the light-flickering darkness. But if he thought the chances of war had been narrowly avoided, he was still to learn that the battle was just about to begin.

'Bring the boats aboard and hoist signal for the pilot, Mr Barr,' Jamie told him. Finis could have pointed out that they were still taking on the cargo and since it was dark the signal would not be seen but his thoughts only showed in a slight hesitation. Jamie read even that. 'We've got to be ready to be one of the first away,' he explained.

By daylight the conditions were ideal. A light breeze was coming down the river and Jamie got his pilot. But before the last few chests were in place, he could see *Wings of America* starting to weigh anchor and raise sail.

'Weigh anchor, Mr Barr,' he ordered to Finis's surprise. They were still attached to a tea-decker. But Finis did not argue. In minutes men were raising the anchor on the capstan, others scurrying aloft to unfurl sail, others to the sheets and braces. The hatches of the *Flying Star* were still open, the master of the tea-decker screaming complaints in Cantonese as he tried to release his securing lines, when Jamie took off, right on the heels of *Wings of America*.

Two hundred feet into the air the sword flew her banners to the rising sun and the greatest conflict ever between two men and two ships was under way.

Chapter Twenty-One

From a distance *Wings of America* looked to be a sight of unqualified grace and magnificence as she ran under full sail on a course south down the China Sea in a fresh north-easterly. She might have been some gigantic, mythical, wave-skimming bird created by the god Aeolus himself, solely for his own and Neptune's pleasure, a creature totally unconnected with the tiny specks of humanity who walked the earth with all their mortal frailties. That was an illusion. From a distance one did not hear the curses, did not see the straining of muscle, the blood and sweat and the tearing out of men's fingernails.

Standing on his quarterdeck, James barked at his first mate Mr Dyson, urging him with instructions for an extra fraction of a knot of speed to be coaxed out of her. On deck, seamen with corn-hardened hands hauled like horses, others aloft using the agility of monkeys and the strength of gorillas. More than a dozen times over several days James had altered course, trying to shake off the *Flying Star*, but every time he had done so the *Flying Star* had not only altered course too but had quickly manoeuvred herself into a position where she could continue to steal some of his wind by holding him partly in its shadow, restricting his speed. He had done everything he could to get rid of her. As there was no moon and with scudding cloud above he had ordered the dousing of all lights at night in the hope that the man he believed to be Eastlake might lose sight of him when he altered course yet again in the dark. But it was not only the stealing of his wind. By covering closely the *Flying Star* was taking advantage of Amy's expert skills and her knowledge of the position of the uncharted reefs since, although they could be distinguished easily enough in daylight by a man aloft noting the discolouration of the water and giving warning, at night it was another matter. So much so that many a cautious master dropped his anchor between sunset and sunrise in certain areas rather than risk going aground.

'Damn and curse him,' James swore as on yet another dawn he looked astern to see the *Flying Star* off his port quarter, close enough to be still interfering with his wind but far enough away for no one on her deck to be identified. But if he was getting extremely annoyed with the unreliable pledge-breaker, Amy could only marvel at Jamie's tactics and say nothing about it. They were both clever and nerveless. But she agonised for him as she no more believed that her son could keep it up than James believed that Eastlake could. As James and everyone else knew, Eastlake had his good days and his bad and these just happened to be a few of his good ones. But although he was certain they would end soon, it did not stop him from getting angrier. Every hour of time was important and, for the sake of these few good days, the man was getting in his way, holding him up.

'What are you doing?' Amy asked him as he ordered wind to be spilled to slow the ship.

'I'm going to give the stupid puke a piece of my mind,' he told her and fetched his large, polished copper loudhailer, waiting for the *Flying Star* to come up.

On board the *Flying Star* where Finis Barr and the crew were being driven every bit as hard, Jamie immediately saw the flapping of sail off his starboard bow and, guessing his father's intention, wasted no time in ordering the same, slowing his ship to keep his distance.

'Who in the hell does he think he is?' James shouted in frustration when he realised his shadower was not going to come up. But neither the wind nor anyone else gave him an answer. For a full ten minutes he waited until he could stand the delay no longer. Shouting to Dyson he had the crew hauling hard again to trim sail and get her back up to full speed. Then, looking grimly determined, he went into the cabin, an anxious Amy following. She watched him study her charts for the position and course and after a few moments he found what he was looking for. He put his finger on an uncharted, submerged reef Amy had previously marked in by hand.

'There,' he said, 'if we alter course, at the present speed we could pass there some time during the night. Am I right?'

Amy did not have to do any calculations or use the dividers to see at once that he was. Neither did she have to be told what James was going to do. He was going to go hell for leather at the reef in the darkness, bear away at the very last minute and let the *Flying Star* go right on to it.

'You can't, James, you can't!' she cried.

'Why can't I?' James questioned, somewhat taken aback by the depth of concern in her protest.

'Because!' Amy argued. 'You just can't! It's immoral!'

'Amy,' James explained patiently, 'there's nothing immoral about it. I'm responsible for the safety of my ship and my crew and the captain of the *Flying Star* is responsible for his. These are the rules of the sea and you know it. We are not his keeper. If he chooses to take our wind and follow our courses exactly without proper navigational care of his own, it's his own lookout.'

That was all true and Amy knew it. There were many instances where one hard-driving captain had tricked his opposition into going aground. It was a hard life. It was what racing and the competition of life was about. In desperation for Jamie, Amy grasped at anything.

'And what if someone gets killed?' she demanded.

'What *is* the matter with you, Amy?' James asked.

'Why should you think something's the matter with me when I'm only trying to be reasonable?'

'But it's not reasonable. In weather like this, no one is going to get killed.'

James knew very well he was behaving badly. He had never condoned the idea of wrecking another man's ship and although he had never said so he regarded it as neither gentlemanly nor good seamanship. But for the sake of making his unbeatable record from China to England he was prepared for once to overlook his principles and say anything to justify himself.

'You'll only have to waste more time standing by to see they're safe,' Amy pointed out in futility.

'I know that, but a few more hours will be a lot better than having to put up with this day after day. Goddamnit, it's not as if the man stands any chance. He must know that himself. But he's trying to spoil my start out of sheer malice and I'm taking no more of him.'

'You're just going to leave him there stranded on a reef?'

'Of course I am if he's safe and acknowledges it. And I can't see him doing anything else. He won't want us standing laughing at his humiliation. He'll probably haul himself off in a couple of days, make his repairs and go on the way he always does. And with no one to blame but himself.'

There was nothing Amy could say. Nothing. But apart from praying she had to find something she could do. In her distress she found it difficult to think.

As darkness fell, distant thunder and lightning rumbled and flashed to the west but it was far away. Above, the sky was clear, the great velvet canopy twinkling brightly with stars. Jamie who had been taking a rest fully clad felt himself being roughly shaken by the strong hand of Finis Barr and was awake in an instant.

'They're changing course again,' Finis told him and Jamie sprang to his feet to get out on deck, giving Finis his orders as he went to harden up his ship as *Wings of America* was doing, going much higher to the wind on a fast reach. On both ships, all hands were called, and yet again men fought hard with sheets and braces, both crews fully occupied. It was then that Jamie noticed something else.

'What in the hell is that?' he shouted to Finis, pointing to *Wings of America*. Being lowered over the stern was what appeared to be a lantern. Obviously on a line, it stopped, swinging under the counter only a few feet above the waves. Finis looked at it but tough as he was there was an element of Celtic feyness to him.

'It's either the eye of a spauldrochie merman or some kind of signal, sir,' he replied but guessed almost at once it was a message from the lovely lady to his captain. So did Jamie and hurried to his charts. His mother was giving him some kind of warning. It could not have been anything else. He studied his position. Clearly marked on his charts were the routes of safe passage he had taken care to learn on his previous voyage to Canton. This new heading was taking him well out of them. He had to make a decision, whether to run off and take the safe route he knew or stick with *Wings of America* and harass his father further. He did not have to think about it for long. The captain would not have been doing this unless it was unsettling him and for Jamie that was an advantage. He would hold his course and keep *Wings of America* in as much of the shadow of the wind as he could.

'Put three lookouts aloft and another on the bowsprit,' he ordered Finis, 'and keep putting down the leadline. All hands will stand by to make the quickest change of course they've probably ever made in their lives. The problem is I can't tell you whether it's going to be to port or starboard until it happens so every man has to stay on his toes and be ready.'

On *Wings of America*, not even James could see the light swinging under his stern, but he too had all hands standing by their belaying pins while all Amy could do was check her position over and over again with the log constantly being put down, hold her breath and pray.

It was three o'clock in the morning when James yelled his orders to Dyson and *Wings of America* suddenly began to bear away and run off. But as quick as the fully alert Jamie was to react, he was hardly quick enough. No sooner were his yards fully swung and he had gone only a little way on when the hull shuddered in a grinding of keel on reef, bringing the hearts of seamen to their mouths. And

234

to Jamie's and Finis Barr's too. If it was only moments it seemed a lot longer as Jamie sprang to the wheel and spun it further out of the helmsman's hands. In that brief eternity they were off, to a cessation of the grinding, and clear, back into deeper water. Nothing could have been closer.

On the afterdeck of *Wings of America* James looked astern in astonishment. He could hardly believe that Eastlake could have been so alive. It was almost as if he had been standing by with all hands, waiting for it. For Amy, whose knuckles were white from grasping tightly at the stern rail, there had been a few moments when she felt she would faint. And now that all her prayers had been answered, she could almost have wept with the overwhelming relief. But she was unable to do either. At the first opportunity when no one was looking she crouched swiftly with a knife and cut the line, letting it and the lantern sink to the sea.

Finis Barr, quickly over his own relief, looked outraged. He thought McBain might have been justified in doing such a thing to John Marsh because of Mrs McBain but not to himself and the rest of the crew. 'And me all this time giving him my respect,' he said. 'God Almighty, he deliberately tried to wreck us! Well, Hurricane Jim or no Hurricane Jim, I'll no' forgive him for that, sir.'

'Good,' Jamie smiled. 'Now you can concentrate on helping me beat him to London.'

'Aye, I will, sir, I will indeed,' Finis promised, 'and it'll give me the greatest pleasure o' my life if we can do it.'

Only seven days after clearing Macao *Wings of America* sighted the Sunda Strait between Sumatra and Java and James might have been a very happy man at the time he had made over the first two thousand miles. Instead, he spent much more time looking aft than he did forward, and with an increasingly worried expression on his face. The *Flying Star* was still no more than a mile behind him. Over and over he secretly and silently tried to will Eastlake into a mortal thirst for his grog but the man refused to oblige him. He even thought of lowering a buoyed case of it over the side as a temptation for him to pick up but decided the gesture would be far too obvious.

In the narrow Strait, the wind fell to a whimper and died but there was no opportunity for what would have been a much welcome rest. From the Sumatra shore came a flotilla of sampans, propelled with vigour by large oars at their sterns. But if they gave the impression of being overeager traders, neither captain was in any doubt that they were pirates. For several hours the crews on both ships were fully occupied in cutting free grappling hooks and clubbing attempting boarders over the skulls with belaying pins before they retreated empty-handed. Then the lightest of breezes began to come in from the south-east.

'Faster, damn you, Mr Dyson!' James roared as the yards were swung and the sheets came on to take every last ounce of advantage of it. And soon, with the breeze filling all the time, the two clippers were heading on a reach south-west into the Indian Ocean. In very little time both vessels were up to good speeds, *Flying Star* still less than a mile behind.

'Ease all sheets, Mr Barr,' Jamie directed, and Finis looked at him in surprise. To do that meant slowing her, but it was not his place to argue. He relayed the order and came aft again with a questioning look on his face. *Wings of America* was already starting to creep further away from them.

'Don't worry, Mr Barr,' Jamie told him, 'I want him to think he's got away. It might help to take the edge off him. We'll also take a course a little further south so he loses sight of us all the quicker. Then over his horizon we'll go again, Mr Barr, and go like hell. Let the crew know in case they think I've given up.'

Suddenly the light flooded into Finis's brain. He was learning more about John Marsh all the time. He had cunning as well as courage. The fox was chasing the hunter. Forget about the love of a pretty woman being the prize. This was an all-in fight now and the longer it lasted the more he was going to like it.

'Aye, sir,' he replied happily and hurried for'ard again.

Amy could feel only a sense of loss and despair as she watched the *Flying Star* begin to fall away. Although in her heart of hearts she knew it had to be inevitable in the end, she still did not want to accept it. It was already hard to believe that over that week Jamie had done what no other captain could have done to James. It had been an incredible performance and she could not have been prouder of him. But that was not going to help him and she tried not to think of what her son might do now, tried not to think of how he might be feeling. Then anger against her child rose in her. It had been utterly foolish of him to attempt putting his father down. She should have stopped him right there and then in Canton when she had discovered him and ended it before it had begun. She felt angry with James too if for no other reason than he was himself. Sometimes she wondered why she loved him.

'Damn you all!' she shouted vehemently before she could stop herself and hurriedly retreated to the cabin.

James who had had the first smile on his face in days looked totally mystified and went after her but try as he might he could get nothing out of her other than an assurance that she was perfectly all right and had simply suffered some minor aberration for which she could give no explanation. To some extent that was understandable. A long time at sea could magnify anxieties out of all proportion, even create fantasies in the mind. But James did not know how close he was in putting her unusual outburst down to an exaggerated worry over their missing son. Neglecting all his other duties he had tea brought for her and stayed with her for a full half watch, gently reassuring her.

A week later it became Jamie's turn to worry. For the very first time since that initial rounding of Cape Horn when everything had seemed so crystal clear, a small cloud of doubt flitted darkly across his mind and from it fell droplets of the possibility of failure. Some of the loneliness that had been kept at bay by his blind single-mindedness began to return. All around in every direction, for further than the eye could see, was nothing but the Indian Ocean. He had no idea where *Wings of America* might be. She could have been behind him. Or far ahead of him. All he could do was drive his ship on in every way he knew how and hope. But hope was not enough. As someone had once pointed out to him at Harvard, hope could be a fickle and deceitful mate. He felt desperate to see a sail, a trail of discarded garbage, a box, a bottle, anything.

'Edge her north, Mr Barr,' he told Finis. 'I have a feeling the wind might be stronger there.'

He was not to be disappointed: the wind was to get stronger all right. Within two days the *Flying Star* was into a cyclone.

'We'll have to take in the skysails and royals, sir!' Finis shouted into his ear.

'Not yet, not yet!' Jamie shouted back and hung on, his ship heeled dangerously over as it rose and plunged to the scream of wind through the rigging and the creaking of timbers and spars. Every moment Finis and the rest of the crew waited in dread for the sudden sound of cracking wood that would bring the great tangle crashing to the deck. It was not until dark was coming on that the anxious Finis and the crew watched in amazement as their captain began to clamber aloft. Captains did not do that. Two hundred feet Jamie went, right to the top of the mainmast, to feel with his hands the tension on the skysail stays. With a bow he could have played a tune on them and he could see rope chafing on a block. He had covered that extra distance by holding her under full sail for all that day but he knew full well that he was pushing her beyond the edge. He came back down on deck.

'Now is the time, Mr Barr,' he said. 'Take in all skysails and royals.'

During the night there were gusts that blew even harder but Jamie would not hear of Finis's suggestion that they take in the topgallants as well. At dawn, it was Finis who found himself being shaken roughly awake.

'Come and look, Mr Barr,' John Marsh was saying in great excitement. 'Come and look. Come on.' But Finis was not bleary-eyed for long as he hurriedly got to his feet and followed his captain on to the deck. The wind had eased considerably but over the heavy sea still running, he looked where Jamie was pointing to the north. On the horizon was a ship and a happy, smiling Jamie handed him the eye glass. Finis raised it, focused, then he too broke into a smile. The skysail masts on both her main and mizzen were dangling and swinging in a mess of stays, shrouds, sheets, braces and halyards. The main topgallant sail was in shreds, ribbons of canvas flying and whirling. And there was no doubt whatsoever she was *Wings of America*. Finis had never really considered the possibility of sighting her again until the whole thing was over. Yet there she was, as if John Marsh had conjured her up by some magic and had made her suffer damage into the bargain.

'Set royals and skysails again, Mr Barr,' Jamie said.

Captain James McBain, at first struck by disbelief at what he saw on his own horizon, passed briefly through the door of despair before he emerged in anger. He had fully expected that Eastlake would have been at least days behind him, the rest of the fleet at least a week. On position he was already headed for his unbeatable record. At times he had touched sixteen knots. In the previous forty-eight hours he had covered six hundred and twelve miles, a feat he had never achieved before in his life. It did him no good to roar at Mr Dyson and everyone else for faster action. The men aloft were fighting for all they were worth to clear the mess, the carpenter standing by with his tools to make repairs. It was unbearable for James to see Eastlake raise more sail and start to move away ahead of him. It was totally mystifying and it was torturing. It was like the nightmares he had had as a boy, feet glued to the ground, unable to move, as some vague but terrifying monster bore down on him.

'It can't be, it can't,' Amy had said on the incredible sighting, then for the very first time she began to realise she had greatly underestimated Jamie's abilities and determination. No longer did she see him as the one who would necessarily fail but she was unable to share her agonising for both with either.

James drove his ship on with what sail he had but it was to be another two days with men working around the clock before repairs were made and she was under full sail again. During all that time

James had been constantly on his feet but if his legs were giving way his mind was not. He had no intention of leaving his deck until he had done everything in his power to make up the time that had been lost.

'Get an armchair and lash it down near the helmsman, Mr Dyson,' he ordered.

'Armchair, sir?' Dyson questioned.

'Dammit, have you gone deaf, Mister?' James snapped at him, and it was soon done. And there the captain sat, shouting, demanding, directing every tiny adjustment to keep his vessel going as fast as she possibly could, cursing men at the wheel if they made the slightest error. Twenty-four hours a day three men were constantly kept busy in taking the log. The duty watches never got a moment's peace. The bosun and his mate worked their fingers raw stitching bolt ropes and clew eyes into new sails on his instructions. For another three full days, no one saw the captain once close his eyes. Soaked to the skin through squalls and spray the armchair was his only living quarters. Amy woke from another fitful sleep and went out on deck to see him still there. Anxiously, she knelt by him. Crystals of brine glistened on his coat and on his unshaven face, making him appear as if he was gradually going grey all over, turning into a ghost.

'James,' she pleaded, 'you can't keep this up. You'll kill yourself.'

'Nonsense, Mrs McBain, we're going well,' the ghost replied and forced a smile for her.

Amy's heart went out to him but she knew nothing she could have said or done would have shifted him. She kept her tears for him hidden. For ten whole days James used his chair for cat-napping now and then but was instantly awake again if he felt any change in the wind or sea or sensed that a sail was not pulling to its full. Then one dawn, knowing he was close to total collapse, he rose.

'Take over and keep her going, Mr Dyson,' he said. 'I'll take a short rest.'

Amy who was back on deck was quickly by his side but knew he would have hated it had she tried to support him with men looking on. Disguising the painful stiffness of his joints, the salt-encrusted figure walked to his cabin with all the dignity he could muster, Amy following closely behind. Within minutes she saw him settled in his bunk, dead to the world. But hardly had she returned to the deck when she saw the bosun coming aft, agitation written all over him.

'There's trouble flared up in the fo'c'sle, Mr Dyson,' he told the first mate with urgency. 'There's going to be mutiny.'

Dyson's face stiffened in consternation. 'I'll get the captain,' was his immediate response.

'You'll do nothing of the kind,' Amy said sharply, stopping him, but it was in sheer desperation that she came to such a quick decision. 'Assemble all hands,' she instructed.

The exhausted off-watch came grumbling and cursing from the fo'c'sle to join the others, rebellious and all to a man looking ready to fight. Dyson did what he could to contain the mob between the mizzen and the main. Then they saw Amy coming for'ard to them and it was as much in surprise at her approach that they quietened and looked at her. Amy stood before them and took in their surly, dark faces. She knew every one of them. Then she raised her voice so that everyone could hear.

'While Captain McBain rests he has given me the authority of master,' she informed them, praying that she might get away with it. 'Is there a man amongst you who wishes to disobey my orders?'

The crew as well as Dyson, who stood with a belaying pin in his hand for protection, were so taken aback by this that not one of them moved, not one of them spoke up. This was not only their navigator who was confronting them but their nurse when they took sick and often their guardian angel who went out of her way to protect them. Amy held the black eyes of a seaman she had guessed to be the ringleader of the trouble. The man was a regular malcontent but she had saved him once from a flogging he had well deserved. The black eyes swivelled away from her challenging gaze.

'Don't you think the captain knows how hard you're all having to work?' she went on. 'Do you think he doesn't know what it's like when he served before the mast himself for so long once? Is there one of you who can claim to have worked harder at their job than he has? Tell me!' But no one told her and she continued. 'You're the best dressed, best paid, best fed, most skilled seamen in the world and you'd do well to be proud of it. But which one of you would take the captain's place? Or mine? Which one of you would bring your ship to shame? Is it a blood ship you'd rather serve on? With Black Douglas for your mate? Getting marlin-spike hash about your bodies for your daily ration? Or on a vessel out to make a time which will not only bring honour to yourselves for the rest of your lives but to the whole of America?'

It was not simply that Amy's speech stirred the better qualities in some of them. No man was going to argue with a woman and risk a put-down in front of his companions, especially by the pretty Mrs McBain. That would have brought blushes to the most blushless of men. For the time the woman claimed to be master, it was better by far to keep their mouths shut and do her bidding.

It was twelve hours before a refreshed James reappeared on

deck to resume driving from his armchair for another long stretch and Amy made sure he knew nothing about the potential mutiny that had been averted. She knew he would have been very angry with her for having exposed herself to the danger alone. But she got no pleasure out of having calmed the situation. There was nothing else she could have done since she did not consider James to have been in any fit state to cope with it, but at the same time she was aware that by her intervention she had helped her husband to the detriment of her son. Never before had she seen James push a ship so hard and there was little doubt in her mind that, once more, the *Flying Star* had been left far behind.

Having flown down the best of the Mozambique current in the Trades, Jamie's confidence was fully restored. Not even his painful struggles as a child to overcome his difficulties could compare with the way he had striven day and night with his ship. And he, too, had faced the threat of mutiny, a problem he had solved with quite a different incentive. Money. A handsome bonus for every man if they co-operated in beating Hurricane Jim. And it had worked. There was no question in his mind as to how he stood as they approached the Cape of Good Hope.

'We go not a mile further than we have to, Mr Barr,' he told Finis. 'The moment we're ready to alter course against the wind, it's all square sails in and no time wasted about it either.'

Only hours later, it was done, the *Flying Star* reduced to fore and aft sail only to claw her way around the Cape against the fresh westerly wind in high, lumpy seas. Jamie himself took the helm and shouted all the orders to bring his vessel safely around on to a starboard tack.

'Flying jib held aback!' he roared to ensure her head was brought round and he would not be caught 'in irons', head stuck directly into the eye of the wind and trapped there. Judging the sea he spun the wheel, yelling for the sheets, Finis there to see it done, men fast releasing to one side and hauling hard and quick on the other. The great clipper came around to a flogging and cracking of staysails as they came across. The wind took them and soon she was heeling over, dipping her spars to the waves, picking up speed again. But hardly had the manoeuvre been completed and Jamie had handed the wheel back to the duty helmsman when the lookout aloft shouted the sighting of sail to port. There was nothing unusual in that. Every East Indiaman coming and going from Europe and America had to round the tip of South Africa. But then the lookout was calling it to be a clipper with skysail rig on a tack to port and converging on them.

There, within view of Table Mountain rising from a haze, the masters of *Wings of America* and the *Flying Star*, both of whom had believed themselves to have left the other far behind, could only look. Not a curse escaped their lips. Both were speechless. Not even Amy could find a word to say. And in no time, every soul aboard down to the cabin boy on both vessels was lining the bulwark rail, staring in silence at the other's ship as they crossed tacks with less than a mile between them. After eight thousand miles, after all the ceaseless, herculean straining, the two clippers were still locked together in their gruelling and deadly combat.

'Jesus goddamn Christ,' gasped an exhausted seaman to himself, and he might as well have been speaking for them all.

Chapter Twenty-Two

On a cold December day in 1851, halfway between the Cherbourg peninsula in France and Plymouth in England and with neither coast in sight, an old Havre packet out of Boston ran up the English Channel before what was nearly a westerly gale with passengers at 'Greatly Reduced Prices'. Her royals and topgallants had long since been taken in but as it was taking two men on the helm to hold her from yawing, her new master, Captain Beriah Gurley, was contemplating reefing her main topsail as well. Having never lost a ship, he had no intention of ruining his reputation now. Although the young John Marsh had once shown him what was possible, he had stuck firmly to his old, cautious ways. And to his beliefs.

'A ship to port, sir,' his first mate had pointed out when they were only four days out of Boston. Gurley had looked to his left and to one of Samuel Cunard's big sidewheelers belching black smoke from its funnel, bound for Liverpool, which was coming up to overtake them. Then he turned back to his mate and glared at him.

'Your eyeballs are off-watch, Mister,' he growled emphatically, 'I see no damned ship.' And the mate quickly learned not to refer to these vessels as ships in front of his captain.

As they went up the Channel, the flag indicating they were for Le Havre flew from the top of the signal halyard and Gurley kept his eyes open for a Havre pilot. After a while he chose to glance astern and at first he thought he was dreaming. Two great white towers were starting to emerge out of the sea.

'What in the hell is that?' he said.

The mate peered at them through narrowed eyes as they grew ever taller, ever closer. They might have been two great mountain peaks of snow, or two strange, enormous white waterspouts reaching for the sky, some terrifying freak of nature charging up the Channel intent on destruction. But after only a few minutes, both men knew they were not.

'God Almighty, sir, they're clippers,' exclaimed the mate.

'You don't have to tell me what they are, Mister,' Gurley rasped. But neither men had ever seen even clippers running under so much sail. There was so much of it the hulls under it could not be seen. That was hardly surprising. Aloft at the very mastheads were small sails on mast extensions to the two-hundred-feet-high skysail masts; sails that did not exist except in the imagination of cartoonists who, in extracting humour out of the extremes these new clippers were going to, had called them 'Angel's Footstools'. And there they were for real. Furthermore, every single incredibly long yardarm, a whole fifteen of them, had its extensions out with big stunsails set out on every single one of them. That was not all. Both ships were carrying a flying jib that ballooned out bigger than any flying jib ever seen before. Nor was that the end of it. An extra yard had been set up at the forward end of the martingale stays under the jib boom itself and on this too was a wide sail, now and then actually scraping the waves before it and obliterating all view of the hull behind. Without them, there would have been little to see. Bow-on under that massive array of canvas the hulls would have looked no bigger than a gull's head sticking out from under a bedsheet.

'It can't be them, sir, can it?' asked the perplexed mate. 'Not from China already?'

He was right to be doubtful. The outcome of the challenge made to Hurricane Jim by the anonymous and mysterious captain was not expected to be known for at least another month. Even then it would have been a very fast time from China. In the United States millions of dollars had been wagered on it. Along Wall Street, thousands of beaver hats. In France, millions of francs. In England, millions of pounds.

'Who the hell else could it be?' Gurley wanted to know. 'Look at them, look at them. They have to be crazed out of their bone-headed skulls. They dip their bows to one decent wave and they'll sail full speed clear to the bottom before they can draw breath. I wouldn't sign on either of the madmen as even a goddamn cook!'

At the news, the passengers who had been huddled in their cramped dog kennel of a saloon poured out on to the deck, grasping at whatever they could find for a safe hold.

'Hold your course!' Gurley barked at the struggling helmsman, afraid that if he did not he would be in danger of being run down and that it would be his own ship that would go to the bottom. And captain, crew and passengers could only look on in wonderment at the awesome sight. As the two great towers came thundering down on them, such was their speed that suddenly it felt as if their packet had gone dead in the water.

'It's the *Flying Star* to port, sir, the *Flying Star*,' the mate called in excitement as he identified her. At first, Gurley was taken aback by that. He knew Eastlake's reputation as well as anyone and had no time for him, but then he remembered hearing that it was John Marsh who had got the job as his mate and it immediately sprang to his mind that Marsh must have done to Eastlake what he had done to him on the return voyage from San Francisco. But he still had a lot of time for the young man. Indeed he had missed him. He ran for his loudhailer, roughly pushing aside anyone in his way. His personal involvement had suddenly made everything different and excitement rose in him too, all thought of criticism gone. But by the time he got back on deck the high towers had swiftly revealed their masts with tier upon tier of sail and were roaring by to either side of him, their sharp bows thrusting white water higher than their bulwarks, their long dark hulls hissing through the waves like streaking demons.

'Mr Marsh!' he bellowed hopefully through his hailer far across the water towards the *Flying Star*. 'Mr Marsh! Captain Gurley here!' But if he was heard everyone on board was much too busy to make a reply and before he knew it he was shouting at a stern and a great tumbling wake, fast fanning out towards him. He soon realised his moment had gone, but he made the very best of its glory. Turning to the passengers he told them with great enthusiasm and pride of how John Marsh, the mate on the *Flying Star*, had come to him with grass growing out of his ears and with clods of New England on his feet but he had picked him out and between Boston and Cape Stiff had turned him into the best able-bodied seaman he had aboard.

'If you ever meet him, you ask him who it was who gave him his chance,' he ended, 'and he'll tell you. Captain Beriah Gurley.' And although there were still things he had to learn, that was to become the most important sea story of Captain Beriah Gurley's life.

On the *Flying Star* Jamie, alias John Marsh, looked not at all like an able-bodied man. His weatherbeaten face had become haggard, a wraith with red-rimmed eyes who no longer slept in a bunk but on his afterdeck so that he would be immediately available and never rest too soundly or too long. And there, many times, in a state of semi-consciousness between sleep and waking, he had struggled to question what darkness of mind had driven him to such extremes. He did not hate and did not want to hate. He had wanted to defeat the captain not to kill him, yet sometimes in his over-fatigue he sensed that was the extent of it and did not like himself. There were even moments because of his own ceaseless efforts when he felt forced to appreciate the strength and skills of his father. He had never imagined it would be like this. It had once all seemed so simple. But he had gone too far to turn back now. If he did there would be nothing left of either John Marsh or James McBain junior. It was the image of walking the earth forever with humiliation leering into his face that kept him battling on for every inch of sea. And although he did not know it, how well Captain James McBain would have understood him.

As *Wings of America* thundered up the English Channel with her enemy to port, James stood by his armchair which had deteriorated badly as a result of constant exposure to the weather. In several places tufts of horsehair stuffing were trying to escape from the cracking and faded leather. And James himself looked every bit as worn. Above the gaunt cheeks, the rims of his eyes were as red-raw as those of John Marsh as he fought to keep concentrating. There were things he had never imagined either, not least the evidence of how a captain like Eastlake could transmute himself into an entirely different creature.

After the Cape of Good Hope, the two ships had lost each other in a storm but that had given neither master any comfort. Rather the opposite. All the way up the Atlantic both James and Jamie had worried themselves witless over where the other vessel might be. Quite independently in their desperation they had thought of every possible way to add extra sail for the times they could run square before the wind and had arrived at the same conclusions. Almost every bit of spare lumber in the carpenter's locker had been used up in making modifications. So it was not in despair or in anger or even in speechlessness when, into the southern end of the Western Approaches, they came within sight of each other again. It was with relief and it was with joy. It meant that the other had not got ahead after all and that they were still undefeated, still in contention, confidence restored, aspirations resurrected.

In her long skirts, a heavy topcoat wrapped tightly around her, Amy came on deck after plotting their position on dead-reckoning and if there was any despair aboard it was in her. She knew only too well that no matter who won the conflict it was herself who would be the loser, and knew too that James would never settle for a draw. He would find some way of avoiding even that. The result had to destroy either her husband or her son and there would be no escaping it. She did not have to be told that if Jamie was defeated she was unlikely ever to see or hear from him again for the rest of her life. Under any other circumstances the passage they had made from Canton after sailing fifteen thousand miles in only sixty days had been so incredible that it would have been the cause for great celebration. Now it meant nothing. Only making the London docks first was of any importance to either of the two men in her life. She looked at James standing by his chair glancing anxiously upwards with his punished face and knew that every single moment he was living in dread of disaster. The ship was far beyond the edge of her limits and any second could have brought the explosion of stays, the terrible cracking and splintering of spars, the ripping and flailing of sail and men diving for cover as mast sections came crashing to the deck. But she had been through that many times already and knew that, while the *Flying Star* held, James would not reduce canvas by so much as a handkerchief's worth. And it would not be long before she was to discover what Jamie had meant by 'the world would be watching'.

'Did you see them, did you see them?' Captain Gurley shouted excitedly over his bulwarks as he spilled wind and the Havre pilot swung to run alongside. '*Wings of America* and the *Flying Star* from China!'

'*Oui*!' a voice just as excited came back. '*Nous les avons vu! Mon Dieu, quel spectacle! C'est incroyable!*'

The pilot to board made a dangerous leap for the packet's rope ladder and the pilot boat immediately headed up across the waves to reach Cherbourg at all speed to take the first news to France. But the clippers had also been sighted and identified by a British pilot cutter which wasted no time in racing for Plymouth. Along both the French and English coasts, by horse, by semaphore and by wire, the news of Hurricane Jim and his challenger running neck and neck up the Channel after fifteen thousand miles swept faster than fire.

'It's a Captain Eastlake,' a harbour master announced after quickly running his finger down the list of clippers and their masters which had been gazetted ever since the *New York Herald* had notified the London *Times* with the story. For a while the name of Eastlake flew as high as that of McBain, but it was not to last.

Further up the Channel, brigs, schooners, cutters and boats of all kinds disregarded the heavy weather as they put to sea in order to get a glimpse of the great event. It was not simply the money that had been wagered. So much mystery had surrounded this challenge. For months curiosity had mounted. For months there had been the wildest speculation as to what might happen, but no one had ever imagined it might be as close as this. After all that time the clippers had appeared locked together as one, the winner *still* to be decided. Interest in what these brash Americans from the New World were capable of had been freshly aroused in August when the Yankee schooner *America* had beaten the cream of English yachts in a ninety-mile race around the Isle of Wight, but that did not compare with this. That had been a little sprint between aristocrats engaged in sport. And only they were sorry at having allowed an American in to embarrass them. This was quite different. This was a marathon. This was real. This was of the people. Newsmen without their own newsboats rushed to ports and jumped on any vessel which would take them out, as did many of the public.

On both the charging clippers, lookouts aloft warned of many kinds of craft ahead, approaching over the waves from both port and starboard. In order to avoid them, both James and Jamie ordered their helmsmen to alter course slightly to head for the gap in the middle and *Wings of America* and the *Flying Star* began to close on each other. In no time both ships were on to the first of the flotilla, several of them, in trying to intercept, in danger of being rammed at full speed and smashed to pieces.

'Where in the hell are they all coming from?' James demanded. 'What in the hell do they think they're doing?'

On the fastest cutters and schooners, helms were put over and sheets let out as they turned and tried to run with the unbelievable sight, if only for a minute since they were quickly left behind. Loudhailer after loudhailer yelled to speak with Captain McBain as he passed by. Ahead, a schooner already running with newsmen aboard manoeuvred itself so that the two clippers would pass either side of it. But as the two ships were closing on each other all the time, it was a dangerous thing to do. There was not much searoom left between the two.

'I represent the London *Times*! Can I speak with Captain East-lake?' a newsman hailed from the schooner's stern as the ships came up on him, and Jamie knew the time had come. With *Wings of America* only a short distance off his beam he could no longer hide himself. With his hailer, the red-eyed wraith dashed to his starboard quarter rail.

'It is not Captain Eastlake!' he hollered down. 'It is James McBain the master here! McBain!'

If the newsman was puzzled by that, Finis Barr was totally mysti-fied as to why John Marsh made such a reply. But his reaction was nothing to that of James, who had also heard it. In a rage he threw himself to his port side with his hailer and yelled to the *Flying Star*, 'How dare you use my name!' then down to the schooner being quickly overtaken, '*I* am James McBain!'

There followed moments of confusion. As the schooner fell fast astern, the voice bellowing to it from the afterdeck of the *Flying Star* was still insisting her master's name was McBain.

'Do you mind me asking what you're doing, sir?' an intensely curious Finis wanted to know. Either it was some new tactic he could not figure or the incessant strain on his captain had finally proved too much.

'I'm giving them the truth, Mr Barr,' Jamie told him. 'If anyone else asks you, you can tell them my name is not John Marsh, it's James McBain,' and he pointed to starboard, 'and that man over there is my father, and I'm his son.'

'Aye, sir,' Finis replied, not believing a word of it, 'and by God will that no' shake him to bring his masts atumble.'

On *Wings of America*, Amy did all she could to avert the direct gaze of her husband's careworn eyes. She knew it could only be a matter of minutes before the revelation came and the shock struck him. There was no telling what he might do. In his tiredness he was half bewildered as it was and grasped at anything that might provide an explanation for Eastlake's behaviour.

'So that's how he did it, is it?' he said to his wife. 'He finally went totally mad and all this time he's been thinking he was me.' Amy could make no comment on that either. Then he called for his eye glass which was hurriedly brought to him. Although Amy felt afraid, she also felt relief that it was almost over. James raised the glass towards his enemy, focused and scanned carefully from figure to figure to pick the madman out. Then suddenly he was looking into a face that might have been his own, standing there at the rail without an eye glass looking right back at him. Stunned, he stood there staring with one red eye stuck to the glass for what seemed to Amy an eternity. Although half of James's brain was trying to tell him who it was, the other half was denying it. There was no sense to it. In his mind, his son had always been a weakling of a boy, at best an indecisive youth whose only contribution to the world, apart from learning Latin and Greek, had been to make known some vague attraction for Chicago and a hatred of the sea. But the longer he looked the more contradictory it became. He knew this could not be his son and knew it could be no one else. Amy, unable to bear the suspense any longer, found herself going to his side.

'You're making no mistake, James,' she said to him. 'It's him. It's Jamie. There's no Eastlake there. Jamie is her master.'

And James lowered his telescope to turn and stare at her instead, unable to speak, his bewilderment complete.

Shortly after, the winter darkness fell and the normally firm jaw of Finis Barr with it. As Jamie convinced him that he had not lost his mind and was indeed who he said he was, the mate felt hot blood rush to his cold, high cheeks in embarrassment. All those unsavoury, lust-laden, lurid thoughts he had had about his captain and another man's older wife had been no more than the innocent relationship between mother and son. He felt disgusted with himself for having got a certain amount of erotic pleasure out of visualising them fornicating on a bunk in the sweaty heat of Canton. His filthy head needed a good scrub-out in the Kirk. But he was not to realise any more than his captain did that he had been right in believing that the attention and the love of the pretty lady was very much at the root of the conflict into which he had been drawn.

A sense of treachery and betrayal coloured the tumbling chaos of James's mind as he fought to clear it and make some sense out of what had happened. For a whole ten minutes an anxious Amy watched him walk the darkness of his quarterdeck in silence. At least one thing became obvious to him. Amy had known about it long before he had. He stopped before her.

'Why?' was his only question.

'Because he is your son,' was all she could think to say in answer.

With the two ships moved so close together that their studding-sail yards almost touched as they rolled, James felt tempted to dash to his rail and for the first time ever curse his son directly to his face. What stopped him was not only Amy's presence but the knowledge that it would destroy his dignity on top of everything else. Still totally at a loss to know how his weakling of a son could ever have become the captain of a rowboat on a river never mind a racing clipper, he nevertheless gathered his senses enough to wrest back some control.

'Mr Dyson!' he boomed and Dyson was quickly by his side. 'Order the master of the *Flying Star* to keep clear and give us searoom. And inform him that the passage of neither vessel will be considered to have been completed until the last ounce of tea has been discharged from her hold in London.'

'Aye, sir,' Dyson replied, and hurrying with the hailer to the rail bellowed his captain's instructions. There was a little delay before the Scottish voice of Finis Barr came shouting back through the darkness under Jamie's direction.

'We are holding our true course! The master demands you give us our water! Away! Away!'

'He is ordering *me*?' an infuriated James roared at Dyson. 'Damn him to hell, Mister!'

Amy, unable to bear it any longer, went to her cabin and sat there in her misery. She knew that neither was going to give the other as much as an inch and every moment fully expected to hear the clash of yardarms then the grinding and splitting of timbers as the two vessels came into collision. It seemed inevitable and such was her own turmoil of mind she felt that if her ship went down she would not want to save herself.

Ashore, printing presses clanked and rumbled for all they were worth as newspapers raced each other to be first to tell the story of the battle taking place between the two American clippers, between two Captain McBains, one the famous and distinguished Hurricane Jim, the other claiming to be his son about whom absolutely nothing was known. But in true journalistic style what the newsmen did not know about James McBain junior they struggled heroically to make up. Alternately he was aged twenty-one and twenty-five, small, dark and nuggety, six feet tall and fair, strong and silent, nervy and blustering, married with four children and a bachelor, wild beyond measure and self-disciplined to a degree. The public could take their pick. Not the bookmakers. Outside in the gas-lit streets, these frantic men, who had accepted wagers on the name of the conqueror being only that of McBain and now on a loser either way, ran from door to door, banging on them to wake up sleeping punters and sort out the confusion.

As the wind began to back to the south-west, James McBain and James McBain junior barked their orders almost simultaneously for sail trim. But no matter how both struggled, neither could gain any advantage and they roared up the English Channel through the night together, both in constant dread of being dismasted. But it was James who was the more disturbed of the two. He simply could not understand what he had done to create such a deadly enemy nor how the boy had acquired the incredible skills and determination which for so long he had believed belonged only to himself. It could have been some eternal nightmare to which there was no end, the stuff of purgatory. But as the wind backed even further to the south and his ship heeled over on her reach, the freezing spray that lashed at his sleepless face was not of hell but of the sea and of reality.

It was not only father and son who did not once close their eyes that night but Amy, and Dyson and Finis Barr too. Now that the end was in sight, seamen aloft found new power to their weary muscles and sinews as they fought tooth and nail with sail and rigging. On deck they heaved on sheets and braces like Trojans. And on that wintry dawn without a moment's rest for hand or head they approached the Straits of Dover. Before them was revealed an endless armada of vessels stretching to the horizon and beyond. Small boats, large boats, craft of every kind had come out from both the coasts of England and France in anticipation of catching sight of the unique contest. Among them, smoke belched from the stacks of several small steamboats, their side-paddles churning. Never before had competing Thames pilots worked so hard at trying to intercept their charges as they tacked again and again, bawling for clearance amidst all the other excited shouting. And when they did turn and run to try to get alongside the clippers, it was leaps of death the pilots made for the swiftly passing rope ladders since *Wings of America* and the *Flying Star* refused to slow any more than the other in order to assist them.

'You have to reduce sail, sir, and now,' both unnerved, red-faced pilots were quick to instruct their respective captains.

'Not until they do,' both masters shot back.

There were several overeager journalists who might have drowned in attempting to board had there not been so many boats surrounding them to pluck them quickly from the freezing water. And in the end, it was the two pilots using hailers who had to agree between them for sail to be taken in – at exactly the same time, so that neither ship would be disadvantaged by it. But if the pilots thought they had assumed full control of these two great clippers they were mistaken. They might have been giving the courses but their masters stood on their quarterdecks continuing to bark orders at their mates for optimum sail trim, both standing by to raise full sail again if the other should do so and to hell with what the pilots wanted.

Running before the wind again, the ships clung inseparably up through the Goodwin Sands and, in unison, slowed again to let the port officials aboard before gathering full speed once more to reach on up the Thames Estuary and into the river. The port health officer had been only moments aboard when he realised that if he had found sickness and directed either vessel to quarantine he would more likely have been thrown back overboard than obeyed.

'Open the hatches, Mister Dyson,' James ordered his first mate to the pilot's and officials' amazement before they were halfway up the river and Jamie, seeing it, ordered the same.

Undeterred by flurries of snow and sleet, swarms of the London public had already collected at suitable spots on the banks of the Thames to view the amazing sight of these two American clippers only sixty-one days from Canton heeled over side by side as they swept up the river with the flood tide at breakneck speed, tea chests already being hauled out on to their decks, boats and sailing barges scattering everywhere before them to give them water. In London itself, others hurried to the East India Docks where, they had learned, the ships would be tying up. They came in barrows, in cabs, in hired coaches and private carriages. Working men, women and children. Clerks from counting houses. Men in tall hats and their fashionable ladies. Shipping men, merchants, shopkeepers, street vendors, Navy men, soldiers and sailors. Almost all had already taken sides. Some for the son, in the English weakness for the underdog and the desire to see a champion floored or because they had taken wagers on the mystery challenger before they had known who he was. Others of more conservative persuasion heavily in favour of the father because they considered it would be an outrage against all moral decency if he were defeated by his own son. None had any reason to spare a thought for Mrs Amy McBain, the wife and mother whose life and spirit was so painfully being crushed to extinction between them.

Again, it was only by agreement between the two frenzied pilots who expected serious collisions at every moment that to strict timing, as if in some ritual conducted to music, much more sail was taken in simultaneously on both vessels, neither giving away as much as a square inch of canvas before the other.

Masts towering high above the warehouses, the ships finally ran into the dock and there bedlam broke out. Pushing dock workers out of the way, hundreds of public hands grasped at the ships' lines to get their favourite alongside all the quicker, stem to stern. Topsides struck hard against the protecting timbers of the dockside and even before the springlines were secured, gangways, planks and anything else they could use to get aboard and get the tea off were thrown up on to bulwark rails. It was useless for either masters or port officials to call for order as ordinary men and women poured aboard each vessel and, like an army of ants, tossed, carried and rolled the chests ashore as quickly as they could move them. Down into the holds they went too with nets and whatever else they could find to haul them out. The scent of fresh tea mingled with the din and the hysteria as each great crowd fought to make themselves the winners. Tartan swirling about his bare knees, a scottish piper scrambled up a mountain of tea chests and there on its peak blew his lungs out on the bagpipes to his troops of combat below, but such was the screaming and the shouting he was hardly heard except by Mr Barr. And through that great cacophony of English delirium the droning and wailing and skirling of his homeland brought tears of emotion to Finis's unrested eyes.

'Oh, listen, sir, oh listen, it's for us,' he choked.

In the crush of bodies and fast-moving tea chests it was hard to tell who had the larger army, and both James McBain and James McBain junior could only look on helplessly. The irony was not lost on them that after having been through so much over fifteen thousand miles their fates and their ends had been taken out of their hands. Amy could not even look. Alone in her cabin she sat hunched over, staring at nothing, but try as she might she could not shut any of it out, could not wish that it had never been.

Empty-handed journalists trying to push aboard were thrown out of the way. Children in danger of being trampled on were swept to safety and put in warehouse doorways. Tall hats accidentally knocked from heads were quickly flattened underfoot before their owners could rescue them. Noses were bloodied and cheeks bruised as several fights broke out between men of opposing sides, but the ceaseless unloading went on.

It was almost dark when Jamie, after all the years his memory could take him back, after all the years of passive submission to the captain's will, after all the years of loss and loneliness and separation and nonentity, at last knew what and who he was. Tea chests were still pouring from the hold of *Wings of America* while he was done and triumph flooded his soul like a blazing light as he shot his arm to the air.

'The hold of the *Flying Star* is empty!' he cried through his hailer and the battle which for him had been engaged on the day that seemed so long ago when he had first rounded Cape Horn was over. Then, unable to help himself, like the child he had once been, he wept.

Chapter Twenty-Three

Not once had Captain James McBain been known to neglect his duties and responsibilities and although he could easily have handed them over to Dyson on some pretence, he did not do so now. No one could have guessed how devastated he was as he concluded his business with the agents and port officials, any more than they would have felt the pains in his joints, since there was not the slightest sign of stiffness in his walk. And if they noticed the faint hunching of his shoulders as in hospitality he ordered them drinks, that was easily excused since it was obvious that the man had long been deprived of sleep. Although most of the journalists were crowding eagerly round his son on the *Flying Star*, James parried the questions of those who came to him with dignity and without the slightest trace of anger, dismay or discomfiture. He even threw in a few comments of his own.

'You might do well to point out to your readers,' he told them, 'that both these vessels are a tribute to the skills of the American craftsmen who built them and an even greater tribute to the American seamen who sail them.'

But all that had been another battle on its own and it was to be quite a different matter when his performance was over and he was able to indulge himself in his true feelings.

For a long time Amy watched him as he sat in silence in his cabin, seeing nothing through his red-rimmed, salted blue eyes. She could not help but be aware of the impenetrable fog of despair in which his sense of failure cloaked him. Not once in all his existence had he come anywhere near to feeling such fatigue and weariness of life. It was as if all his fame and past successes over so many years had suddenly been blotted out and were of no account. The only wonder was that with his total physical exhaustion on top of all else, nature had not already taken her usual course of mercy and swept him into the arms of oblivion. But perhaps some part of his mind was warning him that there lying in wait for him was only a re-enactment of his struggle and defeat.

By contrast, on the *Flying Star*, it was the stimulation of his new

255

self that kept Jamie on his feet, but in case he might himself blush in the telling he had given Mr Barr the honour of explaining to the newsmen what had happened to Captain Eastlake.

'Oh, the rogues and bloody cut-throats,' Finis had told them, 'looked as innocent as wee babes they did and tricked him on to their junk in broad daylight right there in the Roads and away wi' him like slit-eyed ghosts before a man could crack a biscuit. May the good Lord deliver him safely from their foul, pirate hands and that it'll no' be the last o' a bowling alley the captain sees for he's meikle fond o' a game.'

'A most unfortunate circumstance,' Jamie managed to add, 'or this honour might have been his.'

That was as great a lie as he had ever told but it was by no means the only one to fall with the snow on that cold, wintry night.

If Amy was numbed and no longer felt either pity for her husband or pride in her son, she was still not an easy woman to sink. She had always known that James was a man of action and that if the sea had been unable to take him, introspection could. For the sake of herself and trying to make things right again, it was in desperation that she gathered enough strength in her tired soul to make her confession.

'I'd hoped and prayed I'd never have to say this,' she said, 'but now I see I must. I cheated you, James, and I'm sorry.'

She was almost trembling with emotion as she watched the surprised and puzzled gaze of the torn eyes slowly rise to her but she had to face them directly and did not look away. There was a pause before he spoke.

'Cheated me?'

'I did it because I thought he deserved it. He is our son, our own flesh and blood. How as his mother could I have done anything else but tried to give him some help? My intention was only to lessen the extent of his own defeat. I honestly didn't think for a minute he would have been able to keep it up. Otherwise I'd never have done it to you. I swear it.'

'What did you do?' James demanded to know. He had felt besieged by treachery as it was on learning that Amy had known before they even left Canton that it was Jamie who was in command of the *Flying Star*, and it had explained much of her strange behaviour on the voyage. He had done his very best to forgive her for that, but now it seemed there was more. And Amy appeared very reluctant to come out with it.

'What did you do?' he repeated.

'If it hadn't been for me we could have been in at least a day ahead, maybe as much as three. Twice I deliberately took us off the best course and that lost us time. Once in the Indian Ocean and once in the Atlantic.'

'*You what?*' gasped James in disbelief as he heaved himself painfully to his feet.

'God knows I was only trying to do my best for both of you!' she cried, and at least that was the truth. It had been for most of her life.

For a full minute in the lamplight James stood stunned, staring at her. But she did not throw herself at his feet to plead forgiveness, did not bow her head in shame, did not even look away. Indeed, her manner was more angry and defiant than repentant. It was her only protection.

'You are telling me,' he said at last to her, 'that after all these years of giving you my trust you deliberately deceived me and made me lose? My own wife? When you knew how important this was to me?'

'But you didn't lose, don't you understand? That's what I'm trying to tell you, even if you do want to strike me down for it. You think this has been easy for me to say? All right, it might have been stupid of me to deceive you and cause you to lose. But in fairness and truth it was you who won. At first I thought it would have been enough for myself to know but I could see it wasn't.'

Amy's last throw had been totally convincing and certainly James was only too eager to believe her. She had just handed him the spade with which to bury his humiliation and the hook with which to retrieve his pride.

'Then they must know it too,' he said, making for the cabin door, outside of which two seamen had been placed on guard to keep out visitors. But he had hardly gone a step when Amy stopped him.

'You breathe a word of it to a single soul and I'll not be here when you get back!' she almost shouted at him and he turned back to her, for several moments struck dumb again.

'It's enough for you and me to know and no one else, James,' she went on, visibly shaking in her attack. 'Are you so insecure a man that you can't be satisfied knowing it was really you who won without having to shout it to the world? Is that how your fame has corrupted your reason? Can you no longer live without crowds waving their flags at you? Let the world think what it damn well likes! It was only a matter of time before someone overtook you if you'd gone on and don't tell me you didn't know it and didn't fear it. But, oh no, you wanted more and you have no one but yourself to blame, so let all that end now. Would you rather it *had* been

Eastlake? Or some young captain you'd never heard of? His name is McBain – James McBain – and you will give him this.'

As if there was not enough in all that to sting James's conscience, his senses and his ego, the worst was still to come.

'Because if you don't,' Amy ended, 'you can start looking else-where for a wife. As from now.' And there was no doubt in James's mind from the way she said it that she meant it. It seemed incredible to him that while it was his wife who had committed treachery and openly admitted it, she had turned it all around to make him the villain. But he was forced to control his anger. Impossible as she was being, life without her was unthinkable. The only comfort he had to cling to was that had it been a fair fight he was certainly the winner, and that fact was starting to sink fully in. That alone made him feel much better.

'You think I'm not big enough, is that it?' he said finally.

'I'm waiting to see,' Amy replied, but she had to be patient for the answer.

'All right,' he said at last, 'we'll let him have it,' and paused before adding, 'under protest.'

'No protest!'

'All right, all right!' James shouted back and, with his legs barely able to hold him up, took to his chair again, feeling it was his own fault that down the years he had taught his wife how to drive as hard a bargain as anyone. But Amy was not finished.

'Now I'm going to fetch him and bring him here so you can face each other and talk like reasonable human beings,' she said, surprising him further.

'Maybe tomorrow, Amy,' he said. 'Maybe tomorrow.'

'No, now,' Amy insisted, and grabbing her winter coat which lay on the cabin sofa, threw it over her shoulders and made her way out without another word.

The well-lit dock was much more ordered but was still busy with the teams of dock workers who had had to be recruited in to get the mountains of tea chests out of the snow and into the cover of the warehouse. Jamie, still on the deck of the *Flying Star* and almost surrounded by visitors, saw the figure coming. He had been expecting her for some time and had kept an eye open for her, only wondering why she was taking so long. What he desired more than anything now was to feel the proud arms of his mother go around him. Excusing himself he went to the top of the main gangplank to greet her. But when Amy reached the bottom she just stood there looking up at him. She did not look happy, as he expected, and he could not make it out. Eventually he made his way down to her and stood before her but no arms came out to him and he was bitterly disappointed by that.

'You did well, Jamie,' she said rather coldly.

'What's the matter?' he asked anxiously.

'That could take nineteen years to explain and I don't have the time,' his mother replied, at once confusing him and taking the wind out of his sails. 'But right now I want you to come and see your father. And if I see or hear the slightest trace of gloating in front of him you'll never again call me your mother.'

It was not difficult for Jamie to guess that the captain had taken his defeat a lot harder than he had ever imagined and for a moment he even visualised his father lying in his bunk, a man destroyed, ready for his deathbed scene. Between that and his mother's attitude he felt guilty and not a little sorry for what he had done.

'I had to do it, don't you understand?' he tried to say.

'Yes, I know,' Amy replied.

There were to be several interruptions with people demanding his attention before Amy got him to return with her to *Wings of America* but she could not have been away as much as ten minutes and was not prepared for the sight when she stepped back into the cabin, any more than Jamie. It was now her turn to be struck to silence in astonishment. James was seated upright at the table, seemingly busy with ship's papers and the wages book. In what must have been the quickest shave and change in his entire career, he was fully dressed in his finest black suit, a large pearl pin gleaming in his cravat-like tie, gold watch chain dangling from his vest, hair brushed and black boots shining. For all the world he might have been a senior captain who had just completed a perfectly normal, short voyage of no importance winding up the last of his ship's business before sporting himself ashore. Gone was the vanquished ghost. He looked up from his work.

'Ah, Jamie,' he said and rose, well concealing his awareness that he was no longer dealing with the boy he had known. Of the two, which had been James's intention, it was Jamie who looked to have had the hard time of it. Standing there with messed hair, uneven patches of stubble, still dressed in his stained and crumpled sea clothes which were almost soaked with melted snow, he looked a wreck and had been made to feel conscious of it.

'Drink?' James offered.

'Thank you,' Jamie accepted, deliberately refraining from adding the 'sir'. If he was not allowed to gloat, which in any case his father had made difficult if not impossible now, he was nevertheless becoming more determined by the moment not to slacken his lines to him and no longer felt sorry for him, which had also been James's intention since he could not have stood that either. Amy, still surprised by her husband's lightning change, could only look on. They were like two tigers circling each other, measuring each other up for signs of weakness.

'I'll not examine too closely,' James said as he poured, 'as to how you managed to get command of a clipper at your age.' And Amy knew she suddenly had to find voice again.

'But I think Jamie and the *Flying Star* are to be congratulated for their effort all the same, James,' she threw as a warning.

'Yes, yes,' James agreed, handing his son his drink, 'it was a fine sail you made of it.'

'You too,' Jamie returned, not to be patronised.

And, together, they toasted each other's ships, both believing themselves to be the victors, both fighting to the last drop in their blood just to stay on their feet. Matchsticks would hardly have been enough to prop their eyelids open.

There followed a brief, stiffly mannered conversation on the record prices the tea was expected to fetch at auction but although that might have been all-fired important at any other time, in this confrontation it was no more than trivia, and James soon turned it to more burning issues.

'I suppose you guessed,' he said, 'that this was the last place on earth your mother and I expected to find you?'

'I make no excuse for that. If you want the truth it was the last place *I* expected to find myself.'

'You have any idea just how much time and money I've wasted looking for you?'

For the first time in his life Jamie found himself able to stand and face the captain as an equal. All the fear he had once had of him was gone. His father was as vulnerable as any other man and he had proved it.

'Don't try to make your own mistakes mine,' he told him. 'You needn't have spent a penny if you'd followed my instructions and had any regard for my wishes.'

'That's enough!' Amy demanded of them both. So alike were they that James might have been talking to himself twenty years younger.

'No, let him clear his air,' Jamie quickly requested of her and James, angered not so much by his son's arrogance as by the feeling that the authority he had held for so long had lost its power and was slipping away from him, did go on.

'Was it for this I spent a fortune on your goddamn education?'

'*Nemo mortalium omnibus horis sapit*, Captain.'

That set James back. Not knowing what it meant and not wanting to admit it, he could find no immediate answer, and Jamie hastened to take advantage of him.

'It means no man can be wise all the time,' he informed him before his father's aching brain had time to respond.

'I know what it means, damn you!' James blazed, and Amy almost threw herself between them.

'I said that's enough!'

James brought himself under control. 'It's all right, Amy, it's all right,' he assured her.

'Don't worry, Mother,' Jamie assured her for himself.

Then James felt his legs beginning to buckle under him and just managed to make the sofa where he sat. 'God knows,' he said, 'all my life I've tried to do nothing but my best.'

Jamie looked at him resting there. Robbed of the stimulus that had previously been holding him up, the sight of the sofa was suddenly more than he could take. And he, too, took to it to sit. Amy looked at them both. And waited.

'What do you think you're going to do now, then?' James asked his son without turning to him, doing his best for Amy's sake.

'I'm thinking of steam, it's the future.'

'Steam? Steam? Goddamn dirty, filthy steam? You ever see a paddle steamer go around Cape Horn? You ever see a paddle steamer bring tea from China? You ever see a paddle steamer go around the world? Where do you think it would pick up its coal? Out of the goddamn ocean? It's so limited it'll be dead in ten years!'

'No, Captain, it's sail that's going to be dead in ten years.'

'You hear this?' James said to his wife. 'You hear this?' and he turned to Jamie again. 'Listen, I'm going to build clippers that'll go so fast they'll make paddle steamers look like burning ducks with their feet anchored in the mud. They'll never be able to compete for passengers, freight or anything else by the time I'm through. So don't think I'm going to let any son of mine make a fool of himself by thinking he's going to a wedding when he's going to a funeral.'

The overwhelming desire for sleep was consuming him. His reddened eyelids felt heavier than lead. The cabin seemed so far away. Yet still he heard.

'It will be your funeral, not theirs,' came the voice of his son, indistinct but with meaning.

'You want to wager on that?'

'I'll wager on that. Every single cent of my primage.'

'Well, that's not that goddamn much compared with what I

could put up,' James somehow managed to mutter, 'but I'll take it.'

Then suddenly, almost as if he had been struck on the head by the blacksmith's sledgehammer, his eyelids came down all the way, his body slumped and he was out to the world. An angry Amy rushed to him, grabbed him by the lapels and shook him. 'James! James!' she commanded but he might as well have been dead. Nevertheless, she was determined to bring him back to the land of the living. The matter was far from finished. The conciliation between father and son she had so desperately hoped for had not been resolved in any way at all. Unable to rouse him she turned to Jamie. 'Help me get him . . .'she started to say before she realised that Jamie, too, had departed for oblivion. Fury swept over her and she rushed to the cabin door and opened it.

'Get me two buckets of water!' she ordered. 'I want two buckets of water!'

They were soon fetched and she carried them in. With full force she hurled two gallons of foul, icy-cold River Thames at the head of her husband and then at her son's. The worn-out bleary eyes of both partly opened with the shock.

'Amy,' moaned James in vague surprise.

'Mother,' Jamie gurgled almost inaudibly in turn.

'Listen to me, listen to me!' she cried in rage. 'You think I'm going to wait another ten years before you see yourselves and start trying to see each other?' But it was all for nothing. The accumulation of stress, deprivations, anxieties, fight and constant struggle over fifteen thousand miles of ocean had finally taken its toll. Before she had even finished their eyes were shut, their ears beyond hearing, both unconscious again. Only wife and mother was still alive to pain and she could bear it no longer.

Chapter Twenty-Four

The leaden light of a winter morning hung over the ships in dock before James awoke. Although someone had thrown a blanket over him, he felt stiff and frozen and far from rested. He opened his eyes to see that his cursed son was no longer there. There was no one but himself. It hurt to move and, as he eventually tried to stand, he knew he would have fallen to his knees and stayed there had he not quickly sat back to give himself more time. Then, after a short while as he tried to collect himself, Dyson came in. James would have given anything to have told him that, in fairness, *Wings of America* had been the conqueror but, having made his promise, he knew he had to be content.

'The galley has a good breakfast waiting for you, sir, if you're ready for it,' Dyson said.

'I'll wait for Mrs McBain, thank you, Mr Dyson.'

'But Mrs McBain isn't here, Captain.'

'What do you mean she isn't here?'

'I didn't see her go myself, sir, but I was told she went ashore last night and hasn't come back. I thought you knew.'

James was hardly aware of the physical effort it took to bring himself to his feet but the sudden stabbing of apprehension saw him quickly up.

'Of course I knew,' he said to cover, 'I'd forgotten.'

With Dyson gone, he made a hurried search, at first unable to tell if any of his wife's possessions were missing. And only minutes later, tall hat firmly on his head, he was striding along the dockside where the snow had thawed and been trampled into slush. That his wife might have joined his son on the *Flying Star* was as much a hope as a suspicion.

Jamie, who had half woken during the middle of the night and had somehow staggered back to the warmth and comfort of his own bunk, felt himself being urgently shaken. Reluctantly he came back into the world and opened his eyes to the bulkhead which had become almost a stranger to him. Feeling a little disorientated, he heaved his body over and saw his father standing there. 'Where's your mother?' he was saying anxiously. 'Where is she? Is she here?'

Jamie swung himself up to sit between the lee boards of his bunk, still half dazed.

'No.'

'Where did she go then? You know where she went?'

'I didn't know she'd gone anywhere. She didn't say anything to me.'

'That's it, then,' James told him, his worst fears confirmed. 'She's gone.'

'What do you mean gone?'

'I mean she's gone. Gone for good. Left. Deserted.'

Jamie started to feel the anxiety gnawing at him too. 'Are you sure?'

'Of course I'm damn well sure. You think after all these years I don't know her? She's gone, I'm telling you. Gone.'

With mounting concern that his mother had washed her hands of him too after all he had done, Jamie felt at a loss to know what to say or do. He gazed at his father who took to a chair and sat there but if he expected some word from him that might give him a lead he was to be disappointed. None came. Instead, after a long silence as Jamie continued to look at his father, to his utter amazement, he saw the tears that came to the captain's eyes and it shocked him. He had never thought that the captain was capable of weeping over anyone or anything. Yet he could feel the loneliness in him, feel his fear, sense his insecurity. They were all emotions he knew only too well and could easily recognise, but it took him a little time to take in that such human frailty could manifest itself in a man who had no heart, who had no soul, whose only godheads were his pride, his incontrovertible word of command, his self-aggrandisement and his wealth, all supported on dubious crutches with the name of duty. It did not so much as enter his head that it was Aunt Dorothea who had so poisoned him. He simply felt stunned, even embarrassed by this unexpected revelation.

It had not been any part of Amy's intention that by walking out she might arouse such self-pity. She did not even give it a thought. She had gone simply because she had reached the end of her tether and could take no more. She had done all she possibly could for both of them and had failed. There was no question in her mind of ever returning to try again, but it would have been to France she would have fled for comfort had she known what was there.

'You want breakfast in bed or do you want to go down?' Hinton Garrison asked his wife in the bedroom of their hotel in Lyons.

'No, no, we'll go down,' Sophia insisted, not wanting to miss out on a moment of her first visit to Europe, even if it was not meant to be exactly a pleasure trip. With Hinton having to attend banking business in England and France, Sophia, with visions of elegant, scented ladies removing their corsets for her husband all over Europe, although she made no mention of the image, refused to be left behind. They had travelled on Samuel Cunard's big steam packet and had arrived in Liverpool from Boston a month before.

'When we get back to England, couldn't we wait there until Amy arrives?' Sophia asked hopefully as she washed and dressed. 'Couldn't we?'

'Unfortunately not,' Hinton replied patiently but firmly. 'It could be at least another month before James gets in and I have to get back, you know that.'

Although Hinton had been as curious as anyone about the mysterious challenge that had been made to James, the more he thought about it the more he had become convinced that there could be no substance to it. It was clearly the work of some troublemaker envious of James and out to damage his reputation, and the newsmen had created the hysteria to sell more newspapers.

'If there was any other captain on earth who could challenge James,' he had assured a worried Sophia, 'we'd have heard about him long before now and he wouldn't have been hiding his light behind anonymity.'

And they went down to the dining room where it was obvious that some great event had taken place while they slept. Dozens of excited French voices were talking all at once and everyone had newspapers. 'Something political you can guarantee,' Hinton informed Sophia's questioning face. 'Every Frenchman is a politician. It's sauce to their mutton. They can't live without it.' Then the waiter came and he asked for confirmation of his assessment so that his wife would see just how knowledgeable he was about French foibles.

'You have not hear, monsieur?' the waiter said in some surprise since they were Americans and he considered they would have been the first to know.

'Hear what?' Hinton enquired.

And within minutes, in English with a bit of French thrown in, Hinton and Sophia got the news of how, in the great tea race from China to England, the famous American captain they called Hurricane Jim had been defeated in record time by his own son. If the ceiling had suddenly come crashing down on their heads it would have had less impact. They were staggered, agape, speechless. The waiter could only guess they had lost a great fortune on the outcome and discreetly retired to the kitchens to give them time on their own.

'It can't be, Hinton, it can't,' Sophia managed to get out when she eventually found voice. 'It has to be some kind of mistake.'

After all the misjudgements he had already made, Hinton struggled to find some kind of logical explanation without putting himself in any deeper but he did not do very well.

'Maybe,' he suggested, 'James had some other son by another woman he never told us about. The result of some indiscretion in his youth.'

'What?' cried Sophia, for Amy, for herself and for every other woman who had been deceived by their husbands.

'We'll go to London,' Hinton declared. 'Now.'

The dash across France to Calais, if it could have been called that, took more than two days, but all the way, although they both tried desperately to find more acceptable explanations for what might have happened, the story as they had first heard it persisted everywhere. At Calais they were to be frustrated by gales that stopped the paddle steamers from crossing the Channel straits to Dover. After dark in their hotel room, the bitterly cold wind rattled the shutters, smoke blew back down their chimney, and their concern for their friends deepened.

'Whoever it was did this to James and Amy,' an upset Sophia reminded her husband, 'you said it couldn't happen. You said it was a lot of nonsense. You said the man who wrote that letter to the papers was a madman.'

'I know what I said,' Hinton told her irritably.

In the middle of the night Sophia shook him, near to a state of hysteria. 'What if it *was* Jamie?' she almost shouted at him. 'If it was Jamie we might be too late! If it was Jamie, James might kill him and Amy might kill him back!'

'In God's name!' Hinton returned. 'James is a man of control like myself and I haven't killed you yet, have I?'

When the weather eased they were first aboard but it still took another full day to cross and get up to London. It was night again when, without wasting a moment, they reached the East India Dock and *Wings of America*, only to be told by a seaman that the captain was ashore, as was Mrs McBain, for James had made nothing of her disappearance to the crew and it was assumed she was simply staying in the city.

'We'll wait,' Hinton said and the seaman lit the lamps for them in the main cabin. And there they sat and waited for what seemed like a hundred nights. It was late when they heard footsteps come towards the cabin door and they rose to their feet in both anticipation and trepidation, not at all sure in what state they might find

James and Amy. They were totally unprepared for the sight that met their eyes as the two men stepped into the lamplight and pulled up with looks of surprise on their voyage-eroded and gloom-laden faces. It had been a long time since the Garrisons had seen the missing Jamie and he looked very different. Both men were similarly dressed in black suits, both held tall hats in their hands, both were of the same height, both had the sea in their eyes and both were unquestionably James McBain. There was no longer any doubt in either Hinton's or Sophia's mind that the story was true but the mystery was not only how Jamie had changed but how father and son happened to be standing there together with no apparent animosity flowing between them, no feeling of difference of rank and stature, separated only by the years. As for the two James McBains, Hinton and Sophia Garrison were the last people in the world they expected to encounter standing there in the clipper's cabin.

'Hinton, Sophia!' James exclaimed and warmly pumped their hands. Sophia felt delighted but she was no longer tempted to throw her arms around Jamie. Now, that would have been like kissing a stranger in the street.

'Had to come to England on business,' Hinton explained hurriedly, dispensing with the truth, 'were passing through London again, heard you were here and took this opportunity.'

'Where's Amy?' Sophia wanted to know before any more could be said, and saw the smiles of reunion fade from both their faces.

'We don't know, Sophia,' James admitted bluntly after a pause.

'Don't know?'

'The truth is she's gone. Left us. It's my own fault.'

'No, Mrs Garrison, it's mine,' Jamie confessed.

'I should have seen it coming but I didn't,' James went on. 'It was probably on the cards for a lot longer than I knew. Or it might simply have been that I refused to see it or wanted to believe she would never do it. Whichever way, it isn't helping us much now. For five days we've been searching London.'

'If only we knew she was safe and well it would be something to be going on with,' Jamie said.

Hinton and Sophia could feel the pain of loss in the tone of both their voices, and in other circumstances would have been amazed over father and son being in such accord. In all the years they had been close friends of the McBains they had never seen it. The irony was not lost on Sophia. This was what Amy had been fighting for all her life and now that it had happened, it had come too late for her.

'For all we know,' James continued, 'she may no longer be in London, not even in England.'

'You must find her, Hinton,' Sophia cried, shaking her husband's fur-collared coat as if he was a magician. 'You must find her!'

'Hold on, Sophia, and listen to what James and Jamie are saying,' Hinton demanded of her and she bit her lip to control her distress for her friend.

'Yes, Sophia, it may not be so easy,' James said.

'She may not want to be found,' Jamie added.

'Not want to be found?' Sophia said in exasperation. 'Of course she wants to be found. Don't any of you understand anything at all about women?'

As much as James and Jamie might have wanted to believe her, it was certainly not how it looked to them. Although Amy had made many female acquaintances in London over the years and wrote to several of them, she had not left a letter or address behind and James could not remember half their names, never mind where they lived.

For the next three days, Hinton insisted on joining James and Jamie in their search, going in and out of hotels, plodding the cold, wet sidewalks of residential London in the hope that the captain might recognise a house or a square where he had dined with Amy in the past. Hinton, although he did not say so, was not amused by the fact that his friend, who could have navigated himself right around the world without sighting as much as a cobble, kept leading them round in circles or got them hopelessly lost. Indeed, had it not been for Sophia, who was strictly directed to stay in the warmth of her hotel where she had nothing else to do but wait and worry, they would have drawn a blank. She disobeyed and took to touring the streets on her own in a cab, simply inspecting the figure of every woman who came into sight, near and far. 'Where now, madam?' the cab driver would ask his furred-up American lady. 'Anywhere,' Sophia would reply, the tip of her nose almost blue from being constantly stuck out either one side or the other.

'Stop! Stop! she shouted suddenly and the cab driver pulled up his horse to see his fare excitedly pointing at the peeling, painted board of a closed-up shop. '*J. Forsythe*', it had once read clearly, '*Wigmakers*'. It made all kinds of bells ring in Sophia's head.

'Wigs!' she squealed, as a valuable alarm in her mind was triggered. 'Wigs!'

'Madam wants to go and buy a wig?'

'Of course I don't want to buy a wig but it's something like it, I know it is!'

'An 'at,' the cab driver suggested patiently. He had seen them all before, the drunks and the strange ones.

'Anat?' Sophia questioned.

'Thems that yer puts on yer head, lady.'

'No, no, no,' Sophia said but starting to run through her head was the vague memory of Amy telling her once about a very nice Englishwoman she had met who had extended an open invitation to stay with her and her husband any time she was in London. At the time it had not meant very much but she was sure Amy had mentioned where they lived and wigs had something to do with it. 'Is there a Wig Street,' she urgently wanted to know.

'Wig Street? Wig Street? Not's as how I's heard of.'

'Wigmaker Street, then?'

'Wigmaker Street? No, madam. Wiggenhall and Wigmore Streets is all I knows.'

'Wigmore, Wigmore!' Sophia screamed with delight as recognition of the name struck her, turning the curious heads of every passer-by. 'Wigmore Street! Take me to Wigmore Street!'

'American,' commented a gentleman, explaining such unladylike behaviour in a public thoroughfare.

The cab driver started to turn his horse around. 'What number, madam?'

'I don't know which number,' Sophia told him impatiently. 'It doesn't matter what number. Any number!'

Anyone else might have rated the chances of finding Amy on the basis of a London street mentioned years ago as close to zero. Not Sophia. She had never come to grips with the interest rates in which Hinton had been involved all his working life, never mind the incomprehensible ramifications of odds. She felt quite certain about it. Even when she reached Wigmore Street, dashed out of the cab, hurried up stoop after stoop and knocked on doors, only to be confronted by the controlled but rejecting faces of one butler after another, her confidence did not wane. While the cab driver took the opportunity to take out the nosebag to feed his horse and a lamplighter lit the street lamps, Sophia went the full length of the street and started down the other side.

'Excuse me,' she had not tired of saying for the umpteenth time, 'I am Mrs Hinton Garrison from Boston, Massachusetts. I'm looking for my friend Mrs McBain and thought she might be staying here.'

The manservant did not blink an eye. He simply opened the door wider, and stepped aside as an invitation for her to enter.

'Is she here, is she here?' Sophia asked as confirmation as she went in but confirmation she did not get.

'If madam would care to wait I'll make enquiries,' was all he said, showed her to a room, gently closed the door and left her. For a few awful moments, Sophia thought she might have walked into some kind of terrible trap, even if a fire was burning in the grate and the room was warm. All kinds of bizarre things happened to people in foreign countries. She pulled aside the curtains and got a little comfort from seeing her cab still waiting outside under a street lamp. The cab driver at least knew where she had gone and was unlikely to go away until he was paid. But it worried her that the manservant had not told her if Amy was there. She had been a fool to walk into a strange house all alone. Hinton would kill her. Then suddenly the door burst open and Amy was rushing towards her in a mixture of surprise and delight, arms already raised. Holding each other in tears of joy, it was some time before they could speak anything but each other's names and before Sophia could make her explanation for being there.

Over an hour later Hinton Garrison, having temporarily separated himself from James and Jamie, returned to his hotel to attend to his wife and report yet another futile day, only to find she was not there. She had left no note and all he could discover was that she had left in a cab earlier in the day. It did not take long for anxiety to be added to his anger. Sophia never did have any sense of direction but if she had got lost, surely she had not forgotten the name of the hotel where they were staying. Or had she? Or had disappearing become an infectious disease? For another full hour he stood, sat and paced the hotel foyer, not once removing his eyes from the entrance and getting more frantic by the minute, vowing to God he would say nothing to her if He would only return her safely. Then Sophia was bouncing in, looking as bright as a button, and he almost ran to her.

'Where in the hell have you been?' he demanded angrily, keeping his voice as low as he could because of the other guests.

'If you say another word to me, Hinton,' Sophia said haughtily out loud, 'I won't tell you where Amy is.'

Knocked back on his heels by that, Hinton looked at her for a moment in amazement. 'You found her?'

'Of course I found her. It was easy.'

Hinton was stunned, and not just because of the good news. His wife's innocent scattiness and dependency on a man to protect and guide her were qualities that had attracted him to her in the first place and he had never tired of them. It made him the complete husband and master who directed every last detail of running his home. Sophia had never even had to pay a bill. Not in all the years he had been married to her had he considered she was capable of going out alone in a strange city the size of London, playing detective and finding what no one else could. He was not at all sure if he liked that.

'Where is she, where is she?' he demanded to know.

'I'm not saying that until tomorrow, Hinton.'

'You're what?' Hinton questioned in disbelief, then aware that everyone in the foyer was looking at them, he took her arm and started to lead her towards the stairs.

'If I tell you,' Sophia told him as they went, 'you'll rush straight off and tell James and Jamie and *they'll* rush straight off to Amy.'

'And why in the hell shouldn't they?' Hinton asked, keeping his voice down.

'Because although I told her how they've become she didn't believe me. I want to give her a little more time to think. But I've got her to agree to see them tomorrow so she can see for herself.'

'I'll go and tell them that, then.'

'Oh, no you won't, Hinton. You want them to be torturing me to death all night? Breathe a word of it before morning and I'll never speak to you again,' Sophia warned, and tripped on lightly up the stairs ahead of him, a satisfied woman.

The following morning, the two tall-hatted, weather-beaten ghosts in their black suits, with apprehensive eyes, gold watch chains and shiny boots arrived at the hotel to pick up Hinton and resume their search. Not once in their time together had they as much as mentioned their recent contest. And not a single word of accusation or laying of blame passed between them. Yet as unhappy as they looked they were not quite in despair and without hope. If they had not yet found a trace of wife and mother they had at least found each other. If they made no comment on that either, both knew it well enough and it gave them each support. Neither had ever been much good at expressing their feelings with words and they did not try to do so now. There was no need. The sharing, the unspoken understanding and the show of respect they got from each other were enough for them.

In the foyer they did not have to wait long. Soon, Hinton, accompanied by Sophia, was coming down the stairs.

'Now, I will be the one to tell them, Sophia,' Hinton had told her, afraid that his wife might show too much exuberance in public.

'Yes, Hinton,' she had agreed obediently, but on approaching James and Jamie she found she could no longer contain herself. Before they even exchanged 'good mornings' she was excitedly blurting it out.

'I found her, I found her!'

'Oh, God,' Hinton muttered resignedly as the few other heads passing through the foyer turned to look at them.

The unexpected suddenness of it left both James and Jamie standing there with blank expressions for a moment before they felt blown over.

'She's perfectly safe,' Sophia added for their comfort.

'It was the greatest of luck, James,' Hinton said in an attempt at reasserting himself.

'Where is she?' James wanted to know, both he and Jamie glancing anxiously around as if expecting to see her suddenly appear there.

'I can't tell you that,' Sophia told them, 'but it doesn't matter. She'll be coming here in an hour.'

'You want the whole damned world to know, Sophia?' Hinton almost hissed aside to her.

'Yes,' Sophia returned defiantly.

'Come to the lounge,' Hinton said, leading the way, but they were not seated there for long. Although James and Jamie could not have been more grateful to Sophia Garrison and said so, the summer had not yet returned to their wintry eyes. Much too impatient to sit there for a whole hour they excused themselves on the grounds of the lounge being too stuffy for them with the large fire and explained they had to take a short walk. They were hardly outside the entrance when Jamie said, 'You realise that just because she's agreed to come here doesn't necessarily mean she's going to stay?'

'I know,' James replied.

'Then what will we say to her?'

'We will simply be reasonable. Your mother has always listened to reason. We will apologise for causing her such distress and explain it was never our intention to hurt her. We will plead that a man cannot be expected to know every working of a woman's mind but that we'll do our best. We'll tell her that she's needed and ask her to come back.'

They walked along, a freezing wind and a lack of conviction swirling about them in the street.

'And what if she won't listen to reason?' a worried Jamie asked.

'We have to give her every chance. She deserves that.'

They walked on while they thought further about that but neither could see exactly what chances there were to offer and the doubts persisted.

'And if that fails?' Jamie wanted to know.

'What would *you* do,' James questioned, 'if a member of your crew who'd signed on for the whole voyage jumped ship in a foreign port and you found them?'

Immediately Jamie saw that and it brought a smile of relief to his face. He should have already thought of it himself. It was the ultimate solution.

'Right,' he agreed. 'So if the worst comes to the worst we just pick her up bodily, carry her back to the ship and keep her there until she comes to her senses.'

'Right,' James confirmed.

It was probably as well that neither Amy nor Sophia had the slightest inkling of their desperate plan or the meeting might never have taken place. As it was, father and son were seated back in the hotel lounge and as nervous as kittens as the moment approached.

Amy, looking more like a famed London beauty than a celebrated American navigator, stopped at the door. She saw her husband and her son rise slowly in unison and stand there side by side, gazing back at her. She began to go forward to them but stopped again. She could tell almost at once that everything Sophia had told her was true. For the first time since Jamie had been born she could tell that these two men in her life had become reconciled. And after all her painful years of trying and praying she had not even been there to see it happen. It seemed incredible, but she could feel their mutual respect for each other in her very soul. Never had she seen two such anxious and silently pleading faces that were as one. All the arguments she had spent most of the night making against returning were scattered to the winds, and all the defences with which she had determinedly barricaded herself in fell around her like broken matchsticks.

'We would like to say,' James began, having to struggle to say anything at all, but it was as far as he got. Amy was rushing to them and holding them both in a tide of tears. And with the tide the last vestige of the poison dispensed so long before was swept away.

Epilogue

On a fine, early summer's day, Finis Barr stood in the curious crowd that had quickly gathered on a wharf on the busy East River, a horde of newsmen among them. If it could not have been compared with the delirium of his own triumphant return much earlier with the McBains on the *Flying Star* and *Wings of America* when New York had gone wild, it was still an event. Being rowed ashore from a newly arrived ship was none other than Captain Eastlake, standing in the boat jutting a massive beard and waving his hat like a returning hero.

'Och, it's done the man no' a bit o' harm,' Finis declared philosophically to a companion. 'He's still got his ears and ten fingers to his hands. And he might even have learned a wee bit o' Chinese.'

That Eastlake was the first known American captain ever to have been kidnapped by Chinese pirates had gripped the public imagination and people were hungry to hear of his experiences in their hands. But there were things that even Eastlake himself did not know. To start with there was not a breath of suspicion of any skulduggery having taken place aboard his ship, and he had absolutely no idea what an unexpected bonus it was for his captors when a wealthy Cantonese merchant paid his ransom, no doubt in order to avoid an international incident which might interfere with trade. But as Jamie had arranged with Lymann Cobb he was about to be released unharmed in any case.

'Captain Eastlake, Captain Eastlake!' called a well-dressed gentleman from another boat that quickly came alongside, and Eastlake gave him his attention. 'I would strongly advise you to tell them nothing sir,' the gentleman called, waving a sheet of paper at him, 'or you will be giving away a fortune. This is a contract which will take you on a lecture tour of all America, sir, to tell them personally of your adventure. You will be famed across the nation, sir.'

Eastlake found such an idea overpoweringly attractive. All his life fame had been escaping from his hands like a bar of slippery soap. And if the truth was that there was little to tell, he could always make a lot of it up. There was no one who could ever contradict him. He could describe the unknown backwater somewhere west of Macao along the South China coast, speak dramatically about the cutlasses at his throat, every day about to be struck down in a pool of blood by the death-hungry, opium-smoking oriental devils. He could escape in the dead of night in the junk, still bound in Chinese handcuffs, and find himself struggling desperately for his life through the surrounding marshes, only to be caught again. The hell of it all. There was only one snag and it was a formidable one.

'I must speak with my wife first,' he said.

'I've already consulted her, sir, and she's in full agreement with it. Mrs Eastlake will be only too happy to accompany us and tell of the torture of her waiting.'

'Then dammit, sir, it's done,' Eastlake told him.

Eastlake's father-in-law, owner of the *Flying Star* who was also amongst the waiting crowd, was a satisfied man. His daughter had her husband back and he knew that the prospect of ever finding her another had been a poor one. Moreover, not only had his new ship shattered a record but such were the prices the tea had fetched that the cost of her building had been fully recovered in that one voyage. If he was sorry about anything it was that he did not have a prettier, much younger daughter who might have attached herself to young McBain and brought him into the business.

In their counting house, business was very much on the minds of Mr Kimball and Mr Jay. As they stood looking out of their window at the goings-on through the great forest of ever-growing masts and rigging they were thoughtful. There was no doubt whatsoever about the elegance of such sailing ships but in a merchant's accounts even elegance had to be closely related to profits. Both felt there had been some kind of message or omen in the fact that it was a steamship which had brought the amazing story of the McBains from London. And they had been saddened at James's retirement ashore after his return. That, too, seemed to herald a change, despite James's assurance that the whole commercial future lay in bigger and faster clippers. Beyond, on the river, the skimming dish of a ferry was puffing and churning its way over to Brooklyn, and there were other even uglier paddlers making their way up and down, not in the slightest dependent on wind and tide for progress. At one of the large receptions following the return of the two now famous clippers they'd had a long and interesting conversation with young McBain about that, and it had worried them ever since.

'I believe that once coal depots are established around the world at suitable locations,' the bright young man had declared with confidence, 'there will be no stopping these new vessels.'

Mr Kimball and Mr Jay continued to look out of their window.

'What do you think?' Mr Kimball said.

'What do you?' Mr Jay returned.

'We gave our full trust to James all these years,' Mr Kimball pointed out, forgetting all the times they had doubted him. 'Should we now put our faith in his son?'

'That is the question,' Mr Jay replied.

'He's very young, only nineteen,' Mr Kimball noted with a tinge of doubt.

'It's the blood that counts,' Mr Jay contributed.

'And is he a prophet?' Mr Kimball enquired.

'That is another question,' Mr Jay said and they looked down in silence as Captain Eastlake was landed and swallowed up by the eager crowd, but both knew what was in the other's mind, Mr Jay leaving it to Mr Kimball to say it.

'We could, of course, put a foot in both camps,' Kimball suggested after a while with a wave of his cigar.

'Back both horses,' Mr Jay added, knowing it was the shrewdest move.

'We'd have to learn new ropes.'

'Pistons and boilers,' Mr Jay corrected.

And in agreement that they would invest half in new clippers under the guidance of James and half in steamships under the advice of Jamie they prepared to set a new course for the future.

It was not by deliberate default that Jamie was not there to see Eastlake's arrival in New York but he would be very relieved to hear of it for it had lain heavily on his conscience ever since Eastlake had walked so innocently into his trap. He would be even more relieved to hear how it had changed the pledge-signing captain's life since it was a secret he would never be able to share with anyone. As it was he was far away, up in Worcester, New England, standing tall-hatted with his mother and father and Dr Amos Drew in the sunshine, waiting for a quite different arrival. It had been Amy's suggestion that they wait in the grounds and have Aunt Dorothea brought to them. Although it was one of the most modern private asylums in America with wide, airy corridors and simple but pleasant rooms, there was no disguising that scent of madness which permeated the atmosphere inside, a foul scent that came from the

breaths of those to whom the quelling drug had had to be adminis-
tered. And no hiding the occasional iron grille over a window.

'She may not come out unless I tell her she's to get something,'
Miss Blossom warned, 'something like a new dress.'

'Promise it to her, I'll see to it,' James told her, eager to get it
over with and be away from there, and Miss Blossom went in
person. As warden she could have directed one of her keepers
instead but as it was Dr Drew who had recommended her for the
position it was her due to see to the business herself. Gone from the
vast figure was the apron and the stick. There were no such punish-
ments here and, to the surprise of many, the inmates were all the
better behaved as a result. In the grounds they walked about freely
but closely watched.

Eventually, Miss Blossom reappeared, leading her Miss Jackson
who was dressed in crimson silk with a large bustle and a hat which
bore a haberdashery of various coloured ribbons. Clutched in the
bony fingers of her right hand was a lace parasol. Her hair was
hennaed and the cheeks of her small, ageing face were heavily
rouged. As she walked, other lady inmates stopped and curtsied to
her as she passed. It was a royal salutation that Dorothea demanded
from them. And as she kept reminding each of them how she had
murdered her sister, her own children, poisoned her niece and her
niece's child and was the living anti-Christ, in fear they did her
bidding.

For some time Amos Drew had suspected that Miss Jackson's
failure to recognise or remember anyone from the past was only a
screen and that she knew perfectly well who everyone was, but just
in case he was mistaken he never once mentioned it, not even to
professional colleagues. He did not want to know the truth since
that might have brought even more pain to the McBains. It was
enough that he himself felt secure with the way things were.

Aunt Dorothea would have walked right past her visitors had not
Miss Blossom stopped her.

'These are your friends, Miss Jackson,' she said, 'and they've
come to see you.'

James looked directly at her eyes as she regarded them with
disdain, trying for Amy's sake to will her to remember, but she did
not meet his gaze.

'Whoever you are, you don't belong here,' Dorothea said to
James and Amos Drew who were standing together then turned to
Amy. 'Why do you come here wearing such a dreadful dress,
madam? Have you no taste? I hope for your sake that neither of
these smelly gentlemen is your husband.'

'Now, now, Miss Jackson,' Miss Blossom warned in case her patient raised her parasol to strike at any of them, and Dorothea glanced at Jamie. For the briefest moment he felt there was a flicker of recognition on her face but quickly concluded he must have been mistaken.

'As for you, young man, whatever your name is,' Aunt Dorothea told him, 'I hope you haven't got the great misfortune to be related to any of them.' And with that she turned and swept away, bringing the meeting to an end.

'She is very happy here,' Amos Drew said.